Cancer of the Lung

Wiley Series in Diagnostic
and Therapeutic Radiology

Luther W. Brady, M.D., Editor

*Professor and Chairman, Department of Therapeutic Radiology
and Nuclear Medicine, Hahnemann Medical College and
Hospital, Philadelphia, Pennsylvania*

TUMORS OF THE NERVOUS SYSTEM

Edited by H. Gunter Seydel, M.D., M.S.

CANCER OF THE LUNG

By H. Gunter Seydel, M.D., M. S.
Arnold Chait, M.D.
John T. Gmelich, M.D.

Cancer of the Lung

H. Gunter Seydel, M.D., M.S.
Albert Einstein Medical Center

Arnold Chait, M.D.
University of Pennsylvania

John T. Gmelich, M.D.
University of California at San Diego

With a Foreword by F. G. Bloedorn, M.D.

A WILEY BIOMEDICAL PUBLICATION

JOHN WILEY & SONS
New York / London / Sydney / Toronto

Library of Congress Cataloging in Publication Data:

Seydel H. Gunter.
   Cancer of the Lung.

   (Wiley series in diagnostic therapeutic radiology)
(A Wiley biomedical publication)
   Includes bibliographies and index.
   1. Lungs—Cancer. I. Chait, Arnold, joint author.
II. Gmelich, John T., joint author. III. Title.
[DNLM: 1. Lung neoplasms. WF658 S519c]
RC280.L8S48   616.9′94′24   75-19155
ISBN 0-471-77849-4

Printed in the United States of America

10 9 8 7 6 5 4 3 2 1

Preface

The past five years have produced an explosion in the knowledge, techniques, and clinical application of radiology in all of its specialties. New techniques in diagnostic radiology have contributed to a quality of medical care for the patient unparalleled in the United States. Among these techniques are the developments and applications in ultrasound, the development and implementation of computed tomography, and many exploratory studies using holographic techniques. The advances in nuclear medicine have allowed for a wider diversity of application of these techniques in clinical medicine and have involved not only major new developments in instrumentation, but also development of newer radiopharmaceuticals.

Advances in radiation therapy have significantly improved the cure rates for cancer. Radiation techniques in the treatment of cancer are now utilized in more than 50% of the patients with the established diagnosis of cancer.

It is the purpose of this series of monographs to bring together the various aspects of radiology and all its specialties so that the physician by continuance of his education and rigid self-discipline may maintain high standards of professional knowledge.

LUTHER W. BRADY, M.D.

Foreword

The treatment of patients with lung cancer presents an unanswered challenge in today's medicine. Despite the progress achieved in the diagnostic and therapeutic management of patients with bronchogenic carcinoma, the cure rate attained is disappointingly low and diagnosis during the early stages is rare. Statistics of patients treated surgically have improved gradually, but they only reflect the better selection of cases treated with curative intent. Unfortunately, this improvement is not evident when the results are computed for all patients with bronchogenic carcinoma seen in one institution.

Medical knowledge has made excellent gains in revealing the pathology, the types, and the metastatic routes of bronchogenic carcinomas, and in identifying other aspects of the natural history of these tumors. Great strides have also been made in developing techniques for diagnosing the disease. Current resources in this field are numerous and refined: x-rays (plain, tomogram, angiogram, venogram); bone, liver, and lung scans; endoscopy and its auxiliary methods (brushing, washing); cytology; punch biopsy; second intercostal space exploration; scalene fat pad biopsy; and thoracotomy. Yet, despite these diagnostic procedures, early discovery of bronchogenic carcinoma remains the exception rather than the rule because the disease is generally asymptomatic until the advanced stages, and there is no practical and efficient system of screening asymptomatic patients.

Great progress has been achieved in therapy of bronchogenic carcinoma, particularly in surgery and radiotherapy. Advanced techniques in surgery and in pre- and postoperative care are rapidly approaching maximum efficacy. With the advent of supervoltage energy rays, radiotherapy has established itself as a therapeutic modality used not only as an adjunct to surgery but also as a curative procedure. Its results are reproducible and, to a certain extent, predictable. The effectiveness of radiotherapy in controlling disease in primary lung tumor and in its lymph node metastases to the mediastinum and supraclavicular area has been proven in a large percentage of cases.

Despite the availability of two such formidable and efficient methods of eliminating local tumor, the cure rate of all patients with a diagnosis of bronchogenic carcinoma remains about 5%. The main reason that the cure rate has been so dismal for this group of patients is that there is still a lack of understanding of some fundamental facts which could aid in launching a successful attack against this deadly disease. Basic knowledge is lacking about: (1) how to diagnose subclinical disease (microscopic or small, undetectable tumor aggregates); (2) how to screen asymptomatic patients efficiently to reach more patients with localized disease; and (3) how to determine the number of cases in which local therapy fails because of disease outside the treated area at the time of diagnosis, or spontaneous modifications of the host-tumor relationship, or the interference with such a relationship by unwise or untimely therapy.

Whatever the reason for treatment failures, the figures show that except for the development of an improved system for selecting patients to receive surgery and/or radiation therapy, there has not been much progress in the cure of bronchogenic carcinoma. Undeniably, the entire therapeutic approach to bronchogenic carcinoma must undergo radical changes, both immediate and long-range in scope.

The immediate goal should include the following: The criteria for selecting patients to receive radical treatment must be more stringent for both radiotherapy and surgery. Since radiotherapy has shown constant improvement in controlling malignant disease in the lung, mediastinum and supraclavicular areas, its use should be extended to earlier stages of the disease. Some form of combined therapy, such as surgery with chemotherapy or radiotherapy, should be undertaken in more imaginative and extensive clinical trials. These combinations could best be applied in anaplastic and centrally placed tumors in the lung hilum. Finally, until a method for curing a greater percentage of patients with lung cancer is discovered, emphasis should be on better palliative therapy for these patients with the shortest treatment producing the least morbidity and the longest, most useful existence. Not only the length of survival, but also the quality of life provided for the patients must be considered.

The long-range goal should be the development of systems of therapy, alone or in combination with current local treatment, aimed at the systemic destruction not only of the gross, clinically detectable tumor, but also of all malignant cells in the body that constitute subclinical extensions of the tumor. This systemic attack on the disease could be direct, using chemotherapy, radiotherapy or a combination of both, or indirect, enhancing either the host's defense mechanisms or the vulnerability of the malignant cells to such immunologic processes.

Chemotherapy is making a concerted effort in this direction with partial success. Some groups of tumors show measurable regression in response to treatment with a combination of drugs. The different types of combination surgery and/or radiotherapy with chemotherapy and/or immunotherapy should be considered the main hope for improvement in the therapy of lung cancer. Together with the discovery of methods to prevent the disease, such combined therapies will help to eliminate an important cause of human decimation, since we must realize the cure rate for patients with bronchogenic carcinoma cannot be significantly improved by surgery and radiotherapy alone.

Despite the limitations of present-day knowledge, there are many patients with bronchogenic carcinoma to whom therapy cannot be denied. Before attempting to treat these patients, all physicians should have current data available, they should know the state of the art in both diagnosis and therapy and should be aware of the natural history of the disease in relation to its pathology and site of origin. This book is directed to such physicians, to serve as a guide in the management of patients and discuss the anticipated results for each stage of the disease according to the therapy used. This information has been compiled and organized in a logical sequence by experienced specialists to be used in a clinical setting. The vast experience of the authors in the management of bronchogenic carcinoma is amply shown in the well-chosen discussions and insightful conclusions. The comprehensive information presented in a book of this scope and caliber should foster a better understanding of this devastating disease and lead toward the ultimate goal: development of new and improved methods of therapy and thereby hasten the cure for bronchogenic carcinoma.

FERNANDO G. BLOEDORN, M.D.

Tufts-New England Medical Center

Acknowledgments

We are most obliged to our photographers and departmental secretaries, especially Ms. Sophia Grzybowski of The American Oncologic Hospital, Philadelphia. The Special Services of the Institute for Cancer Research, Philadelphia, have been of invaluable help. Our thanks go to Lawrence Anderson and his coworkers. The expert photographic and administrative assistance of Douglas Danner, San Diego, is gratefully acknowledged. Without him Chapter 4 could not have been completed.

We have striven to acknowledge the many authors and publishers of scientific journals, papers, and books who have generously allowed us to employ copyrighted material. We hope that any neglect in this respect will be forgiven in the same generous spirit.

H. GUNTER SEYDEL
ARNOLD CHAIT
JOHN T. GMELICH

Philadelphia, Pennsylvania
La Jolla, California
August 1975

Contents

Cancer of the Lung

Chapter One

The History of Diagnosis and Treatment of Cancer of the Lung

The first issue of the *New Series of the Transactions of the College of Physicians* was published in 1850 and contained an article entitled "Cases of Cancer of the Lungs and Mediastinum" by Dr. William Pepper,[18] an outstanding physician of the Pennsylvania Hospital. He surveyed the data about lung cancer that had been gathered up to that time and stated: "Such cases were viewed as mere matters of medical curiosity not known to be in any degree influenced by medicine and too rare to be of much practical importance." He emphasized "the rarity of the affection and exceeding great difficulty which attends its diagnosis," and said that there was reason to believe this disease occurred much more frequently than was commonly supposed and might escape detection entirely in a great majority of cases. Of the 3 patients reported by Dr. Pepper 2 were women 20 and 27 years of age, the other was a 20-year-old man.

Probable cases of thoracic or pulmonary neoplasm were mentioned as early as 1761 by Morgagni;[14] however, the first commonly accepted case of primary lung cancer was reported by Bayle[2] in 1810. The author described his attendance at the autopsy of a 72-year-old man who died in 1805 and was found to have a mass "the interior of which resembled brain" at the root of the left lung and in the lung itself. The patient also had small tuberculous cavities in the remainder of the lung, numerous brainlike masses in the liver, and movable, subcutaneous bodies similar to the internal tumors.

To my knowledge, the first reported patient in the United States is mentioned in the *U. S. Medical and Surgical Journal* of August 1835 and later reported verbatim in the *Boston Medical and Surgical Journal* of December 1835. A Dr. Hall[6] of Newark, New Jersey described the clinical symptoms in this 40-year-old man: "He had been ill for many weeks, and on examination the following symptoms were manifest—emaciation, extreme pain on pressure in the region of the diaphragm, great debility, prostration, and difficult respiration. Tongue red at the edges, moist, with its papillae erect in the centre. No pain in the head, but at times complains of dizziness, with cramps in the arms, feet and legs. Pulse 120, full and quick, but in ten or fifteen minutes, intermitting, slow, and weak, becoming in a few minutes again full, with a flush on the cheek, and when the face was flushed the breathing was most difficult. When the pulse was weakest, the greater was the pain in the region of the diaphragm. Bilious and dark-colored discharges from the bowels, which we learned from the attending physicians were alternately constipated and relaxed through the whole of his illness."

The patient died the following day, and the autopsy is reported by Dr. Hall as follows: "On raising the sternum, we found it adhering firmly to the mediastinum by a preternatural enlargement, so as to require the use of the scalpel, to detach its whole length. At the superior extremity of the sternum, the tumor was small, compared with its magnitude at its termination—for as we approached the pericardium, the morbid appearances increased; the morbid mass was of a pyramidal shape, with its base resting on the pericardium, and its top running a small space above the superior portion of the sternum. The superior and anterior portion of the pericardium, and the inferior portion or base of the tumor, were so firmly attached, that it was not possible to detach them only by dissection. The tumor was, from its anterior to its posterior surface, two inches in thickness, at its base gradually tapering to its top, and from one lateral extremity to the other, between four and five inches, and running to its superior termination tapering, giving the mass a sort of cuneiform shape. When detached it weighed three pounds (avoir-dupois). It was of a pale red color generally, with interstices of a pale yellow, occasionally slightly vascular, heavier than water, and resembled in its general appearance the glands of the mammae; the left lobe of the lungs adhered extensively to the tumor, at its posterior and superior portion, and at the inferior extremity of the right and middle lobes they were both found strongly adhering to the tumor immediately above the right superior portion of the pericardium. The right lobe was also adhering to the pleura at the second rib near its centre, extending round from thence to the spinal column; in other respects the lungs were sound and manifested a healthy appearance. In the cavity of the thorax were effused seven pints of serous fluid, slightly tinged with blood; the pericardium contained a small quantity of effused fluid, not exceeding two ounces. The heart at its superior extremity was slightly inflamed; pleura costalis sound; diaphragm inflamed slightly; stomach and intestines were healthy, and no symptom of inflammation was discovered in either. Spleen, paler than usual; the vessels of the pancreas engorged with grumous blood; liver slightly enlarged; the gall-bladder flaccid and empty; the renal glands, ureters, urinary cyst, manifested no diseased appearance; the encephalon with its contents was not examined."

The symptoms of prostration, flushing, tachycardia, and diarrhea fit the clinical picture of a carcinoid tumor, although at the time of this report the histologic diagnosis of tumors had not been introduced into medical practice. As in other case descriptions in the earlier part of the nineteenth century, treatment was usually limited and unsuccessful, and the gross pathology is confusing. Cancer of the lung was clearly a necropsy diagnosis, as shown in a review of the nineteenth century literature by Onuigbo.[16] Cockle[3] reported that a Dr. Baron may have been the first to diagnose lung cancer during the life of his patient, who was initially examined in 1819 but not reported in the literature until 1865. Differential diagnosis in the early nineteenth century was usually between aneurysm, tuberculosis, and lung cancer. Dr. Pepper[18] wrote: "In a vast majority of cases it [lung cancer] entirely escapes detection owing to the great difficulty which attends its diagnosis."

Metastatic disease as a presenting symptom was reported by Greene[5] in 1843 in a patient who had metastatic lung cancer deposits in the frontal brain lobes. The astute physician also noted that such deposits do not produce pain. Another extrathoracic finding was described in 1869 by the Swiss ophthalmologist Horner,[7] who reported the first patient with the syndrome which bears his name.

The scientific basis for the diagnosis of lung cancer was greatly enhanced by Virchow[21] in Germany, who applied the concept of cellular pathology to the histologic study of tumors. No longer was it permissible to grossly describe "encephaloid" lesions, and histologic examination became a routine feature of postmortem examination. In 1857, Quain[19] was one of the first to describe the microscopic appearance of malignant cells

in lung cancer and the spread of these tumors along the bronchial tree and in pulmonary veins. A report on the first series of patients with histologically confirmed cancer of the trachea and bronchi was published by Langhans[12] in 1871. Thus, clinical diagnosis and histologic diagnosis on postmortem examination developed gradually following the introduction of the stethoscope by Laennec in 1834. The attempts at clinical diagnosis before death were frustrated by the difficulty of diagnosing lung cancer by auscultation and percussion.[1]

On November 8, 1895, Wilhelm Conrad Roentgen discovered roentgen or x-rays, and a few months later, in April 1896, F. H. Williams[24] of Boston demonstrated one of the first chest x-rays of a patient with pulmonary tuberculosis at a meeting of the Association of American Physicians. The exposure was made with a Crookes' tube and a Wimshurst electrostatic machine: "The lungs are easily penetrated, the ribs, clavicles and vertebrae are in marked contrast to other portions of the thorax. Against the lower part of the right lung the outline of the upper portion of the liver is distinctly seen, and the rise and fall with the respiration easily follows. Between extreme inspiration and expiration the liver moves vertically about three inches." The application of radiographic methods to the diagnosis of diseases of the thorax was the most

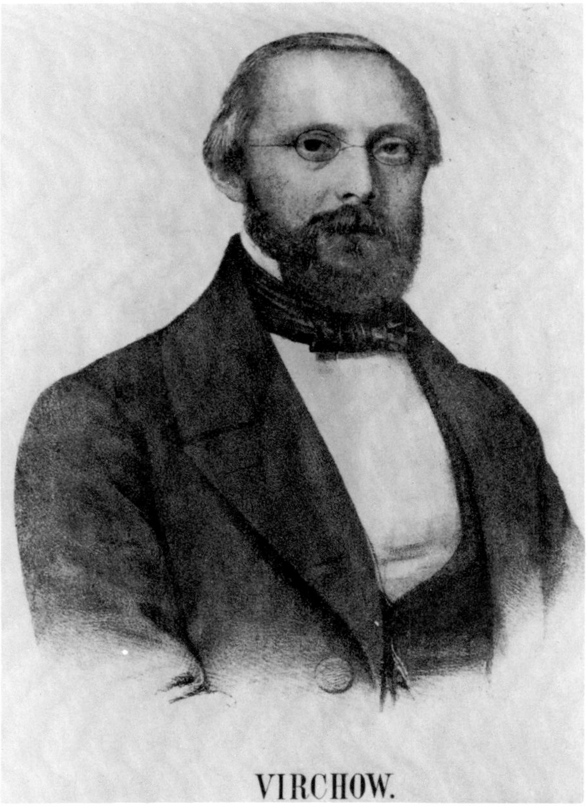

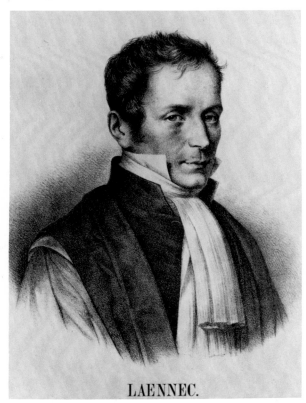

VIRCHOW.

Fig. 1. Rudolf Virchow (1821–1902). (Used with permission of the library of the College of Physicians of Philadelphia.)

LAENNEC.

Fig. 2. Rene Theophile Laennec (1781–1826). (Used with permission of the library of the College of Physicians of Philadelphia.)

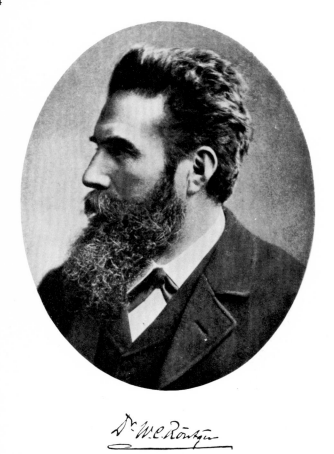

$\mathcal{D}^r \; \mathcal{W.C.Rontgen}$

Fig. 3.   Wilhelm Konrad Roentgen (1845–1923). (Used with the permission of the library of the College of Physicians of Philadelphia.)

important early development in diagnosing of bronchogenic carcinoma during the patient's lifetime.

Other technological advances occurred toward the end of the nineteenth century, and on April 23, 1895 Kirstein[10] first observed directly the vocal cords and the bifurcation of the trachea, thus marking the birthday of direct laryngoscopy and heralding the development of bronchoscopy, described by Killian[9] in 1898. Thoracoscopy followed in 1912, and bronchography in 1922.

Thus, the methods of clinical diagnosis, radiographic and histologic examination of specimens combined to allow a more accurate and earlier diagnosis of lung cancer in the twentieth century. Although Flint[4] prophesied as early as 1866, "It is possible that the microscopical characters of cancer may be discovered in the sputum," and although the first identified cancer cells were described in the sputum in 1875, it was not until after World War II that Dr. George N. Papanicolaou[17] developed cytologic examination of sputum specimens to its present technical perfection. His first examination

of tumor cells in a patient with lung cancer was reported in 1945.

As expected, treatment in the early reports of necropsy material was entirely symptomatic and unsuccessful, and included the use of sal soda and senna, sulfate of quinine, wine whey, brandy toddy, and other tonics (Hall[6]). Small bleedings were believed to afford temporary relief but could not be repeated often.

The first intrathoracic operation, described in 1889, changed an attitude that was dramatized by Salter[20] in his lectures: "With regard to treatment, gentlemen, I need not tell you that I have nothing to tell you." In that year a simple thoracotomy was performed for a localized lung abscess. In 1895, Sir William Macewen, Regius Professor of Surgery at the University of Glasgow, actually removed a lung, a portion of the chest wall, and a lung tumor by repeated cauterization. The patient survived and was alive as late as 1940.[22] In 1911, Kümmell[11] reported the first successful total pneumonectomy for cancer. The patient subsequently blew out his bronchial stump and died of "septic suppuration." The surgeon reported that "the danger of a lung operation can be lessened; namely, by instituting a gradually increasing pneumothorax." X-Rays of the thorax accompanied this report, and an overpressure apparatus was not used. Twenty-two years later, Dr. Evarts A. Graham of Memorial Hospital in New York performed the first resection of a whole lung for cancer, including in his procedure a thoracoplasty and the implantation of seven gold-shielded radon seeds into the stump of the hilum, the site of a suspected residual metastatic node. Although this patient also blew his bronchial stump, with subsequent empyema, he survived the operation and continued practicing as a physician for many years afterward.[23]

Although x-rays were used therapeutically a few years after their discovery, the practical application of radiation therapy in the treatment of lung cancer was not possible until 1928, when the radium element pack at Memorial Hospital in New York was first used clinically. This device contained 4 g of radium and was the forerunner of megavolt therapy equipment, which forms the basis of modern therapeutic radiology. One of the first reported results of radiation therapy for histologically confirmed lung cancer was published by Ormerod,[15] who reported a series of 100 consecutive cases of inoperable lung cancer, most of which were treated by interstitial implantation during exploratory thoracotomy; 4 of these patients survived for 5 years or more.

The palliation of lung cancer by chemotherapy followed shortly after the introduction of nitrogen mustard in the treatment of malignant disease, and was reported by Levine and Weisberger[13] in 1955. More recently, manipulation of the immune status of patients with lung cancer has been used in treating patients with bronchogenic carcinoma by Israel and Halpern[8] with some encouraging results.

"What is past is prologue" is as true in cancer of the lung as it is for the Archives of the United States of America. The survival rate among patients with lung cancer remains poor. The possible rate of cure has been raised from 0% 150 years ago to about 3 to 5% of all patients diagnosed as having bronchogenic carcinoma in 1973. On the other hand, although cancer of the lung used to be described as a rare disease, it has now become a major killer of men in the United States. Treatment remains unsatisfactory in spite of all the technical advances our modern age has achieved. Hopefully, the past will prove the prologue to successful elimination of the mortality rate from bronchogenic carcinoma, if not to its complete extinction.

REFERENCES

1. Addison, T.: On the difficulties and fallacies attending physical diagnosis in diseases of the chest. *Guy's Hospital Rep., Second Ser.* **4**:3–36, 1846.

2. Bayle, G. H : *Recherchés sur la phtisie pulmonaire.* Gabon, Paris, 1810, pp. 24, 34.

3. Cockle, J.: *On intrathoracic cancer.* J. Churchill, London, 1865, pp. 16, 61–84.

4. Flint, A.: *A practical treatise on the physical exploration of the chest, and the diagnosis of diseases affecting the respiratory organs,* 2nd ed., H. C. Lea, Philadelphia, 1866, pp. 489–495.

5. Greene, S.: Encephaloid tumours in the brain and lungs. *Dublin J. Med. Sci.* **24**:282–283, 1843.

6. Hall, L.: Case of tumor in the chest. U.S. Med. Surg. J. 13:2–3, August 1835. (Reported verbatim in: *Boston Med. Surg. J.* **13**: 295–297, December 1835).

7. Horner, F.: Uber eine Form von Ptosis. *Klin. Monatsbl. Augenheilk.* **7**:193–198, 1869.

8. Israel, L., and Halpern, B.: Le corynebacterium parvum dans les cancers avances. *Nouv. Presse Med.* **1**:19–23, 1972.

9. Killian, G.: Über, directe Bronchoskopie. *Muench. Med. Wochenschr.* **45**:844–847, 1898.

10. Kirstein, A.: Autoscopie des Larynx und der Trachea. *Arch. Laryngol. Rhinol. Berl.* **3**:156–164, 1895.

11. Kümmell, L.: Totalresektion einer Lunge wegen Karzinom. *Zbl. Chir.* **38**:427–428, 1911.

12. Langhans, W.: Primaerer Krebs der Trachea und Bronchien. *Virchow's Arch. Pathol. Anat. Physiol. Klin. Med.* **53**:470–484, 1871.

13. Levine, B., and Weisberger, A. S.: The response of various types of bronchogenic carcinoma to nitrogen mustard. *Ann. Intern. Med.* **42**:1089, 1955.

14. Morgagni, J. B.: De sedibus et causi morborum. Lavanii Typogr. Acad., 1761, Lib. II, ep. 22 (quoted by Pepper[18]).

15. Ormerod, F. C.: The pathology and treatment of carcinoma of the bronchus. *J. Laryngol. Otol.* **52**:733–745, 1937.

16. Onuigbo, W. I. B.: Lung cancer in the nineteenth century. *Med. Hist.* **3**:69–77, 1959.

17. Papanicolaou, G. N.: Diagnostic value of exfoliated cells from cancerous tissues. *J. A. M. A.* **131**:372–378, 1946.

18. Pepper, W.: Cases of cancer of the lungs and mediastinum. *Trans. Coll. Physicians Phila. N.S.* **1**:96–110, 1850.

19. Quain, F.: Encephaloid tumour involving the heart and lungs. *Br. Med. J.* **44**:902, 1857.

20. Salter, H.: Clinical lectures on diseases of the chest. Lecture I. Primary cancer of the lung. *Lancet* **2**:1–4, 1869.

21. Virchow, R.: *Cellular pathology.* J. Churchill, London, 1860, p. 479.

22. Watson, W. L.: Radical surgery for lung cancer. *Cancer* **9**:1167–1169, 1956.

23. Watson, W. L.: *Lung cancer.* C. V. Mosby, St. Louis, 1968, p. 10.

24. Williams, F. H.: A notable demonstration of the x-rays. *Boston Med. J.* **134**:447, 1896.

Chapter Two

The Incidence of Cancer of the Lung

B ronchogenic carcinoma was a medical curiosity 150 years ago. It has now achieved the dubious distinction of being the number one killer among malignancies in United States males. The statistics of the American Cancer Society[1] for 1975 indicate that 81,100 patients are expected to die of lung cancer, and 63,500 of these will be male. Of the 83,000 new cases that will be diagnosed, 67,000 will be male. For comparison, the next most frequent malignancy in the male, cancer of the prostate gland, killed 17,200 patients in 1971 of 35,000 newly diagnosed cases. In the United States, of the 69,600 female patients newly diagnosed as having breast cancer, there were 30,750 deaths, approximately triple the female death rate from bronchogenic carcinoma in this country. United States vital statistics for 1967[9] reveal 310,983 deaths from cancer in that year, a record second only to heart disease, the cause of death in 720,892 patients. The percentage of cancer deaths expressed in relationship to the total number of deaths was 16.8%. Death from bronchogenic carcinoma accounts for nearly 20% of all cancer deaths in the United States; thus approximately 3.5% of all U.S. patients die of this disease. Disregarding the obvious differences in populations that might die from one disease or another, lung cancer causes death in as many patients as do highway accidents or influenza and pneumonia.

Although underreporting and early death from infectious disease were mainly responsible for the apparent rarity of lung cancer in the nineteenth century, the statistics of the U.S. Bureau of the Census[2] indicate a precipitous rise in the frequency of bronchogenic carcinoma in male patients since about 1935 (Fig. 1). This increase is greatest for the nonwhite male population.[4] Racial differences are also evident in national trends in bron-

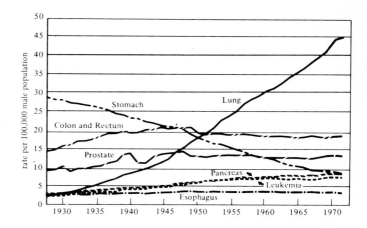

Fig. 1. Male cancer death rate by site, United States, 1930–1969. (Courtesy of American Cancer Society, Inc.)

chogenic carcinoma, with significant differences in the incidence of lung cancer in male and female Japanese and Chinese as compared to U.S. whites (Table 1).[7] The relatively uniform incidence of lung cancer among females of all races except Maori women, who are heavy cigarette smokers, is very evident.

If male lung cancer mortality had been eliminated, there would have been no increase in the U.S. male cancer rate over the past 10 to 20 years. At present lung cancer accounts for 32% of the male cancer rate in the United States and for 43% in England, Wales, and Scotland.

The increase in longevity in the U.S. population earlier in this century is not the only factor contributing to the frequency of lung cancer, although there is a

TABLE 1. AGE-ADJUSTED DEATH RATE PERCENTAGES BY SELECTED PRIMARY SITE AND SEX: JAPAN, TAIWAN AND U.S. WHITES, 1960–1961[7]

Primary Site	Japan Males	Japan Females	Taiwan Males	Taiwan Females	U.S. Whites Males	U.S. Whites Females
Buccal cavity and pharynx	1.32	0.59	4.73	2.10	4.58	1.26
Esophagus	6.95	2.26	6.97	1.58	3.26	0.78
Stomach	69.50	36.80	21.86	11.93	11.46	5.81
Intestines (except rectum)	2.79	2.88	3.02	3.34	13.24	13.31
Rectum	4.27	3.44	2.74	1.40	5.97	3.80
Liver and biliary passages	15.07	9.46	—	—	4.66	4.53
Pancreas	3.02	1.88	—	—	7.78	4.63
Lung, bronchus, and trachea	9.97	3.67	7.73	4.00	31.36	4.69
Breast	—	3.76	—	3.80	—	21.38
Uterus, all parts	—	15.51	—	16.32	—	11.52
Ovary, fallopian tube, and broad ligament	—	1.57	—	—	—	7.35
Prostate	1.43	—	0.59	—	12.84	—
Bladder and other urinary organs	2.05	1.03	—	—	5.18	1.80
Leukemia and aleukemia	3.35	2.56	—	—	7.84	5.05

higher incidence among older patients (Fig. 2).[6] Langston[5] reported that the increase in mortality from cancer of the lung has been less for patients 40 to 44 years old since about 1945, for those in the 45 to 49 age group since 1950, and for those 50 to 54 years since 1955. These statistics may indicate a prospect for slowing the rate of increase in male mortality from bronchogenic carcinoma, with the patients who were born around the turn of the century showing the highest rate. If this wave of high-risk patients passes through our patient population, a possible decrease may be forecast for the future. It should be noted here that this study applies only to patients seen in a U.S. Veterans' Administration Hospital; similar studies are not available for other population groups.

Another significant factor in the incidence of lung cancer is the ratio of male to female patients in the United States. Between 1950 and 1967 this ratio increased from 6:1 to 5:1.[1] Since then, however, the rate of increase has been higher in the female population.

Although possible etiologic factors will be dealt with in the next chapter, major differences in incidence are noted among histologic subgroups of lung cancer. According to a study published by Vincent et al.,[8] 60% of the male patients with lung cancer had epidermoid carcinoma, whereas only 9% had adenocarcinomas. The data for female patients showed epidermoid carcinoma in 14% and adenocarcinoma in 49%. This suggests that the rapid increase in the incidence of lung cancer among female patients may be limited to epidermoid and oat cell carcinomas.[10]

The economic impact of lung cancer in this country can only be estimated, since accurate figures of the cost of treatment are not available. It is difficult, however, to underestimate this impact when one considers the relatively small change in survival rate and the rapid increase in incidence since earlier this century. A U.S. Public Health Service report[3] indicates that there were approximately 300,000 cancer deaths in the United States in 1963. The direct cost for hospitalization, nursing care, physicians, and other services and medications exceeded $1.5 billion in 1969. The indirect cost is even greater when one includes the loss of earnings during the illness and the loss of earnings during the balance of the normal life expectancy of these patients, many of whom had been stricken in a productive phase of their lives. Taking all these factors into consideration, the total cost of cancer to the U.S. economy is approximately $15 billion. Thus, each cancer death may represent an expenditure of about $5000 in direct services and $50,000 in loss to the economy as a whole. At current rates of inflation, the cost of cancer to our economy may amount to as much as 2% of the gross national product. Bronchogenic carcinoma accounts for a major portion of this loss of the most important resource of our country: the lives of our citizens.

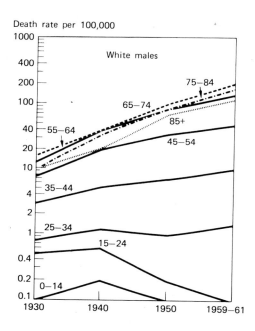

Fig. 2. Trends in death rate for malignant neoplasms of bronchus and lung in white males, United States, 1930–1961. (Copyright 1972 by the President and Fellows of Harvard College.)

REFERENCES

1. *1975 Cancer Facts and Figures.* American Cancer Society, New York, 1974.

2. *Current Population Reports—Population Estimates,* U.S. Bureau of the Census, Washington, D.C., 1968.

3. *Health Economic Series No. 6. Estimating the Cost of Illness,* United States Department of Health, Education and Welfare, USPHS Publication No. 947–6, May, 1966.

4. Henschke, Ulrich K., et al.: Alarming increase of the cancer mortality in the U.S. black population. *Cancer* 31:763–768, 1973.

5. Langston, H. T.: Lung cancer—future projection. *J. Thorac. Cardiovasc. Surg.* 63:412–415, 1972.

6. Lilienfeld, A., Levin, M., and Kessler, I.: *Cancer in the United States,* Harvard University Press, Cambridge, 1972.

7. Segi, M., and Kurihara, M.: *Cancer mortality for selected sites in 24 Countries,* No. 4 (1962–1963), Department of Public Health, Tohoku University, Japan, 1966.

8. Vincent, T. N., Satterfield, J. V., and Ackerman L. V.: Carcinoma of the lung in women *Cancer* 18:559–570, 1965.

9. *Vital Statistics of the United States,* USPHS, National Vital Statistics Division, Washington, D.C., 1967.

10. Wynder, E. L., Mabuchi, K., and Beattie, E. J.: The epidemiology of lung cancer. Recent trends. *J. A. M. A.* 213:2221–2228, 1970.

Chapter Three

The Etiology of Cancer of the Lung

Tobacco was introduced to Europe during the reign of James I of England (1603–1625), who was also James VI of Scotland (1567–1625). In a treatise entitled "A Counterblast to Tobacco," he described smoking as "a custom dangerous to the lungs, and in the black stinking fumes thereof nearest resembling the horrible Stygian smoke of the pit that is bottomless." Three and a half centuries later, in 1964, another counterblast to tobacco was published, a report by the U.S. Surgeon General[14] that summarized evidence implicating smoking as one of the major contributing factors in the development of lung cancer and other serious threats to health. Since then, additional information linking smoking to lung cancer has come to light. A study of major importance deals with the mortality rate in Swedish twins.[4] Death rates of cigarette smoking patients were compared with those of twins who did not smoke. There was no excess mortality among the smokers born between 1886 and 1905. Among twins born between 1906 and 1925, however, there was a higher death rate among the smokers.

This study forms one of the links between smoking and lung cancer, and other demographic studies support the thesis that cigarette smoking is a major factor in the development of lung cancer. The disease is rare among nonsmoking Seventh Day Adventists.[4] The incidence of lung cancer among British physicians who stopped smoking is decreasing, while an increase is evident among the male adult population in the United Kingdom[13] (Fig. 1). The correlation of decrease in cigarette smoking with a lower incidence of lung cancer is statistically significant. Another prospective study linking cigarette smoking to the development of lung cancer comes from Japan:[9] in a study of 265,118 adult males who were followed, the death rate of the cigarette smokers from lung cancer was four times higher than that of the nonsmokers.

Retrospective studies have shown a dose-response relationship between cigarette smoking and lung cancer[19] (Fig. 2) and prospective studies have confirmed this relationship. A study by Graham and Levin[8] indicates that lung cancer risk in smokers approaches that of nonsmokers after abstention from cigarette smoking for 10 years, and that the risk also declines in patients who have smoked for 30 or more years.

The likelihood of developing lung cancer is related to both the amount of smoking and the length of exposure. Evidence is also being accumulated that smoking not only causes cancer of the respiratory and upper digestive tracts, but that there is also an increase in cancers of the esophagus and bladder among tobacco smokers.[7] It has been estimated that in male patients who never smoked the total mortality rate from lung cancer may be reduced to 10% or 20% of its present rate, and female mortality may be cut to approximately 50%.[5]

Pre-malignant changes introduced into the bronchial mucosa of smokers who died of accidents and other causes not related to cancer have been described in detail by Auerbach et al.;[2] the resulting changes after cigarette

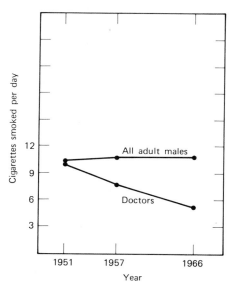

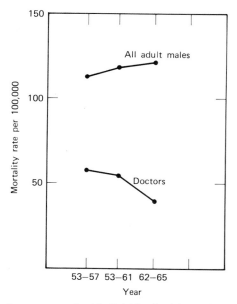

Fig. 1. Cigarette smoking and lung cancer: time trends of smoking and lung cancer mortality for all adult males in the United King-dom compared with British physicians. (Reprinted with permission from reference 13.)

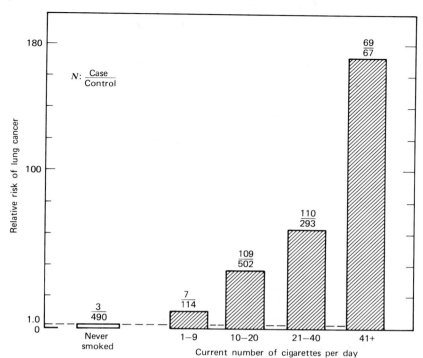

Fig. 2. Relative risk of lung cancer by number of cigarettes smoked: 408 male lung cancer patients and 2272 controls in New York, Los Angeles, and Houston, 1966–1971. (Reprinted with permission from reference 19.)

smoking, such as squamous metaplasia, carcinoma *in situ*, and invasive carcinoma show a significant relationship between inhaled cigarette smoke and carcinogenesis in the bronchial mucosa. Auerbach et al.[3] also have produced carcinoma *in situ* in dogs, following inhalation of cigarette smoke through a tracheostomy tube. Correlating evidence indicates that patients who use snuff, an unlit form of tobacco, develop an aggressive type of squamous cell carcinoma in the buccal mucosa, since the snuff is usually placed between the cheek and the jaw. The paper used to make cigarettes is considered a major irritant in producing bronchogenic carcinoma, but this action is absent in snuff users. Similarly, cancer of the tongue, lip, and larynx are related to cigar or pipe smoking. Alcohol consumption and nutritional disturbances may be further contributing factors in lung carcinogenesis in man.

One does not have to be an active smoker to be exposed to the carcinogens in tobacco smoke. Anybody who has driven in a car with several smokers is aware of the concentration of smoke in the air, and we may do well to remember the words of John Stuart Mill: "The liberty of the individual must be thus far limited. He must not make himself a nuisance to other people." One writer has gone so far as to suggest that smoking should be made a criminal offense unless carried out among consenting adults in private.[15]

Although the results of attempted efforts at public education about the effect of tobacco on health have been negligible, and there has been no significant change in cigarette consumption during the last 10 years,[16] cigarette manufacturers have changed the type of tobacco used in cigarettes, have added filters, and so on. The tar and nicotine content of best-selling cigarettes have decreased since 1955[7] (Fig. 3), and the smokers of filter cigarettes have a lower risk of developing lung cancer than those who smoke nonfilter cigarettes[19] (Fig. 4).

Further reduction of the carcinogenic activity of tobacco tar may occur as knowledge increases about the nature of the oncogenic substances in tobacco, since the development of tobacco substitutes or selective breeding of tobacco may also reduce cancer risk. It is unlikely, however, that tobacco products that can be inhaled with complete safety can ever be produced. It may be worthwhile to consider the cost of lung cancer in economic terms, the money paid by taxpayers, employers, and relatives of patients, to develop a more rational campaign against the health hazards of cigarette smoking.

Occupational factors that contribute to the development of bronchogenic carcinoma are listed in Table 1.

The hydrocarbons present in gasoline and diesel engine exhaust that cause widespread pollution in our society comprise some of the occupational hazards of

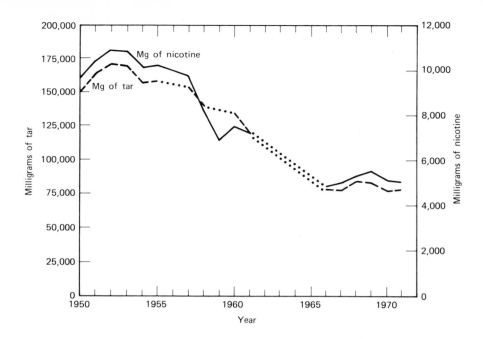

Fig. 3. Annual consumption of tar and nicotine for a person 15 years and over, United States, 1950–1971. Data are not available for years where the broken lines are used. (Reprinted with permission from reference 19.)

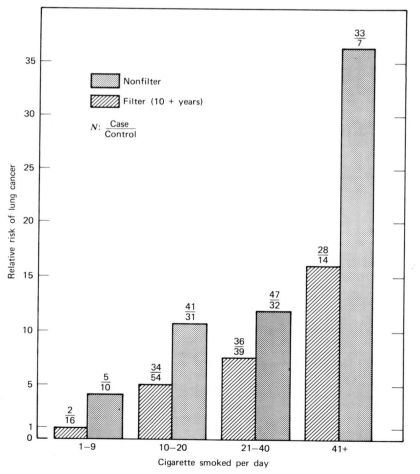

Fig. 4. Relative risk of lung cancer among current male smokers by number of cigarettes per day in New York City, Los Angeles, Houston. Controls matched by age. (Reprinted with permission from reference 19.)

TABLE 1. WORKER GROUPS WITH SPECIFIC RESPIRATORY CANCER HAZARDS[10]

Agent	Worker Groups
Asbestos	Asbestos miners, textile workers
Arsenic	Manufacturers, handlers, and users of arsenical insecticides; arsenic smelter workers; taxidermists; sheep dip workers; copper smelter workers
Chromium	Chromate manufacturers including plant maintenance workers; chrome pigment handlers
Nickel	Nickel-copper matte refinery workers
Iron	Iron ore (hematite) miners; Iron foundry workers
Radioactive substances	Radioactive ore (pitchblend) miners; miners of nonradioactive ores working in radioactive mines
Isopropyl oil	Isopropyl alcohol manufacturers
Coal tar fumes	Coke oven operators; gas house retort workers
Petroleum oil mists	Paraffin pressers; mule spinners; metal lathe workers and drillers

certain populations. Recently a new occupational hazard was found among workers in a manufacturing plant which produced chloromethyl methyl ether, in whom a prevalence of oat cell carcinoma was observed.[6]

Other tumor-producing substances such as mustard gas, may be involved in causing bronchogenic carcinoma, as was shown in a Japanese study[17]: a high incidence of lung cancer was found in relatively young patients on an island where a poison gas factory which produced mainly mustard gas was operated by the Japanese army from 1929 until 1945. Although factory employees who were not engaged in the production of mustard gas had a 0.3% incidence of lung cancer, the rate increased almost 10 times for 274 men who were involved in the production of mustard gas and who inhaled high concentrations of the poison for prolonged periods of time. This explains the lack of an increase in bronchogenic cancer among military personnel exposed to mustard gas in World War I, when smaller doses of the gas were inhaled. Occupations in which exposure to chemicals or fumes has been associated with increased risk of developing lung cancer, such as newspaper workers, painters, and carpenters among others, also implicate the previously mentioned chemical categories as potentially carcinogenic to the respiratory passages.[11]

Radioactive materials such as radon gas in radium mines, radioactive pitchblend, and the like have been related to the development of lung cancer, and the risk may be expressed as one lung cancer/million persons per year/rad of exposure. The average internal dose required to produce one lung cancer is 1.3×10^5 g rad.[1] Cigarette smoking produces an even higher rate of lung cancer, for example, among uranium miners who smoke.[20] It is worth noting here that the survivors of the atomic explosions in Hiroshima and Nagasaki have shown a large increase in bronchogenic carcinoma.[18] A comparison between this group and a group that was out of the city on the day of the blast indicates that the rate of lung cancer was increased beyond normal expectations in persons exposed to a dosage of 90 rads or more of atomic radiation. The ratio of observed to expected deaths ranges from 2.5 in the autopsy series to 1.6 in the group that was examined clinically.

Among the medical conditions that predispose to lung cancer, possibly in association with carcinogenic agents, a British study shows a higher rate incidence of lung cancer in patients with chronic bronchitis (5.89/1000) than in those without this condition (2.54/1000). In the same study, cigarette smokers with chronic bronchitis had almost double the rate (7.12/1000) of bronchogenic carcinoma as compared with cigarette smokers without bronchitis 3.61/1000); nonsmokers had an incidence of only 0.35 cancers/1000 patients.[12]

In summary: a correlation exists between the development of squamous cell and oat cell carcinoma of the lung and exposure to a number of carcinogenic agents such as coal tar fumes, metals, and radioactive substances. In some countries, cigarette smoking seems to be a major contributing factor in the development of bronchogenic carcinoma. A decrease in exposure to these carcinogenic agents may lead to a great reduction in the incidence of bronchogenic carcinoma, especially in males.

Although unions, legislators, and others are attempting to deal definitively with the occupational hazards leading to a predominance of lung cancer among exposed workers, smoking remains an elusive factor in the prevention of this type of cancer. Doll[5] states the case well: "Whether an individual smokes or not is a personal matter which he alone is entitled to decide. The smoker runs the risk and, although he may also influence others by example, there is no reason to suppose that his example must necessarily carry more weight than informed education and the example of others. The individual, however, is entitled to know the facts and to be free from pressure to smoke, merely for the sake of others' gain. The primary responsibility lies with the medical profession, who must first obtain the facts, not only about the effect of smoking on health but also about its power of addiction, then explain the facts to the public, and finally set the example of practicing what they preach."

REFERENCES

1. Archer, Y. E., and Ludim, F. F.: Radiogenic lung cancer in man: exposure effect relationship. *Environ. Health* **1**:370–383, 1967.

2. Auerbach, O., Stout, A. P., Hammond, E. C., and Garfinkel, L.: Changes in bronchial epithelium in relation to cigarette smoking and in relation to lung cancer. *N. Engl. J. Med.* **265**:253–267, 1961.

3. Auerbach, D., Hammond, E. C., Kirman, D., and Garfinkel, L.: Effects of cigarette smoking on dogs, II. Pulmonary neoplasm. *Arch. Environ. Health* **21**:754–768, 1970.

4. Brass, A.: Tobacco and health. Report of the Scottsdale Research Conference. *J. A. M. A.* **15**:1879–1880, 1970.

5. Doll, R.: Practical steps toward the prevention of bronchial carcinoma. *Scott. Med. J.* **15**:433–447, 1970.

6. Figueroa, W. G., Raszkowski, R., and Weiss, W.: Lung cancer in chloromethyl methyl ether workers. *N. Engl. J. Med* **228**:1096–1097, 1973.

7. Ghori, G.: Smoking and cancer: research in etiology and prevention at the National Cancer Institute. *Cancer* **30**:1340–1343, 1972.

8. Graham, S., and Levin, M. L.: Smoking withdrawal and the reduction of risks of lung cancer. *Cancer* **27**:865–871, 1971.

9. Hirayama, T.: Huge Japanese study adds to smoking death link. *J. A. M. A.* **220**:654–655, 1972.

10. Hueper, W. C.: Epidemiologic, experimental and histological studies on mental cancers of the lung. Acta Unio Int. Cancrum **15**:424–436, 1959.

11. Moss, R., Scott, T. S., and Atherley, G. R. C.: Mortality of newspaper workers from lung cancer and bronchitis 1952–1966. *Br. J. Ind. Med.* **29**:1–14, 1972.

12. Rimington, J.: Smoking, chronic bronchitis and lung cancer. *Br. Med. J.* **2**:373–374, 1971.

13. Schneiderman, M., and Levin, D.: Trends in lung cancer. *Cancer* **30**:1320–1325, 1972.

14. Terry, L.: *Smoking and Health*, U.S. Department of Health, Education and Welfare, Washington, 1964.

15. Tinker, J.: Should public smoking be banned? *New Sci.* **59**:313–315, 1973.

16. *The Health Consequences of Smoking. Report to the Surgeon General,* Washington, D.C., 1971; U.S. Department of Health, Education and Welfare, USPHS Publication No. HSM-71-7513, 1972.

17. Wada, S., Nishimoto, Y., Miyanishi, M., Kambe, S., and Miller, R. W.: Mustard gas as a cause of respiratory neoplasia in man. *Lancet* **1**:1161–1163, 1968.

18. Wanebo, C. K., Johnson, K. G., Sato, K., and Thorslund, T. W.: Lung cancer following atomic radiation. *Am. Rev. Respir. Dis.* **98**:778–787, 1968.

19. Wynder, E.: Etiology of lung cancer. *Cancer* **30**:1332–1339, 1972.

20. Yesner, R., Gelfman, N., and Feinstein, A.: Epidemiology of small cell carcinoma of the lung. Presented at the XIth International Cancer Congress, Florence, 1974.

Chapter Four

The Pathology of Cancer of the Lung

John Gmelich, M.D.

The standardization of various classifications of lung tumors and their terminology is necessary for proper communication, for without this there would be no way to accumulate interpretable data. Correlations could not be established with subsequent determination of the natural history, prognosis, and possible etiological factors. In 1924, Marchesani divided 26 cases of lung cancer, a large series at that time, into four cell types: basal, polymorphocellular, keratinizing squamous, and cylindrical.[120] Over the next quarter century, new, diverse, and contradictory terms proliferated to describe new tumor types.[171,196] To eliminate the contradictions and to establish order, the World Health Organization (WHO) established a classification system provided by an international committee of scholars, and published a historical synopsis of its evolution.[100]

Dr. Leiv Kreyberg, chairman of the group, had based his classification on an epidemiological separation of tumor types.[99] Epidermoid and anaplastic small cell carcinomas were classified as group I and correlated with cigarette smoking, whereas most of the remaining epithelial lung tumors were group II and believed to be unrelated to cigarette smoking (Table 1).

The Veterans Administration Lung Cancer Chemotherapy Study Group (VALCCSG) first modified (Table 2) the forthcoming WHO classification (Table 3).[200] In the VALCCSG classification bronchioloalveolar carcinomas are not a separate entity, but are included within the class papillary adenocarcinoma. Thus, many classification systems have minor differences reflecting individual preferences and use the WHO classification system as a standard of reference.[190]

The practical application of the WHO classification is the assessment of variables within the tumor, which are then subdivided into more than 29 types. The monograph is simply an illustrative manual, with guidelines as to initial separation; however, the greatest deficiency is that of the individual pathologist.[50] A study by the VA Lung Study Group has shown a marked inter- and intraobserver variance in determining subtypes of lung cancer. The present method is a gestalt photorecogni-

TABLE 1. KREYBERG CLASSIFICATION

Group I	Epidermoid carcinoma
	Small cell anaplastic carcinoma
Group II	Adenocarcinoma
	Bronchioloalveolar
	Carcinoid
	Mucous gland tumors
Others	Large cell undifferentiated
	Combined
	Sarcomas

TABLE 2. THE VETERANS ADMINISTRATION LUNG CANCER CHEMOTHERAPY STUDY GROUP (VALCCSG)

Type	Class
Squamous cell carcinoma	10
With keratin	1a
With intercellular bridges	1b
Without keratin bridges	1c
Small cell undifferentiated carcinoma	20
With oat cell structure	2a
With polygonal cell structure	2b
Adenocarcinoma	30
Acinar	3a
Papillary	3b
Poorly differentiated	3c
Large cell undifferentiated	40
Combined carcinoma	50

TABLE 3. HISTOLOGICAL CLASSIFICATION OF LUNG CANCER WORLD HEALTH ORGANIZATION CLASSIFICATION

I. Epidermoid carcinoma
II. Small cell anaplastic carcinoma
   1. Fusiform cell type
   2. Polygonal cell type
   3. Lymphocytelike (oat cell) type
III. Adenocarcinoma
   1. Bronchogenic
      a. Acinar, with or without mucin formation
      b. Papillary
   2. Bronchioloalveolar
IV. Large cell carcinoma
   1. Solid tumors with mucinlike content
   2. Solid tumors without mucinlike content
   3. Giant cell carcinoma
   4. Clear cell carcinoma
V. Combined epidermoid and adenocarcinoma
VI. Carcinoid tumors
VII. Bronchial gland tumors
   1. Cylindromas
   2. Mucoepidermoid tumors
   3. Others
VIII. Papillary tumors of surface epithelium
   1. Epidermoid
   2. Epidermoid with goblet cells
   3. Others
IX. "Mixed" tumors and carcinosarcomas
   1. Mixed tumors
   2. Carcinosarcoma of embryonal type (blastoma)
   3. Other carcinosarcomas
X. Sarcomas
XI. Unclassified
XII. Mesotheliomas
   1. Localized
   2. Diffuse

tion process correlated with microphotographs illustrated in the manual. Perhaps a more objective method for interpreting carcinomas could be used, such as the morphological measurement of nucleus, cytoplasm, cell size, chromatin patterns, nucleolar presence, and cytoplasmic characteristics as mentioned by Reagan, Patten, and Ng, in their descriptions of carcinomas of the cervix and uterus.[142,151] Although they are rudimentary, some measurements will be discussed to help interpret and delineate some subtypes in the WHO classification system.

Some authors have attacked the terms used to describe different carcinomas, and this may reflect strong preferences of objective criteria. Although the presence of squamous pearls, intercellular bridges, and keratin are objective criteria,[198] stratification resembling the epidermis, dense cytoplasmic margins, centrally placed nuclei, and other variables are more subjective. The use of special stains and histochemical techniques to determine the presence of one of several mucopolysaccharides or of keratoprotein, varies with each institution. Some pathologists believe that the keratin stain does not show prekeratin adequately and would abolish this method, while others believe that it is useful in distinguishing keratin from necrotic debris.[2] The mucin stain to determine mucopolysaccharides, suggested by the WHO Committee, is an Alcian green without specific detail as to pH. Advances in the chemistry of mucins have not been used on a large scale to determine various mucin types within adenocarcinomas of the lung.[144,173]

Additional problems in interpretation are the effects of therapy. Chemo- and radiation therapy distort the original appearance of numerous tumors and are responsible for particular artifacts, such as pyknosis or karyorrhexis of the nucleus, induction of keratin formation, and a peculiar distribution of mucopolysaccharides within the nuclear membrane. Other artifacts extremely useful in interpretation and relatively consistent in some tumors are the crush artifact in bronchial biopsies of oat cell carcinoma, and the basophilic staining of reticulum fibers in regions of necrosis. The basophilic deposition represents DNA material by special histological stains and electron microscopy. Although this is characteristic of oat cell carcinomas, it can occur in any tumor undergoing lysis. Keratin induction can be caused by numerous agents, even to the point of confusion, such as is shown by the presence of keratin pearls with a benign cytologic appearance located subcutaneously in metastatic epidermoid carcinoma of the head and neck in radical neck specimens.[158]

It is important for nonpathologists to be aware of the principles used in classifying lung cancers. Type designation is based upon the most highly differentiated tissue tumor type available. Modifying adjectives or modifying clauses are used to specify either degree of differentiation or mixture of various types. Special classifications, such as epithelial tumors showing both epidermoid and adenocarcinoma, are listed separately, and designated in the WHO monograph as combined epidermoid and adenocarcinomas. However, other terms have been employed with specific names for similar tumors.[2,82] The term adenosquamous carcinoma is used by some to refer to this mixed carcinoma when both components are malignant and equally represented. Although adenoacanthoma has been used to designate benign squamous components in an adenocarcinoma, some might illadvisedly use the term mucoepidermoid, which is reserved by the WHO Committee for surface tumors and counterparts of salivary gland tumors. If a tumor is composed primarily of one well-defined type, with an additional small proportion of cells of another type, the best means of classification is according to the dominant type with annotations referring to minor variants.

The degrees of differentiation are expressed in grade. Although Broders has elaborately specified a grading system of 1 through 4, a simpler, more practical system uses modifying adjectives rather than numbers.[29] Thus a well differentiated carcinoma would be Broders' grade 1; a moderately well differentiated cancer would be Broders' grades 2 and 3; and a poorly differentiated tumor would be grade 4. In a pathological diagnosis other modifying terms such as *in situ* and invasive may be used to delineate a primary carcinoma. The TNM system for lung cancer reflects the growth stage and can be incorporated into the final diagnosis.[6] Further qualifications may include general or specific localization and may be related to a specific structure, such as a mucous gland or a specific cell type. Recent advances in electron microscopy have shown several cells of origin in adenocarcinomas, especially those of the peripheral type. Histochemical determinants have been used to separate several types of adenocarcinomas from similar morphological counterparts, as described in "sugar" tumors of the lung.[80,111] Thus, future qualifying statements may routinely include the electron microscopic appearance of cells, as well as histochemical determinants to specify tumor type.

EPIDERMOID CARCINOMA

Epidermoid carcinomas had been said to originate most frequently in the central bronchi, that is, the first two bronchial divisions including the lobar bronchi. However, studies not based on autopsy material indicate a more peripheral origin within the intermediate bronchi, the 18 segmental or tertiary bronchi. Subsegmental bronchi are usually defined as the visible branches, and the periphery of the lung refers to distal lung parenchyma in which bronchi cannot be identified by the naked eye. Rigler studied the evolution of bronchial carcinomas radiographically and observed that tumor growth was not symmetric.[153] Peripheral tumors extended eccentrically in a centripetal direction into the lobar bronchi. Garland et al. retrospectively reassessed the radiologic origin of lung cancer and found a shift in distribution from the main bronchus to the subsegmental area.[60] His origin data differ from previous information: main bronchus 11%, compared to older data of 32%, lobar and segmental origins 58%, com-

pared to 48%, and subsegmental origin 31%, compared to 14%.

Over 50% of all tumors were found to arise in the periphery of the lung in two studies using surgically removed specimens.[160,187] To better identify the tumor origin, the lungs were dissected along the plane of the bronchial tree. One analysis revealed that >50% of epidermoid carcinomas originated beyond a segmental bronchus (Fig. 1a). All these studies dealt with radiologically visible lesions, so that the carcinomas were very large.

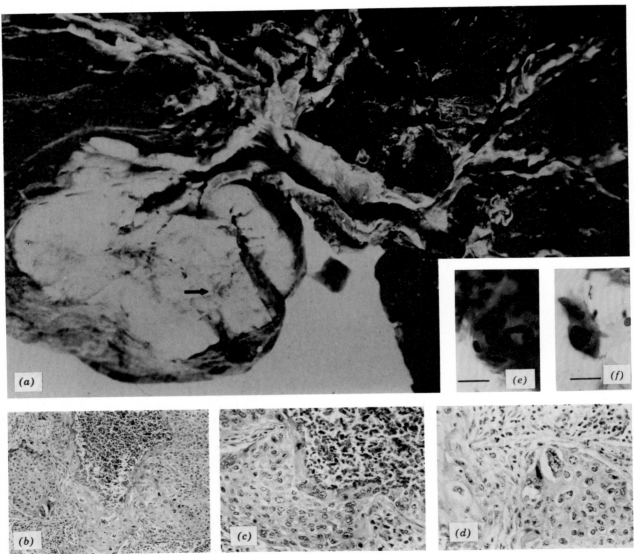

Fig. 1. (a) A 7.0 cm bulky epidermoid carcinoma involves three subsegmental bronchi and extends toward a segmental bronchus indicating a subsegmental origin. Note distal atelectasis, pneumonia, and parenchymal involvement with a round pushing margin. Early central necrosis and cavitation (arrow) are present. (b) Nodular sheets of moderately well-differentiated epidermoid carcinoma abut a central necrotic region. X80. (c) Stratified tumor cells mimic growth of epidermis and exfoliate necrotic cells (tumor diathesis). X200. (d) Marked anisocytosis, hyperchromatic irregular nuclei, and dense rigid cytoplasmic borders can be seen. X200. (e) Lamellated concentrically arranged cells depict formation of a keratin pearl. X400. (Line equals 20 μ.) (f) An irregular, hyperchromatic enlarged nucleus dominates a large, irregular polyhedral cell of epidermoid carcinoma. X400. (Line equals 20 μ.)

Studies of radiologically negative, often asymptomatic patients, drawn from either high-risk patients or those with a suspicious or positive cytology indicate more peripheral origin for many bronchogenic carcinomas. The increased ability to biopsy, brush, selectively irrigate, and visualize the more peripheral airways with the smaller, more flexible fiberoptic bronchoscope has considerably altered the cure rate, resection rate, and detection of epidermoid carcinoma[90,148,202] (Table 4).

These studies reaffirm the Auerbach findings and re-emphasize the wide distribution of mucosal alterations, the coexistence of precancerous changes, carcinoma *in situ*, and invasive carcinoma, and the presence of synchronous and metachronous multiple epidermoid carcinomas.[10-12,34,166]

Additional information may be gained by using other techniques, such as transcutaneous transpleural needle biopsy, which may allow a definitive tissue diagnosis of peripheral lesions beyond the range of the fiberoptic bronchoscopes.[28,203]

The gross appearance of epidermoid carcinoma varies with the stage of its development (Figs. 1a,2a,3a,b,4a). The earliest lesions may be difficult to discern grossly, and may be represented only by slightly thickened mucosa, granular and irregular in outline. The thickness of the mucosa, the granularity of the surface, the volume of the altered mucosa increase, and the transition from minimally to markedly involved mucosa becomes more apparent with increasing growth of the carcinoma. Loss of the usual longitudinal and circular mucosal folds or grooves, loss of the commonly present light reflex or mucosal sheen when viewed through a bronchoscope, and the loss of the usual surface pits designate fully developed *in situ* and early invasive carcinoma (Fig. 4a). Small pits on the surface normally present are the pores or mouths of the mucous glands, and their obliteration is the macroscopic counterpart to the histological replacement of normal ductal and glandular epithelium with effacement of ducts and acini (Fig. 4c). This represents a contiguous extension of the surface alteration and may be solely intraepithelial. However, the basal portions of the completely effaced glandular acini are frequently the site of early invasion (Fig. 4b).

These changes relate not only to invasive cancer, either in a distant site or more usually in the adjacent perimeter either distal or proximal, but also exist in the absence of a more advanced lesion. It is to be hoped that the bulky, nodular gray-white, partially obstructing lesion of invasive epidermoid carcinoma will become a thing of the past.[30] The earliest lesions are plaquelike, relatively sessile, and involve only a portion of the circumference of the bronchus. Later there is circumferential involvement in a sleevelike manner with a proximally projecting, exophytic tongue of tumor (Figs. 2a,3a). Occlusion of the bronchus is first partial, then total, but rarely is there any significant bronchial compression prior to extension through the basement membrane. A nonobstructive 4mm carcinoma was shown to be invasive in one study. This early invasion is in contrast to the biologic behavior of papillary carcinomas of the surface mucosa and the unusual pedunculated variant of epidermoid carcinoma.

After extension through the basement membrane, the submucosa internal to the cartilaginous plates is effaced and the tumor has ready access to the lymphatics and blood vessels. The loose areolar tissue of the bronchovascular ray offers little resistance to contiguous, centripetal axial spread. Except in the most distal lung parenchyma the direction of lymphatic flow is toward the hilum, and this plus the mechanical efforts of respiration help the migration of carcinoma centrally. Tumors limited to the mucosal aspect of the cartilaginous plates without significant encroachment of the bronchial lumen produce neither a mass effect to distort the bronchial contour nor a significant distal air-trapping, common radiographic manifestations of early carcinoma. Newer bronchographic techniques that include the insufflation of tantalum or other heavy metals combined with magnification films to detect minor surface alterations of the mucosa within the bronchus may greatly increase radiologic detection of very early carcinoma.[54,58]

Transmural involvement is followed by involvement of the more peripheral lung parenchyma (Fig. 3b). The biologic behavior of individual tumors has been correlated with the growing margin of a tumor mass: a round, pushing margin indicates a better prognosis in medullary carcinoma of the breast, in contrast to the stellate, crablike edges of infiltrating ductal carcinoma. In the lung, well-differentiated tumors often use the preexisting lung architecture for structural support for neoplastic growth. This is commonly observed in bronchioloalveolar carcinoma, and the pneumoniclike tumor growth merges

TABLE 4

	Resections	Total	DOD[a]	New Primaries
Pearson et al.[145]	14	20	0	0
Woolner et al.[197]	15	15	2	0
Lerner et al.[104]	4	4	0	0
Melamed et al.[124]	5	12	1	1
JHH[b46]	8	9	1	1
	46[c]	60	4[d]	2

[a] Dead of disease.
[b] Johns Hopkins Hospital statistics reported at Short Course, International Academy of Pathology, February 1974.
[c] Resectability rate = 76%.
[d] Mortality rate of those resected = 9%.

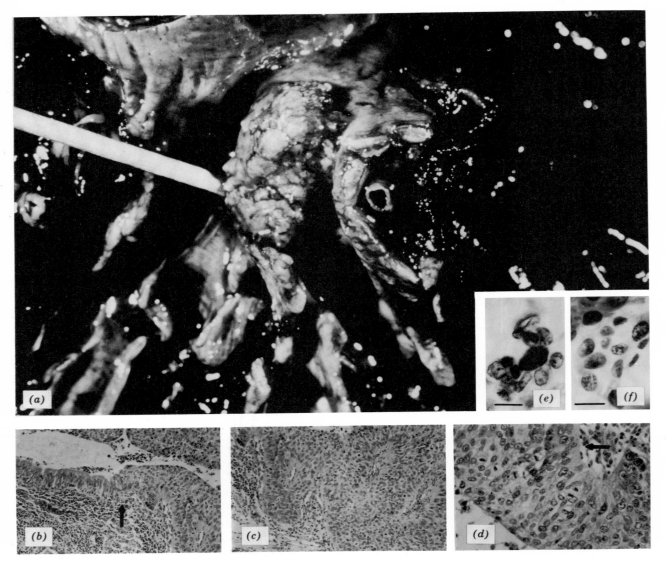

Fig. 2. (a) An exophytic centripetal extension of a proximal epidermoid carcinoma projects thumblike into a sublobular bronchus. Subtle distal mucosal changes of dysplasia and carcinoma *in situ* are hidden. Note the pebbly, irregular pearl-white surface and intact cartilaginous plates. (b) An abrupt zone of transition (arrow) between normal respiratory mucosa and carcinoma *in situ*. The absence of a dysplasia zone indicates a lateral margin of invasive carcinoma. (c) Increased thickness of the mucosa produces an uneven, ragged, dull surface. (d) Nonkeratinized cells exfoliate from the surface. Note intact basement membrane (arrow). X200. (e) Most tumor cells contain vesicular nuclei with uneven, irregular nuclear membranes. Only the central cells exhibit markedly hyperchromatic nuclei. (Line equals 20 μ.) (f) Vesicular malignant nuclei predominate. Cytologic differentiation between nonkeratinizing epidermoid carcinoma and poorly differentiated adenocarcinoma would be difficult without the hyperchromatic, irregular nucleated carcinoma cell. (Line equals 20 μ.)

gradually with the frequently associated "golden," obstructive or endogenous lipid pneumonia (Fig. 5a). This subtle transition is shown by gradual changes in the color and firmness of the pneumonic regions. Less well-differentiated tumors push away and compress rather than utilize preexisting lung parenchyma.

The surface of epidermoid carcinoma is gray-white, dry, rough, and granular, with poorly defined, round peripheral margins (Fig. 2a). This contrasts with the yellower, glairy mucoid surface of adenocarcinoma with its multilobulated margin. Epidermoid carcinomas usually cavitate and microscopic and gross necrosis is common. The center of the lesions becomes soft and cheese-like and is readily expectorated through the bronchial tubes. Cavitating epidermoid carcinoma can be diagnosed cytologically because of the large amount of necrotic material, highly keratinized cells, and necrotic tumor cells that are cast off.

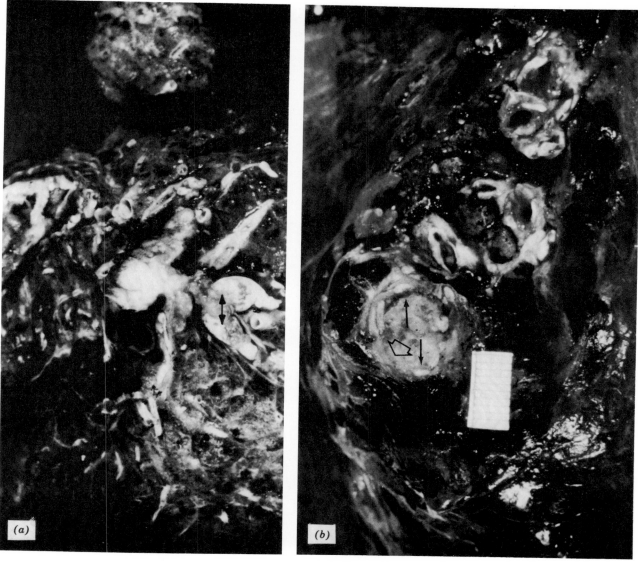

Fig. 3. (a) A V-shaped fingerlike growth (double arrow) occludes several segmental bronchi without parenchymal extension. (b) Peripheral section of epidermoid carcinoma, mainly intraluminal, with intact cartilaginous plate (single full arrows) and mucosal and transmural extension (single empty arrows).

The major blood supply of primary and metastatic carcinomas within the lung is by the bronchial arteries. Pulmonary arterial contribution can only occur if the supporting framework of the lung is not dissolved by tumor growth. Although intramural bronchial growth can cause distortion of bronchial arteries, total obstruction is rare. Cavitating carcinoma can be suspected when the cavity is located in an unusual site for aspiration and there are no clinical signs of sepsis. Radiographic and macroscopic observations demonstrate that the interior of the cavity is occasionally furrowed or ribbed like that of a ship's bulkhead. This correlates with the preservation of the bronchovascular rays at the periphery of the cavity. Also, the surface of this cavity differs from an abscess cavity in that it is frequently thick, granular, and shaggy in contrast to the thin shiny epithelial lining of healed abscess cavities.

A significant degree of vascular invasion is not readily seen in most epidermoid carcinomas. Arteriographic studies in human and animal carcinomas by Delarue reveal that the vascular network of malignant tumors is similar structurally to unorganized capillary and precapillary systems.[40] This explains the absence of distinct elastic lamina and the poor histological separation be-

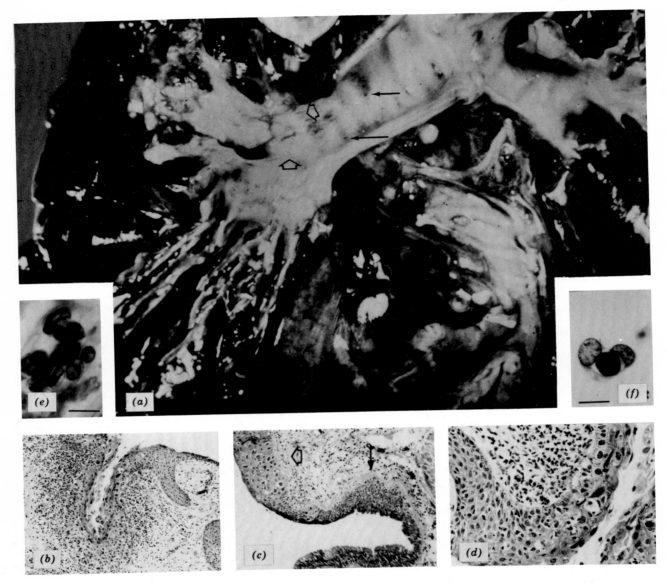

Fig. 4. (a) Subtotal luminal occlusion with eccentric subcircumferential mural involvement by epidermoid carcinoma. Mucous gland pores (full arrows) are seen proximally. Obliteration of pores, longitudinal striations, and irregular advancing front of thickened altered mucosa show carcinoma *in situ* (open arrows). (b) Epidermoid carcinoma *in situ* extends into the mouth of a mucous gland. The base of a gland is often the site of early invasion. X80. (c) Zones of hyperplasia and dysplasia (full arrow) merge with carcinoma *in situ* (open arrow), forming a zone of neoplastic transition. X100. (d) The lumen of the gland duct contains desquamated keratotic tumor cells. Eventually the duct of the bronchial submucosal mucous gland will be totally obliterated. X200. (e) Tumor cells are exfoliated in tissue sheets. (Line equals 20 μ.) (f) Cytologic pattern known as pseudocannibalism or tumor cell phagocytosis shows loss of polarity with possible loss of surface contact inhibition. (Line equals 20 μ.)

tween arterial and venous elements within malignant tumors.[82] Elastic stains are used to show the internal and external elastic lamellae of the pulmonary artery, the external elastic lamella of the pulmonary vein, and the internal elastic lamella of the bronchial artery. However, the study by Hukill and Stern indicates that routine elastic stains cannot show clearly the type of vasculature present within malignant tumors and do not help clarify the presence or absence of vascular invasion.[82] Instead of infiltrating, as is typical in adenocarcinoma, the contiguous, pushing growth pattern of epidermoid carcinoma may also affect the degree of vascular invasion.

The interval between the invasion of carcinoma and that of lymphatic dissemination can only be deduced from studies of simple versus radical lobectomies and appro-

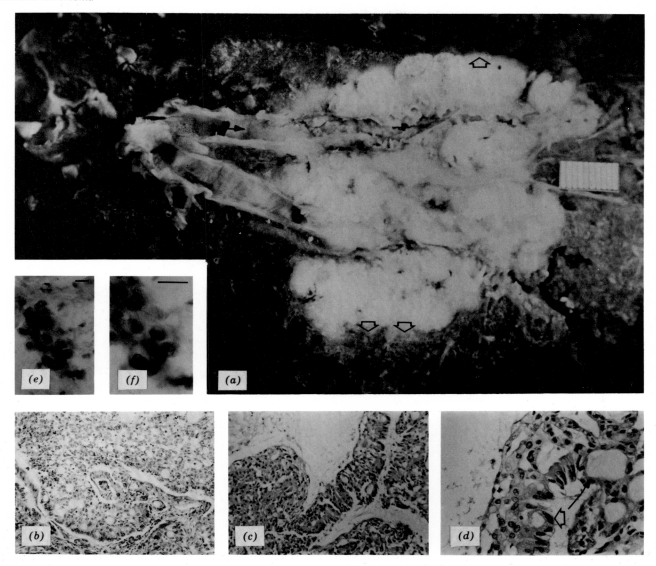

Fig. 5. (a) A 6 cm midcentral, lingular adenocarcinoma showing transegmental extension, pleural involvement (open arrow), lobulated margins, subtle pneumoniclike filling of adjacent parenchyma (double open arrows), and replacement of bronchial mucosa (full arrow). The latter suggests that the site of origin is cartilage-bearing bronchi, and thus a bronchogenic carcinoma. (b) A moderately well-differentiated adenocarcinoma replaces lung parenchyma. In this portion of tumor, there is no use of preexisting alveolar septa for growth. (c) Acinar pattern can be seen in the linear sheet of tumor. Some mucous is present. (d) Gland acini filled with mucin (full arrow) and individual intracytoplasmic mucin vacuoles (open arrow) are present. (e) Overlapping cells form papillary clusters of 6–8 cells each. (f) Granular cytoplasm, prominent nucleoli, and nuclear molding of cells at periphery of cell cluster confirm the diagnosis of adenocarcinoma.

priate lymph node dissections. Lymph nodes are frequently free of tumor metastases, even when the tumor has reached an appreciable size. An uncommon source of blood-borne metastases is the secondary involvement of the venous system through angiolymphatic communications, which may develop after massive metastatic replacement.

Auerbach provides a good description of the histological variants of precursor carcinoma lesions.[8,9] The earliest carcinomas are *in situ*, with Bowenoid-like changes within the respiratory mucosa (Figs. 2b,2c,4c). The precancerous reactions within the mucosa are of two types: basal cell hyperplasia or squamous metaplasia. Auerbach suggests that changes differ depending upon the stimulus; if the stimulus is carcinogenic, it produces atypia of either basal or squamous cells. Atypia is difficult to define, and many terms have been used by various authors to describe both histological and cytological changes of precancerous lesions. The histological changes of basal cell hyperplasia and squamous metaplasia with subsequent atypical squamous and basal cell metaplasias of varying degrees are comparable to the dysplasias of the uterine cervix. These terms are only important because they designate the evolution from a precancerous to a cancerous process. At first, the lesions appear microscopically as an increase in the width of the mucosa related to an increase in the cell layers, particularly those of basal cells. This reaction is similar to acanthosis of the skin. Hyperplasia is accompanied by squamous metaplasia, with loss of the usual ciliated columnar respiratory cells. In addition to the loss of ciliated cells, goblet cells are no longer present. This is in contrast to changes in chronic bronchitis, also believed to be related to tobacco smoking. Here there is an increase in the number of goblet cells or mucous metaplasia, and a great increase in the volume of the bronchial mucous glands in proportion to the thickness of the wall of the bronchus, the Reid index.

Saccomanno showed the temporal sequence cytologically,[156,157] and Auerbach[8,9] indicated the physical sequence within the tracheobronchial tree in the development of precancerous lesions to invasive carcinoma.

Two variants of epidermoid carcinoma include those with a pedunculated intrabronchial lesion and those associated with peripheral scars. Pedunculated carcinoma is extremely rare, is usually attached to the bronchial wall by a relatively narrow stalk, and frequently occludes the bronchial lumen early in its development.[106] Obstruction and subsequent pneumonia may lead to early detection. These tumors are macroscopically and microscopically similar to those usually seen in the oropharynx and larynx.

Peripheral epidermoid carcinomas can be related to diffuse or focal scars. Focal scars usually are related to old granulomatous disease, healed pneumonia, and infarcts, whereas diffuse scarring in the form of honeycombing, as described by Meyer and Liebow,[126] is associated with the highest reported incidence of squamous carcinoma in pulmonary scars. Most studies show a predominance of adenocarcinoma and oat cell carcinoma associated with scars.[187] Epidermoid carcinoma can rarely be observed in the extreme periphery of the lung in association with honeycombing and subpleural bullous formation.[42,126] This is more common in adenocarcinoma. Transpleural invasion with the peripheral epidermoid carcinomas is common, and with proper therapy involvement of the chest wall does not mandate a poor prognosis. Squamous carcinoma is rarely seen in pleural effusions. Approximately 15 to 20% of scar carcinomas are truly invasive epidermoid tumors. Squamous metaplasia and atypical bronchiolar epithelial proliferation of the squamous type are seen frequently in association with honeycombing, the end-stage of usual interstitial pneumonia.

Well differentiated epidermoid carcinoma mimics the tissue organization and cytoplasmic specialization of the skin's epidermis. Cytologic characteristics of keratin formation and tissue characteristics of intercellular bridges are typical of this neoplasm. The replacement of pale yellow by porcelain-white mucosal color is the gross correlate of microscopic keratin formation. Intercellular bridges correspond to desmosomes seen with the electron microscope, and tonofibrils are the connecting filaments. This type of membrane connection is analogous to spot welding and is one of three forms of membrane connection between cells.[139] Histologic reflection of this intercellular junction type is a pattern of tightly adherent cells growing frequently as small nests or sheets. The overall growth pattern simulates that of epidermis growing in a stratified arrangement, mixed with whorling features that are associated with the production of keratin pearls. A three-dimensional representation of pearl formation is well described by Naib.[129]

Poorly differentiated tumors retain some of the above characteristics, but are recognized primarily by the overall growth pattern of stratified cell masses. Variations of cell growth include pseudogranular formation due to central necrosis with subsequent desquamation of the central cells, and a pseudosarcomatous appearance due to elongation and spindling of tumor cells invading the stroma, where they are mixed with a desmoplastic fibrous tissue host response.[106] If the tumor is poorly differentiated or is one of these variants, other regions of the tumor should be examined for the usual histologic features and many sections should be used for a positive identification of an *in situ* component, and thus the tumor's origin.

Usually great difficulty arises in defining poorly differentiated epidermoid carcinomas; therefore, the WHO Committee suggested less rigid terms, such as large and small cell anaplastic carcinoma. Cell size in epidermoid carcinoma varies considerably; cell shapes vary from polygonal to round or spindle-shaped. Poorly differentiated forms should show neither keratin formation nor intercellular bridges. The small cell forms are usually difficult to distinguish from anaplastic small cell carcinomas. There is a gradual histologic and cytologic transition in both small and large cells of epidermoid carcinoma to those of small and large cell anaplastic tumor varieties. Patton et al. discussed the difficulties of distinguishing between large cell carcinomas and poorly differentiated epidermoid and adenocarcinomas.[141] A similar statement can be made in regard to small cell carcinomas. Thus the variable quoted incidence of large cell carcinoma in different series relates directly to the rigidity of criteria in separating poorly differentiated forms of epidermoid and adenocarcinoma from large cell carcinomas. A decrease in the inter- and intraobserver variation may be possible by using cytologic parameters comparable to those used by Reagan and Ng.[151] Even the crude cytomorphologic ranges illustrated in the Figures may be helpful.

The cytologic and histologic similarities between anaplastic small cell carcinoma and small cell, poorly differentiated epidermoid carcinoma suggest that oat cell carcinoma represents a variety of epidermoid carcinoma. This is debated in the literature and will be discussed in detail in the section on oat cell carcinoma.

ADENOCARCINOMA

The WHO classification divides adenocarcinomas into bronchogenic and bronchioloalveolar carcinomas. Those of bronchogenic origin are subdivided into acinar or papillary with and without mucin. Bronchioloalveolar and papillary carcinomas are combined in the VACCLSG study, since separation was thought to be unreliable.[200] Acceptance of bronchioloalveolar carcinoma as a specific subtype of adenocarcinoma has been debated in the literature;[22,42,103,119,121,131,190] even the term bronchioloalveolar carcinoma was chosen to indicate an uncertainty of cell and site of origin.[110] Bronchioloalveolar carcinoma is defined as a well differentiated adenocarcinoma arising in the periphery of the lung behind cartilage-bearing bronchi and using preexisting lung parenchyma for growth. There is little invasion of the substance of the lung, and the tumor metastasizes by lymphatic and aerogenous spread. Additional criteria include a relatively bland cytological appearance of individual cells, lack of other glandular or acinar patterns, that is, characteristics of less differentiated carcinomas, and the lack of a desmoplastic reaction in the lung at the periphery of the tumor mass.[189] However, these criteria are nonexclusive and the possibility of metastatic adenocarcinoma from one of several sites should be eliminated. This type of tumor differs significantly from other types of lung adenocarcinomas: since there are no extrathoracic metastases in 25% of reported cases, metastases are limited to the thorax in another 50% of cases, and only 25% of cases have extrathoracic spread.

Electron microscopic studies have shown several different cell types within macroscopically similar bronchioloalveolar carcinomas.[3,36,64,65,104] Type II alveolar lining cells or granular pneumocytes contain typical lamellated cytosomes in the apical portion of their cytoplasm and microvillae on their luminal surface. Ciliated cells have specialized basal bodies located adjacent to the luminal surface, numerous mitochondria, and various membrane and nonmembrane bound granuoles. Nonciliated bronchiolar cells or Clara cells with membrane-bound secretory granuoles are believed to be the production site of surfactants.[47] Cells that are electron microscopically found to contain mucin, frequently in an apical cytoplasmic position, represent goblet cells of respiratory mucosa. These cell types have been described in bronchioloalveolar carcinomas composed of either a single cell line or mixtures, the latter often representing a composite of cells from the bronchiolar mucosal surface. Kulchitsky's cells (K cells) are also located in the bronchiolar mucosa, but are not a proliferating cell type in bronchioloalveolar carcinomas. The proliferation of Kulchitsky's cells will be discussed later.

Histochemical determinations of mucin have been done on a variety of bronchioloalveolar carcinomas with diverse results. Mucicarmine, Alcian green, and p-aminosalicylic acid usually stain goblet cells; only PAS stains granular pneumocytes, which are typically unreactive after diastase digestion. Histochemical advance should allow better separation and thus support histologically observed differences within bronchioloalveolar carcinomas or tumors (BATs). Recently described pure Clara cell bronchioloalveolar carcinomas are rare, without any indication of special histologic characteristics. Alveolar cell carcinomas (ACC), an appropriate term for granular pneumocyte neoplasms, histologically resemble benign reactive proliferations of these lining cells, that is, desquamative interstitial pneumonia.[3] The former are grossly multiple, nodular, and focal, the latter diffuse and uniform. Cells in ACC are not uniform, are slightly larger, and have cytologic criteria of malignancy. Central interstitial fibrosis characterizes individual nodules in contrast to diffuse fibrosis, an end-stage result of desquamative interstitial pneumonia (DIP). The biologic behavior of this variant should be investigated, since it may be significantly different from the more common BATs derived from cells of bronchiolar surface epithelium. Occasionally mucorrhea, which is clinically attributed to some BATs, may reflect those tumors with a large goblet cell population. Obstruction of bronchioles by occluding tumor proliferation results in obstructive or "golden" pneumonia because of the loss of normal alveolar clearance. Mucopolysaccharide material released from necrotic tumor cells or within viable cells may be mixed with fat-filled macrophages or Type III pneumocytes. Inspissated mucin devoid of cells within acini or alveolar ducts should prompt an etiological search. An unusual variant of bronchogenic carcinoma, colloid carcinoma, may produce copious mucin similar to carcinomas originating in the breast or colon. Neoplastic proliferations of membranous pneumocytes (Type I alveolar lining cells) have not been described. A possible explanation for this is that Type I and Type II alveolar lining cells are not separate entities but represent the same cell in either an immature or specialized state of development.

There is a remarkable histological resemblance between some cases of bronchioloalveolar carcinoma and a viral sheep disease known as jaagsiekte. The viral etiology of pulmonary adenomatosis has been demonstrated by its production in sheep experimentally induced by cell-free transfer. The possible viral etiology of bronchioloalveolar carcinoma has been suggested by the presence of viral-like nuclear inclusions in BAT and DIP.[36,137] Although a viral origin is not excluded, electron microscopic studies show that these inclusions are not viral but are infoldings of the nuclear membrane with inclusions of cytoplasmic material. The incorporation of cytoplasmic material within nuclei is commonly found in many neoplasms, including various adenocarcinomas, and is prominent in malignant melanoma cells.

A spectrum ranging from noninvasive bronchiolar epithelial proliferations to invasive bronchioloalveolar carcinoma has been produced in cigarette-smoking dogs.[72] Structural changes associated with invasion are destruction of alveolar structure, formation of confluent cell masses, and partial thickening of the interstitium by fibroblasic cells representing a stromal desmoplastic reaction. Invasion into the interstitium is by subtle penetration of the proliferating lining cells (Fig. 6d). Benign cytologic correlates include the preservation of cilia and terminal bars whereas malignant cells exhibit loss of cytoplasmic specialization and nuclear criteria of malignancy. Although ciliated cells have been shown in some human bronchioloalveolar carcinomas, it is doubtful that they represent neoplastic cells with invasive potential. Cellular proliferations of the acinar and papillary types may have mixed squamous cell foci, but no combined carcinomas are described. The destruction of the alveolar structure is histologically similar to regions of atypical bronchial epithelial proliferation observed in humans.

There are three distinct types of bronchiolar epithelial proliferations, acinar or glandular, squamous, and carcinoid associated with either focal or diffuse fibrosis in human lungs. Tumorlets, an appealing but less precise term, or carcinoid atypical proliferations are found in almost one-third of bronchiectatic lungs associated with central peribronchial fibrosis.[109,194] Intramucosal and peribronchiolar carcinoid proliferations seem unrelated to fibrosis and represent a proliferative hyperplasia of unknown etiology. All three cellular types of proliferation can be found around focal peripheral zones of fibrosis. Focal fibrosis may be related to old granulomatous disease, infarcts, healed pneumonia, or even to fibrotic tracts secondary to penetrating wounds of the thorax.[199,]

Honeycombing represents an end-stage in chronic interstitial pneumonia (Figs. 7a,b). This form of diffuse fibrosis has numerous, diverse etiologies. Similar architectural derangements resulting in interstitial fibrosis are related to many other diseases such as farmer's lung and allied hypersensitivity reactions, eosinophilic granuloma, sarcoidosis, and aged lungs. Usually in these conditions, the interstitial fibrosis is intimately related to a small bronchiole, and results from the porous revision of the partially destroyed bronchiolar wall similar to that in the Aschoff-Rokitansky sinuses in the gallbladder. This should be distinguished from the Canals of Lambert, which are normal accessory bronchioloalveolar connections.

Although any type of interstitial fibrosis may support any of the cellular proliferations,[69] the acinar or glandular type is the one most frequently associated with peribronchial fibrosis, and squamous proliferations are usual in the diffuse honeycombing process. The combination of squamous and acinar cells is most common. Proliferations can be so widespread and of such cytologic deviation from the norm as to be indistinguishable from minute scar carcinomas.

Regions of honeycombing have been associated with cellular proliferation in 40% of human lungs surgically removed for carcinoma.[69,126] Some regions of fibrosis have cellular proliferations and, in cigarette-smoking dogs and some BATs, cellular proliferations occur prior to fibrous thickening of the interstitium. Although fibrosis and cellular proliferation are related, some aspects of the disease origins, the etiologic relationships, and the biologic significance are still unknown.

How significant is the degree of central fibrosis in a peripheral well differentiated adenocarcinoma? If there is a perceptible fibrotic component, some would exclude the possibility of bronchioloalveolar carcinoma; others would argue that no distinction should be made between adenocarcinomas.[85] The degree of central fibrosis varies with the initial macroscopic manifestation of bronchioloalveolar carcinoma. It is frequently small in the pneumonic form, large in the single nodular type and varies with each nodule of the multiple nodular type; the earliest nodules are often the most fibrotic (Fig. 6d).

Abundant anthracotic pigment is often found within the central fibrotic region and may be the result of condensation of a large amount of lung parenchyma and the obstruction to drainage of lymphatics, with loss of one of the usual exit mechanisms of pigment-bearing macrophages.

Does focal central fibrosis represent a preexisting scar

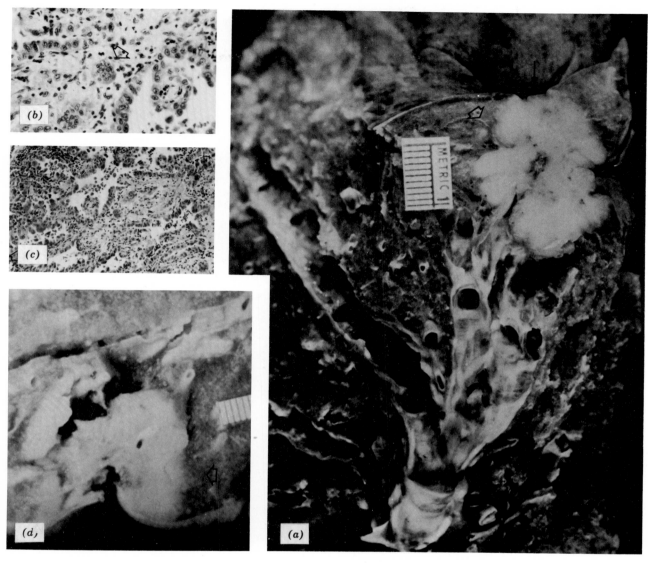

Fig. 6. (a) A 3.0 cm peripheral adenocarcinoma has caused retraction of pleura. There is no evidence of anthracotic pigmentation or fibrosis. Note the subtle pneumonic involvement laterally (open arrow). (b) A peripheral adenocarcinoma involving basal (small) and lateral (large arrow) pleurae extends centripetally toward cartilage-bearing bronchi. Note the central pigmented, depressed scar and lobulated margin of tumor and pneumonic spread (open arrow). (c) A low columnar, glandular epithelium partially lines thickened, preexisting alveolar architecture. The perpendicularly arranged epithelium often grows intraluminally as papillary tufts (open arrow). X80. (d) Interstitial invasion (open arrow) is one of the best criteria for malignancy. X200.

or an induced desmoplastic host response? The smallest scar carcinomas have been documented incidental to studies made to determine the origin of lung carcinoma or to determine relationships between atypical bronchiolar epithelial proliferation and zones of fibrosis (Fig. 8a). New data show unusual host responses to some bronchioloalveolar carcinomas. Intravascular proliferation of bronchioloalveolar carcinoma results in hyalin-like nodules with massive stromal proliferation of cells that appear in some cases to be fibroblastic and non-epithelial. These nodules are centered upon blood vessels, either veins or arteries, and frequently have a stellate margin because of the extension of the fibroticlike process along bronchovascular rays or secondary lobular septa. Upon examination, the material is unlike hyalin, amyloid, or collagen. The lesions are not infarcted and, although they are based on blood vessels, they are not necrotic. The interstitial widening is unlike metastatic tumors, including the propagation of intrapulmonary mesotheliomas, which are clearly associated with and

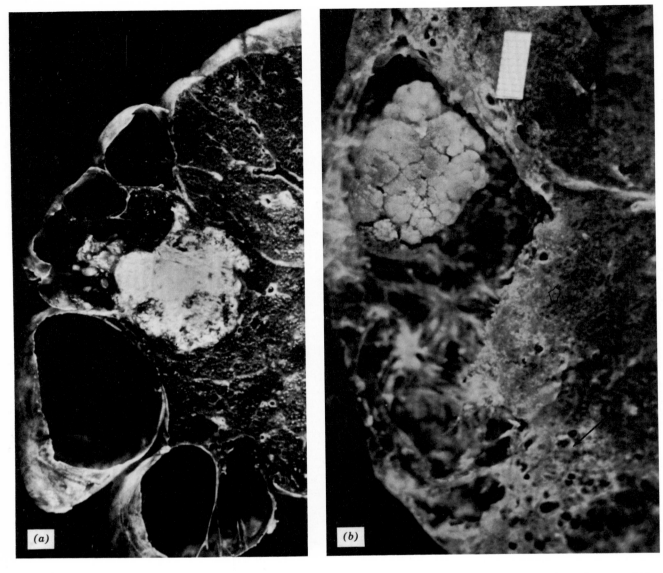

Fig. 7. (a) Apical bullous emphysema with subjacent honeycombing is the origin of a peripheral bronchioloalveolar carcinoma. Note the small fingers of carcinoma projecting into the bulla. (b) A lobulated, polypoid peripheral bronchioloalveolar carcinoma is attached by a thin stalk and floats free within a large honeycombed space. Around the borders are zones of finer honeycombing (full arrow) and pneumoniclike growth of carcinoma (open arrow).

best recognized by foci within lymphatics rather than blood vessels.[1]

Special stains such as elastic stains show that the lumina of both arteries and veins are filled with abundant intercellular material. With elastic stain, the nodules are unlike the elastosis seen centrally in scar carcinoma; superficially they resemble localized amyloidosis or end-stage or "burned-out" plasma cell granuloma.

Intravascular metastases within the lung are rare. After choriocarcinoma, probably the most common, are primary sarcomas within the heart with multiple metastases in small arteries and arterioles and with secondary extravascular extensions into lung parenchyma.[184] Rare examples of intravascular dissemination have occurred in gastric adenocarcinoma, adenocarcinoma of the gallbladder, and melanoma. Hepatoma and renal cell carcinomas often invade and sometimes propagate along the inferior vena cava and can cause a lung embolus.

Secondary involvement of pulmonary veins is common and occurs either by direct extension from a massively replaced lymph node or through lymphaticovenous anastomoses that may represent the mechanism of entry into Batson's paravertebral plexus. The normally numerous bronchial and pulmonary venous anastomoses are en-

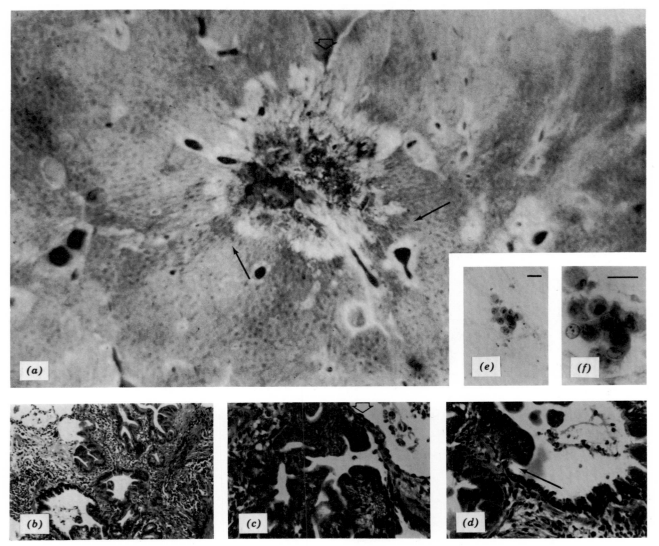

Fig. 8. (a) A small peripheral scar adenocarcinoma with distal loss of lung volume, pleural involvement (open arrow), depressed central anthracotic scar, and lobulated margin with disseminated metastases. Note the pneumonic foci and traction (scar) emphysema (full arrows). (b) A dense fibrous scar supports a well-differentiated adenocarcinoma growing as a papillary carcinoma. Note the interstitial inflammatory infiltrate. X80. (c) The junction (open arrow) between normal alveolar walls and the extension of adherent neoplastic cells. X200. (d) Normal respiratory mucosa is encroached upon and replaced by neoplastic epithedium (full arrow). This represents lateral growth and is not the origin of the carcinoma. X200. (e) Frondlike or papillary cluster of tumor cells has some cells projecting at right angles to a central core. (f) Varying sized vesicular nuclei, multiple micronucleoli, and cellular overlap characterize a well-differentiated peripheral adenocarcinoma. X400.

hanced by metastases and with bronchial venous drainage directly to the right atrium, secondary tumor dissemination can occur.

Attempts to correlate vascular invasion with metastic potential and prognosis have failed. Chemotactic and tumor inhibiting factors correlate better with metastasis than evidence of neoplastic proliferations within blood vessels.[76,135]

Poor clinical prognosis may not necessarily follow vascular invasion as suggested by some cases of IVBAT (intravenous bronchioloalveolar tumor). This entity was introduced by Dr. Liebow at the San Diego Session of the California Tumor Tissue Registry[112] and was referred to in an article on deciduosis.[48]

Neoplastic interstitial infiltration is one mechanism of metastatic spread, since the interstitial tissue space connects with the first recognizable lymphatic channels at the level of respiratory bronchioles. Larger peribronchial, septal, or subpleural lymphatics are clearly separated from veins because of their valves. Aerogenous spread of carcinoma by seeding via the airways is commonly associated with BATs, occasionally with other types of primary neoplasms and rarely with aspiration of metastatic carcinoma cells.

Experimental tracheal installation of tumor cells results in aerogenous seeding of the lung and, in addition to contiguous growth, may represent one method of disseminating mucosal surface lesions resembling viral papillomatosis. Although it is often difficult, determination of an *in situ* component in primary adenocarcinoma of the lung is most reliable and can be shown by transmural destruction of a bronchus or may, as in BAT, be related to the largest, centrally sclerotic peripheral nodule. A

histologic or cytologic inconsistency in usual pulmonary adenocarcinoma without a desmoplastic pulmonic response should stimulate a search for other primary sites.

Of the neoplasms which have been demonstrated to metastasize intrabronchially, adenocarcinoma of the colon is most common, but adenocarcinoma of the kidney does so in a higher proportion of cases. Although it is usually associated with breast and prostate carcinomas, lymphangitic spread is frequently the initial route of dissemination of leukemic and lymphomatous processes.

BATs cavitate and, unlike epidermoid carcinoma, Hodgkin's disease, and some metastatic tumors, are usu-

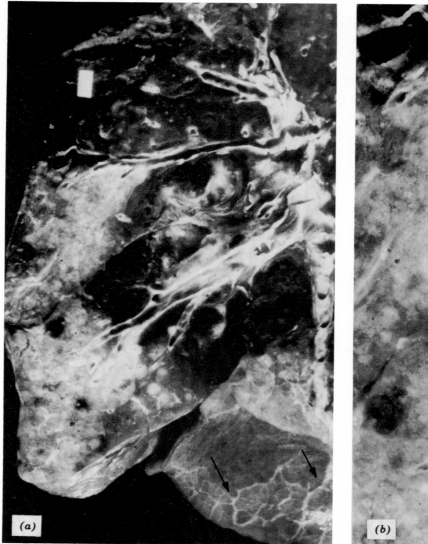
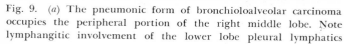
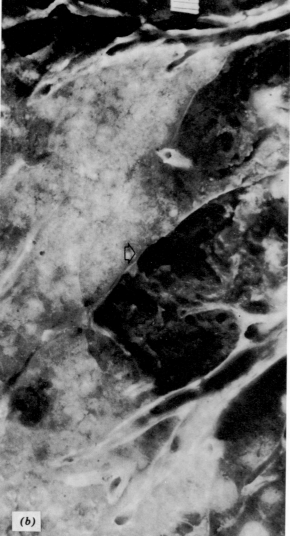

Fig. 9. (*a*) The pneumonic form of bronchioloalveolar carcinoma occupies the peripheral portion of the right middle lobe. Note lymphangitic involvement of the lower lobe pleural lymphatics (full arrow). (*b*) Pneumonic foci and multiple tumor nodules involve pulmonary parenchyma. Note the unusual, smooth wall cavities within the regions of consolidation (open arrows).

ally not visible on x-ray. The cavities are small and multiple and possess a margin of viable neoplastic cells (Figs. 9a,b). As in all benign or malignant papillary tumors, psammoma bodies can be found and are believed to represent laminar mineral incrustations on the necrotic stroma and peripheral cells of the papillary frond.[143]

The term bronchogenic adenocarcinoma is reserved for glandular or papillary cancers that arise from visible bronchi with destruction of lung parenchyma and that usually excite a desmoplastic response (Fig. 5a); tumors that originate in bronchial glands should be excluded. Mucin production varies considerably. The cytological detection rate and origin within all the ramifications of the bronchial tree are comparable to those of epidermoid carcinoma. Although many adenocarcinomas contain a few giant cells, the term giant cell carcinoma should be reserved for a different kind of tumor.

Although goblet cell hyperplasia in the surface mucosa and hypertrophy and hyperplasia of mucosal glands are associated with chronic bronchitis, adenocarcinoma

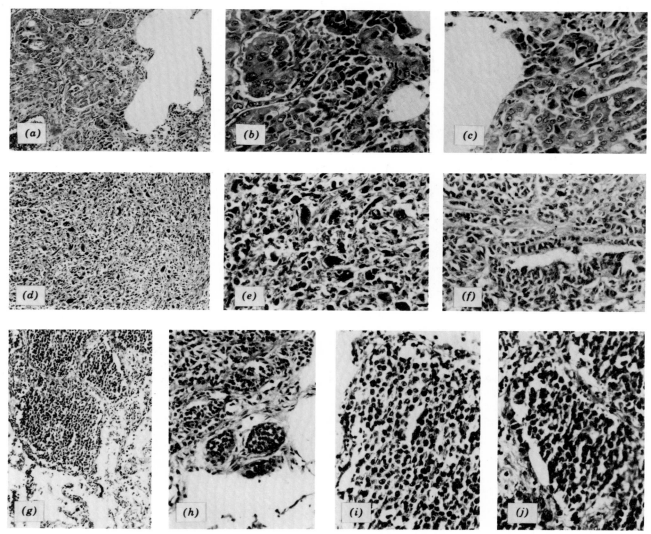

Fig. 10. (a) A poorly differentiated adenocarcinoma growing within the distal lung parenchyma. X100. (b) Neoplastic cells fill alveolar lumina in a pneumonic fashion without necrosis of alveolar septa. X250. (c) Neoplastic cells spread into alveolar duct but do not use alveolar septa for growth. Although alveolar septa are not destroyed this histological pattern is not a bronchioloalveolar carcinoma. X250. (d) A giant cell carcinoma destroys all preexisting lung structure. X80. (e) Varying shapes and large size of the anaplastic cells often suggest sarcoma rather than carcinoma. X200. (f) Poorly differentiated adenocarcinoma with linear growth of cells similar to Indian filing and abortive acinar formation. X200. (g) Pneumonia-like growth of undifferentiated cells replaces lung without destruction of alveolar septa. X80. (h) In contrast to the large cell anaplastic carcinoma (Fig. 10g), cell nests incompletely surrounded by septa use alveolar septa for growth. This is typical of peripheral carcinoid tumor. X200. (i) Lack of cell nests, larger cells, and cell pleomorphism typify large cell anaplastic carcinoma. X200. (j) Similar to small cell anaplastic carcinoma, a fast growing large cell carcinoma maintains intact alveolar septa. X200.

appears to be epidemiologically unrelated to cigarette consumption.

LARGE CELL CARCINOMA

This classification includes carcinomas composed of large cells $>20\mu$ without glandular, papillary or acinar forms and lacking keratin production or demonstrable intercellular bridges. Frequently, the cellular proliferations are solid nests of neoplastic cells with or without intracellular mucin or clear cytoplasm. The presence of intracellular mucin without glandular formation is of questionable diagnostic value, because many various mucopolysaccharides are normally located in the epithelial cells of mucosal surfaces in diverse organ systems throughout the body. The distinguishing of large cell carcinoma from poorly differentiated adenocarcinoma is difficult and the rigidity of the interpretation relates ob-

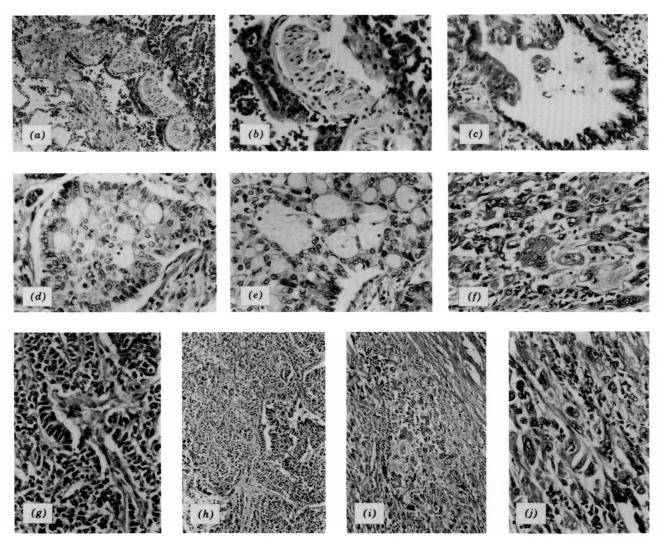

Fig. 11. (a) A well-differentiated bronchioloalveolar carcinoma uses alveolar septa for growth (upper right). X80. (b) The respiratory mucosa are replaced by carcinoma (lower right), with communicating tumor ducts through the muscle coat. X250. (c) Papillary fronds of tumor focally replace the lining mucosa of a terminal bronchiole. X200. (d) A moderately well-differentiated acinar bronchogenic adenocarcinoma fills a terminal bronchiole. X200. (e) Mucin may be free in between tumor cells or may reside in giant cytoplasmic vacuoles. Free mucin within alveoli should prompt a search for neoplastic cells. X250. (f) Multinucleated giant tumor cells and large bizarre cells with vacuolated cytoplasm suggest that many giant cell carcinomas are poorly differentiated adenocarcinomas. X200. (g) A poorly differentiated adenocarcinoma has a growth typical of adenocarcinomas with tumor cells aligned perpendicularly to a basement membrane. X200. (h) The lower power of Figure 11g reveals destruction of all previous lung parenchyma. X80. (i) A desmoplastic reaction (upper right) surrounds an inflammatory infiltrate and permeates a giant cell carcinoma (same tumor as in Figs. 11 f and 11j). X80. (j) Bizarre spindle and polyhedral cells of giant cell carcinoma mimic myosarcoma cells. X200.

served incidences of this carcinoma type in different series.[141]

Intracellular mucin has been shown in another variant, giant cell carcinoma[78] (Figs. 11f,i,j). Large multinucleated tumor cells $>50\mu$ and up to 500μ with abundant cellular phagocytosis dominate the structure. Spindle-cell metaplasia and pseudosarcomatous appearance are common and may be misinterpreted. This frequently peripheral carcinoma in older individuals has a prognosis equal to that of small cell anaplastic carcinoma.[70,91,104,125,130,149] Its incidence varies in different reports, and a 10% incidence appears inappropriately high.[74]

The presence of gynecomastia is evidence that gonadotrophins are secreted by some large cell lung carcinomas.[56] The differential diagnosis of giant cell carcinoma includes primary or metastatic choriocarcinoma in the lung parenchyma. There may be a relationship between some of the giant cell carcinomas of the lung and reported cases of pulmonary choriocarcinomas.[16] Embryological basis for tests of choriocarcinomas in the lung may be misplaced portions of thymic tissue within the lung or the totipotential of pulmonary mesenchymal cells. Other findings that support these concepts include carcinoidlike neoplasias of the thymus and malignant lymphomas resembling granulomatous thymomas within the lung parenchyma.[88,116,155] There is also a relationship between large cell carcinomas and pulmonary osteoarthropathy, since immunoreactive studies show that some large cell carcinomas contain human growth hormone.

The clear cell variant of large cell carcinomas is determined by the absence of mucopolysaccharides. These carcinomas may or may not contain PAS-positive diastase-sensitive granules in the clear or watery cytoplasm. If the neoplasms contain mucopolysaccharides and PAS diastase-resistant glycomucoproteins, these should be classified as large cell carcinoma with mucin. Metastatic tumors and adrenal and renal cell carcinomas must be considered in the differential diagnosis in addition to the benign variant of clear cell carcinoma or sugar tumor. Sugar tumors, so named because of their high carbohydrate content, were first reported by Castleman and Liebow in 1963; 12 cases were described in 1971.[111] Recent electron micrographic studies differ about cell origin; some believe it represents a variant of the Kulchitsky cell, others think the cells are similar to pericytes or smooth muscle cells. The histological criteria used in the differential diagnosis include PAS-positive cells within anastomosing cords lined by thin-walled, wide vascular channels without necrosis or mitosis. This is in distinction to renal cell carcinoma, which has narrow, thick-walled vascular channels with regions of necrosis

and abundant mitotic activity.[111] There is some resemblance to the clear cell form of leiomyoma as shown in the uterus and stomach.[80]

COMBINED CARCINOMAS

This classification should be used for those carcinomas that demonstrate well-differentiated foci of both epidermoid and adenocarcinoma. The WHO schema does not state specifically the relative quantities of each component. Some pathologists maintain that each component must be present in a significant quantity, that is, about 50% each.[2] Small foci of squamous metaplasia may be present in well differentiated bronchioloalveolar tumors, thus these tumors should not be classified as combined; these are sometimes called adenoacanthomas, similar to uterine carcinomas. Most pathologists classify adenosquamous carcinoma as equal to combined carcinomas. These tumors are extremely rare if each is required to have a major component. There is no information to warrant either a prognosis or treatment different from that of the usual bronchogenic adenocarcinoma because of the rarity of these tumors.

CARCINOID TUMORS

These epithelial neoplasms are called tumors, since histological differentiation between benign and malignant is considered unreliable so that inference to the biologic behavior of an individual tumor is unpredictable. The same reasoning is used in classifying some of the bronchioloalveolar cellular proliferations, the BATs. These tumors are composed of specialized neurosecretory cells first described by Kulchitsky as normal components of the gastrointestinal tract mucosa. These cells are located not only in the major bronchi but also in the far periphery of the lung in respiratory bronchioles.[23,24] They have a basal site in the mucosa and are concentrated near the necks of the bronchial mucous glands. Histological, histochemical, and electron microscopic similarities lend support to the paracrine system suggested by Feyrter.[53,138] A third nervous system is present in all structures derived from the primitive entodermal canal that is distributed as neurosecretory cells among the mucosa to promote hormonally an intrinsic function of these organs. To date, no better hypothesis for the existence of these cells has been formulated.[26]

The sequestration of fragments of bronchial mucosa or mucous glands by the peribronchial fibrotic process in bronchiectasis with subsequent proliferations of Kulchitsky cells results in the central form of carcinoid ABEP (atypical bronchioloalveolar epithelial proliferation) or tumorlets.[108,194] Intramucosal hyperplasia associated with central carcinoids was described in one patient in whom K cells were later shown electron microscopically in the bronchiolar mucosa and peripheral carcinoid tumors.[52,61] Hyperplasias of K cells and multiple carcinoid tumors of the gastrointestinal tract, some gastric in origin, have also been described.

The commonly shared argyrophilic- and argentaffin-staining properties of these widely distributed cells and another system of cells that may be derived from the neural crest tentatively implies some embryological relationship.[191] Recent histochemical studies of bioamines have shown a histochemically distinct amyloid and also confirmed that these neurosecretory cells share identical properties and should be included in the APUD (amine and amine precursor uptake and dicarboxylation) cell system. Tumors of these cells or apudomas include carcinoids, chemodectomas, carotid body tumors, pituitary adenomas, medullary carcinoma of the thyroid, and pheochromocytomas and also Werner's syndrome or pluriglandular adenomatosis, and Sipple's syndrome or medullary carcinoma of thyroid, pheochromocytoma and parathyroid adenoma.

To date, the paracrine and APUD systems are in complete agreement in the gastrointestinal, respiratory, and urogenital tracts but there are still differences in the dermal and mammary areas.[144]

The differential diagnosis of carcinoid tumors includes hemangiopericytoma and chemodectomas. Differentiation of endocrine tumors by differences in their cytoplasmic neurosecretory granules is not decisive. The peculiar U-shaped configurations and apposition of endoplastic reticulum in carcinoid tumors differentiate these two intrapulmonary neurosecretory tumors. The choice interstitial location of primary pulmonary chemodectomas adjacent to and with a blood supply from pulmonary venules, and the cell ball pattern of circumscribed cell nests, clearly shown with reticulin staining, separate these histologically from the similar carcinoid tumors.[98]

The reticulin stain separates the walls of the labyrinth between which the anastomosing cords or trabecular columns of K cells proliferate. Hemangiopericytomas show an angiocentric, loose lamellar pattern with the reticulin stain. The pericytes are outside the basement membrane of the small vascular cores in contrast to the cells of hemangioendothelioma.

The macroscopic presentation of central carcinoids varies from pedunculated polyps to smooth-surfaced nodules with little intrabronchial intrusion and mainly extrabronchial extension.[32] Usually, there is a large intrabronchial, obstructive mass with distal pneumonia and bronchiectasis. The transmural and extrabronchial extension accounts for the rarity of surgical cures by endobronchoscopic removal. The abundant bronchial arterial supply has been shown by injection techniques, so that one might expect brisk bleeding after biopsy or attempts at snare removal.

The histologic pattern and site of origin are often related and a spindle-cell variant reminiscent of neurofibroma is commonly found in peripheral carcinoids, whereas mosaic and trabecular patterns are seen in central carcinoids (Figs. 12c,g,h,i,j). Histologic criteria have been studied in an attempt to forecast biologic behavior.

Acinar structures with mucin do not relate to biologic behavior but do reflect the potential development of two divergent cell lines from a multipotential precursor cell. Glandular participation in carcinoid tumors has been shown previously in the gastrointestinal tract, and histological transitions to possible adenocarcinoma have been seen in the vermiform appendix.[96]

Hyperplasia of the bronchial cartilaginous plates, described in lung carcinoma, is often seen in carcinoid tumors.[73] This reflects the slow growth of the neoplasms and relates to the bulk of the intrabronchial mass. Grading of nuclear changes does relate to metastatic potential; however, variations in nuclear grade are considerable in individual tumors.[63] The degree and histologic pattern of extrabronchial growth are the most reliable criteria for correlation with biologic behavior. The size and degree of bowel wall penetration by carcinoid tumors relate to prognosis in the gastrointestinal tract.[71] The formation of a pseudocapsule of compressed lung parenchyma and the tight nesting of cells relate to a benign course. Ribbon patterns, rosettes, loss of delicate vascular stalks, loss of cellular cohesion, and foci of necrosis characterize central carcinoids that metastasize.[62]

SMALL CELL CARCINOMA

Documentation of the site of origin of many small cell carcinomas has not been possible because of the few available surgical specimens. This connotes the poor success of surgery in treating this third most common type of lung cancer. At autopsy, two features characterize the gross appearance (Fig. 13a). A collarette of peribronchial lymph nodes impressively enlarged with metastatic tumor is frequently associated with a sunburst appearance of the tumor metastases in the lung parenchyma. The feathery parenchymal margins are due to massive involvement of the lymphatics and interstitial tissue planes by the stellate dissecting growth of small cell carcinoma. Often the multiple submucosal metastases due to intramural and lymphangitic spread with subsequent ulceration of the overlying mucosa do not allow definitive localization of the neoplasm's bronchial site of origin in autopsy material. This difficulty is compounded since the primary

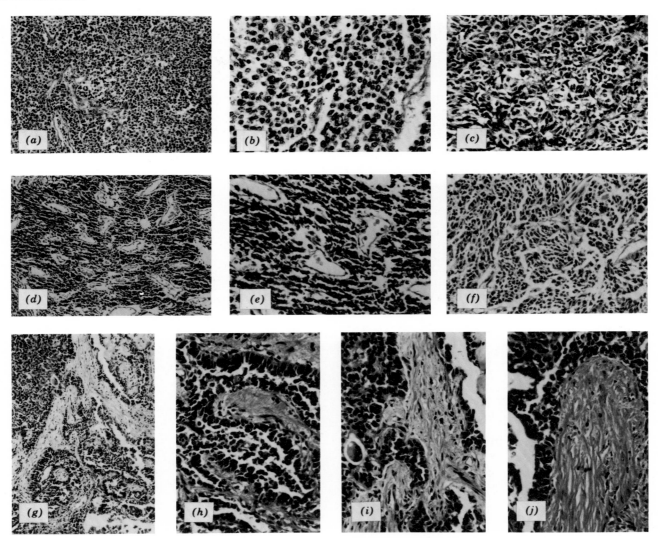

Fig. 12. (a) Large cell anaplastic carcinoma with a highly cellular structureless pattern. X80. (b) Loosely aggregated nests of large cells contain hyperchromatic variable nuclei. X200. (c) Tight cell clusters frequently surrounded by supporting septa which contain abundant capillary networks. Cells may assume a spindle shape, are more cohesive and often larger than the small cell (oat cell) anaplastic carcinoma cells in Figure 13f. X200. (d) Loss of cellular cohesion, absence of small tight cell clusters, and few thin capillary networks characterize small cell anaplastic carcinoma. X80. (e) Larger sinusoidal vessels supply large, poorly cohesive cell clusters (small tumor neoplasms are frequently smaller in size than their metastases. Microscopically, the *in situ* component as seen in epidermoid carcinoma is rarely identified.

as in Fig. 12d). X200. (f) A striking similarity exists (cf. Fig. 13c) to peripheral carcinoid tumor. This strengthens the argument that some small cell anaplastic carcinomas are malignant variants of carcinoid tumors. X200. (g) Centrally located carcinoid tumor has a fibrous pseudocapsule (upper right). X80. (h) Carcinoid tumors use the stromal septa for growth and exfoliate cells without necrosis, in contrast to oat cell carcinoma. X200. (i) Permeation of the fibrous pseudocapsule allows carcinoid cells to line the outer wall in an epithelial manner. X250. (j) Cells line and project into previous air spaces, a feature not seen in chemodectomas. X250.

Most small cell anaplastic carcinomas arise in lobar and segmental bronchi, which may be related to the many Kulchitsky cells around the mucous gland ducts. Some carcinoid ABEPs are located peripherally, and rare evidence of small cell anaplastic carcinomas arising peripherally together with scars has been documented.

At first, because of the similarity of cell size and shape and the frequent hemogenous enlargement of lymph nodes, some small cell carcinomas were thought to be lymphomas of the mediastinum. Similar errors in interpretation have occurred in metastases of other small cell carcinomas, such as lobular carcinoma of the breast.

The subtypes of the WHO classifications of small cell carcinoma illustrate the varying cell shapes—round, fusiform, polygonal—and histologic patterns of growth.

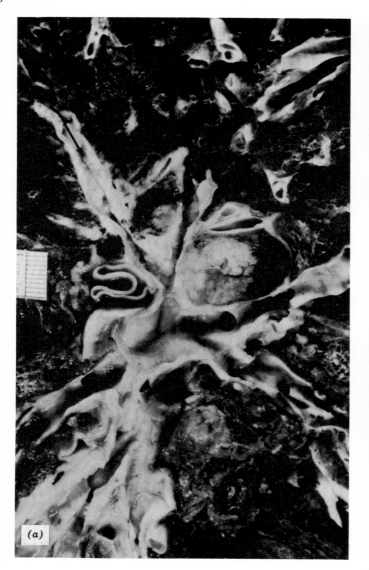

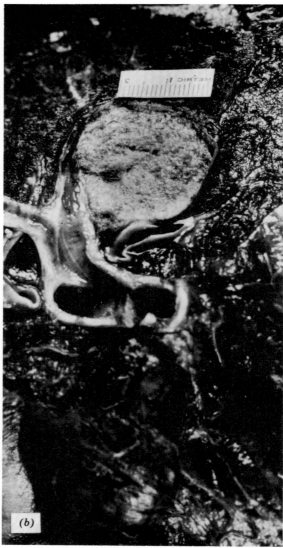

Fig. 13. (a) A collarette of tumor-bearing peribronchial lymph nodes often dominate the gross appearance of small cell anaplastic carcinoma. The site of origin may not be located, since bronchial submucosal metastases are numerous. (b) A pushing tumor margin and a cleavage artifact between the neoplasm and the adjacent lung parenchyma delineate large cell anaplastic carcinoma. Similar features are seen in primary and metastatic sarcomas.

All types have cells $<15\mu$ in diameter, but may have varying amounts of cytoplasm and nuclear chromatin. Nuclear contour is related to cell shape. Histologic patterns frequently relate to cell type and interlacing bundles, ribbons, and rosettes as well as to diffuse, loose lymphocyticlike infiltrations that occur.

Occasionally, small foci of either squamous or glandular differentiation (WHO IV 4) can be found. They have no effect on biologic behavior and may be compared to the acinar foci seen in carcinoid tumors. Squamous metaplasia of the overlying bronchial mucosa occurs in carcinoids but not as a mixed component of the tumor. Squamous differentiation within small spindle-cell forms

has led some to believe that small cell carcinoma is histogenically similar to epidermoid carcinoma. However, proponents of the Kulchitsky cell origin[25,75] cite evidence of neurosecretory granules in small cell carcinoma similar to those in carcinoid tumors. Oat cell carcinoma represents the malignant variety of carcinoid tumors in the neoplastic spectrum of Kulchitsky cells. The dispute continues and a unifying concept of histogenesis has been proposed: all divergent cell lines of growth are from a totipotential reserve basal cell, and either mono- or polycellular neoplasms result because of variation in degree of specialization or dedifferentiation.

Many pathologists do not see a significant histologic

difference between nuclear grade IV carcinoids and oat cell carcinoma, and rare examples of mixtures of well-differentiated carcinoid tumors with small cell carcinoma and regions of apparent transition lend credence to this theory. Additional evidence results from the large number of different hormonally directed polypeptide syndromes associated with oat cell carcinomas.[15,193]

Necrosis is common in small cell carcinomas in contrast to carcinoid tumors and primary lymphomas, and may represent a means of passively transferring the various polypeptide hormones. The relationship of steroid-like hormonal syndromes such as an ACTH type of syndrome to small cell carcinoma may reflect stimulation of an end organ by polypeptide hormones. Similar syndromes have been described with carcinoidlike neoplasms arising in the thymus, whereas myasthenia gravis, a hormonally opposite syndrome caused by the presence of lymphorrhages, has not been correlated with one specific cell type.[92] Disorders of growth hormone and pulmonary osteoarthropathy thought to be related to steroidlike hormone-producing neoplasms frequent in large cell carcinomas, are rarely found in small cell carcinomas. Release of nuclear DNA in zones of necrosis results in Feulgen-positive basophilic staining of the reticulin network of the tumor and is typical but not pathogonomic, since this can occur in any necrotic, highly cellular neoplasm. Although necrosis is rare in carcinoid tumors, when it does occur a local thrombosis can often be identified as the ischemic agent. Macroscopically detectable necrosis or cavitation occurs rarely in oat cell carcinoma after radiation therapy.

The lack of cohesive cell growth as shown in WHO IV 3 is similar to the histologic growth pattern of lymphosarcoma (Figs. 12d,e). The lack of a desmoplastic response of the lung and infiltration without destruction or distortion of preexisting structures such as mucus glands, bronchial cartilage, or alveolar septa may be the histological reflections of both rapid growth and loss of host response. This may explain the lack of amyloid or bone formation, or structural calcification that is seen in slow-growing carcinoid lung tumors. Binucleated cells, giant cells, and bizzare mitosis rarely seen in some carcinoids are not usually related to small cell carcinomas.

This infiltrative or dissecting growth pattern suggests a poor prognosis that is shared by large and small cell carcinoma. At least 95% of small cell carcinomas show extrathoracic spread at autopsy, and over 30% have bone metastases on routine aspiration studies. Metastases by the hematogenous route are often the first clinical signs of the disease. Alveolar aerogenous dissemination similar to that in BATs is rare, although the reason for this lack is still unknown. Dissection along interstitial planes provides ready access to alveolar capillaries, but secondary hematogenous entry may be a more likely means of vascular entry.

The epidemiologic relationship of small cell carcinoma to radioactive ores and to tobacco inhalation is well established. Although either may produce a carcinogenic or synergistic effect, the host response to such carcinogenic stimuli is shown in the studies of Saccomanno et al.[157] In a reappraisal of the effect of quantity cigarette smoking and histological type of carcinoma, in a VACCLSG study, Yesner was able to correlate only small cell carcinoma with the cigarette habit.[201]

The cytologic identification of oat cell in the sputum is generally associated with finding two to three adherent cells either linearly or in a phagocytic profile. In addition to the larger cell size, the difference in chromatin content and appearance, and their nonspherical shape allow differentiation from lymphoma or inflammatory infiltrates.

BRONCHIAL GLAND TUMORS

When origin from bronchial mucous glands can be shown, these tumors should be classified separately since their prognosis is better than that of bronchogenic carcinomas. These tumors are the bronchial counterparts of major and minor salivary gland tumors (see Table 5). Malignant counterparts demonstrated in the lung include acinic cell tumor,[49] adenoid cystic carcinoma,[77,143,181] and mucoepidermoid tumor.[13,123,136] They differ little in gross appearance, arise in lobar and segmental bronchi, and the prognosis parallels those of salivary gland tumors. Benign proliferations comparable to benign mixed tumor or pleomorphic adenoma are not

TABLE 5. BRONCHIAL MUCOUS GLAND TUMORS[a]

I. Adenomas
    A. Pleomorphic adenoma (mixed tumor)
    B. Monomorphic adenomas
        1. Adenolymphoma
        2. Oxyphilic adenoma
        3. Other types including tubular, basal cell, and clear cell
II. Mucoepidermoid Tumor
III. Acinic Cell Tumor
IV. Carcinomas
    A. Adenoid cystic carcinoma
    B. Adenocarcinoma
    C. Epidermoid carcinoma
    D. Undifferentiated carcinoma
    E. Carcinoma in pleomorphic adenoma (malignant mixed tumor)

[a] Adapted from Thackray, A. C. and Sobin, L. H.: *Histological Typing of Salivary Gland Tumors*, International Histological Classification of Tumors, No. 7, WHO, Geneva, 1972.

included in this group but are represented in the mixed tumors classification. To my knowledge, some of the rarer forms of monomorphic adenoma in the lung have not been described.

Bronchial adenoma is a misnomer and a collective term that includes carcinoid, mucoepidermoid, and acinic cell tumors, as well as adenoid cystic carcinoma.[182] The two cell types of adenoid cystic carcinoma are duct lining cells and myoepithelial cells. Nearly half of these carcinomas metastasize late, and 10-year survival rates differ considerably from 5-year rates. Acinic cell and mucoepidermoid tumors vary considerably in their degrees of differentiation. Metastasis is rare and cannot be predictably correlated with degree of differentiation. Acinic cell tumors are derived from serous cells; mucoepidermoid tumors are of three cell types: squamous cell, mucus secreting cell, and intermediate or transitional cell.

All types are usually covered by intact bronchial mucosa and project into the bronchial lumen as polypoid masses. Often, secondary bronchiectasis and obstructive pneumonia cause clinical symptoms and may prompt early resection. Adenoid cystic carcinomas infiltrate frequently in perineural tissue planes and are the most common to ulcerate the bronchial mucosa. Of the so-called bronchial adenomas, the metastatic rate is nearly 50% in adenoid cystic carcinomas, 20% in central carcinoids, and is rare in acinic cell and mucoepidermoid tumors.

Hyperplasias and adenomas of the bronchial mucous glands are rare but give rise to unusual histologic findings.[46] When mucus dissects into the interstitium, it incites a plasma cell reaction that may be so intense that the epithelial proliferation, comparable to mucoceles of the lip, can be overlooked. Similarly, abundant plasma cells can mask the presence of metastatic renal cell carcinoma. If the carcinoma is a spindle-cell variant, misinterpretation of plasma cell granuloma and fibroma is possible.

Although bronchial gland adenocarcinomas occur, little is known of their behavior or frequency.

SURFACE TUMORS

Papillary tumors of the bronchial mucosa can be epidermoid, mucoepidermoid or adenocarcinomatous, and are listed in their order of frequency.[81,15,105,167,169,170] The mucoepidermoid type should be separated from those of bronchial gland origin and should not be confused with inflammatory or reparative polyps of the bronchi. These tumors proliferate mainly in the bronchi, with little invasion of the bronchial wall or the distal lung parenchyma. When they are small and focal, the term transitional cell papilloma may be used. The epidermoid type does not, however, differ much histologically from the proliferations of juvenile papillomatosis. Isolated masses are more common in older patients, although papillomatosis of both trachea and bronchi that resembles the lesions of juvenile papillomatosis can occur. The usual lingering clinical course of the multiple lesions may be lengthened by endobronchial curettage, but recurrence of the tumor and associated pneumonias are frequent. Although the prognosis is usually good, upon recurrence the tumors become more aggressive and invade the bronchial wall and the lung parenchyma, paralleling the behavior of the papillomas and papillary carcinomas of the urinary bladder.

Juvenile papillomatosis occurs early in life and often mainly affects the larynx with subsequent involvement of trachea and bronchi. Little success has been reported with any kind of therapy, although autovaccination has succeeded in prolonging the course of the disease. Thus this lesion may be viral in origin.

Microscopically, all surface tumors are similar; the delicate fronds of connective tissue are covered by well-oriented epithelium without much cytologic variation in cells of normal mucosa. The epithelium can be purely epidermoid or adenocarcinomatous, or mixtures of goblet cells can be dispersed throughout a predominant epidermoid growth as in mucoepidermoid tumors. Microscopically, single stalks without branching or multiple infoldings with appreciable arborization may look like fronds or delicate fingerlike projections. The more complex structure of the larger projections resembles villous adenomas of the intestine.

MIXED TUMORS AND CARCINOSARCOMA

This class includes all tumors in which epithelial and connective tissue can be identified in the composition of the neoplasm. Clearly definable separations of some subtypes do not exist, and modifications to the present schema have been suggested.[31,39,74]

The most common proliferation of mixed elements is misnamed pulmonary hamartoma. This tumor is composed of bronchial epithelium, adipose tissue, and hyaline cartilage, is the most common benign lung tumor, occurs in approximately 1 out of 400 adult lungs, and represents 8% of radiologic coin lesions.[112] No description of congenital origin or recording of this lesion in infancy exists. Gradual enlargement has been demonstrated in successive x-rays. Distribution relates to any cartilage-bearing bronchus, and central ones may present as polypoid endobronchial proliferations.[146] No malignant transformation has been described. Some believe these tumors are fibromas or fibroadenomas, but they are probably the bronchial counterpart of benign mixed tumor or pleomorphic adenoma of the salivary gland.[20] When there is a scanty epithelial component, these tumors may be confused with true chondromas of the lung.

Carcinosarcomas of the embryonal type are classified separately and are also called pulmonary blastomas.[19,21,35,38,84,132,172] Although all carcinosarcomas have a better prognosis than bronchogenic carcinomas, the term blas-

toma alone implies a benign lesion. Central and peripheral locations in the lung are described. Endobronchial variations similar to the other carcinosarcomas have also been reported.

Blastoma has a distinctive microscopic appearance, with stellate and small polygonal cells of connective tissue loosely arranged to resemble embryonal mesenchyme in which glandular structures with a definite two-layered clear cell arrangement are embedded (Fig. 14g,h). There is a lack of condensed reticulin fibers around these glands. Although many accept the bigerminal origin of

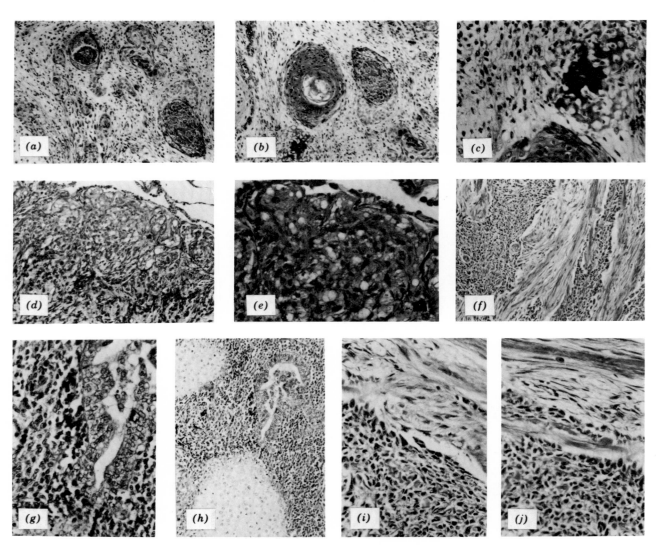

Fig. 14. (a) A mixed malignant tumor with both carcinomatous and sarcomatous elements. X80. Islands of keratinizing epidermoid carcinoma and malignant cartilage (lower left); (b) pearl formation X100, and (c) malignant osteoid (upper right). X200. (d) A malignant primary chondrosarcoma fills alveolar spaces and destroys preexisting lung structure. X80. (e) Abundant myxoid intercellular material may be confused with intracellular mucin. X200. (f) Frequently misdiagnosed as fibroma or leiomyoma, plasma cell granu-

lomas are the most common tumor in children. X80. (i) Fibrous trabeculae separate the cellular islands. X200. (j) Plasmacytoid lymphocytes, plasma cells, and histiocytes comprise the cellular infiltrate. X200. Transitional zone with histiocytes assuming spindly and fibroblastic form. (g) So-called pulmonary blastoma contains vacuolated double-cell layered glands, X200, and (h) zones of cartilaginous differentiation, X80.

peripheral lung parenchyma, as demonstrated by Waddell in transplants into vitreous tumor of the eye, the inclusion of tissue from dorsal myotomes has not been eliminated as a possible source of embryonal carcinosarcomas.[185]

Transitions are recorded between these distinctive blastomas to less characteristic mixtures of epithelial and connective tissue elements.[86] Thus elements of blastoma, rhabdomyosarcoma, squamous carcinoma, and chondrosarcoma can all be found in one tumor. Although the bronchial counterpart of malignant mixed tumor or carcinoma arising in pleomorphic adenoma is not now a separate class, it may represent those carcinosarcomas with an epidermoid rather than an adenocarcinomatous element mixed with various forms of sarcomas (Fig. 14a,b,c).

True sarcomas occur in the lung less frequently than carcinosarcoma.[83] To make this diagnosis one should exclude a metastasis from another primary site and the lack of an epithelial component. The majority of sarcomas described within the lung parenchyma are myosarcomatous or fibrosarcomatous in origin.[67,120] Rarer osteogenic primary sarcomas,[152] malignant mesenchymomas,[87] and primary chondrosarcomas[127] (Fig. 14d,e) have been described. These lesions resemble their soft tissue counterparts and, despite the frequently poor prognosis when they originate elsewhere, these tumors generally are easier to treat than primary bronchogenic carcinomas. These tumors may arise in the periphery of the lung with intrabronchial extensions or may occur centrally. Often, they have a pseudocapsule formed by compressed adjacent lung parenchyma and are distinctly separated from the lung. Occasionally, hemorrhage or necrosis will produce an arc or halolike linear space around the mass that can be filled with air to produce the radiographic air crescent sign more frequently identified with fungal or Echinococcus disease.

Hemangiopericytoma and Ewing's sarcoma usually extend into the lung from their origin in the chest wall.[14,17,51,147] Rare hemangiocytomas may be primary in the lung, and the use of reticulin stain is very effective in distinguishing this neoplasm from others.[128] Periodic acid Schiff test stains small granules in the cytoplasm of Ewing's sarcoma cells and aids in separation from reticulum cell sarcoma.[162] In Kaposi's sarcoma,[37,168,179] interstitial and septal proliferations occur with eventual alveolar involvement. Visceral involvement occurs and, in autopsy studies, the lung is often involved.[7]

Involvement of the interstitium by cellular infiltrates occurs in eosinophilic granuloma and infectious mononucleosis.[107] These dissimilar cellular infiltrates are easily differentiated from the early septal involvement of Hodgkin's disease and other lymphosarcomas.[93,97,165,193]

Lymphomatoid granulomatosis is characterized by an atypical lymphoproliferative angiocentric infiltrate with necrosis, vasculitis, and granuloma formation.[113,114] This and lymphoid interstitial pneumonia (LIP) rarely develop into lymphoma.[115] The latter is associated with Sjögren's syndrome and dysproteinemia. The lack of significant cytologic irregularities and the polymorphous composition of the infiltrate, as well as the lack of pleural and bronchial wall involvement, provide criteria for the separation of pseudolymphoma and LIP from true primary lung lymphoma.[66,160,161]

Misinterpretation of sclerosing hemangioma is rare, but electron micrographic studies conflict as to whether this represents a vascular or an epithelial neoplasm[68,79,109] (Figs. 15,a,b,c). Plasma cell granuloma can be differentiated from the more inclusive term of postinflammatory tumors because of a well portrayed spectrum of histologic characteristics and different clinical setting[18] (Fig. 15f,i,j).

Rare mucosal melanomas are described, and amelanotic melanomas may sometimes be difficult to diagnose if they are solely interstitial or lymphatic in distribution in the lung.[4,159,177] The melanocytic system is also derived from the neural crest, and melanocytes are rarely identified in the bronchial mucosa.

The most common neural tumor is benign cell myoblastoma, although rare neurofibromas and schwannomas have been described.[33,57,59,134]

Mesotheliomas rarely occur as primary intrapulmonary neoplasms; they metastasize via the lymphatics and grow along tissue planes. Although the predominant pattern is stromal or fibrous, epithelial components are almost always present. The three histologic subtypes of mesothelioma relate to the adaptability of mesothelium and are classified as epithelial or tubulopapillary, mesenchymal or fibrous, and mixed or bimorphic. A more frequently encountered difficulty is the differentiation between the epithelial type of mesothelioma and secondary tumors of the pleura, especially primary lung and bronchioloalveolar tumors.

Macroscopically, mesotheliomas are either localized or diffuse. The localized type commonly presents as an ovoid, pedunculated mass attached to either the visceral or parietal pleura. These are well-encapsulated, firm and, on cut surface, gray-white to tan with a whorled pattern similar to that in fibromas or neurofibromas. Occasionally, mesotheliomas are red, hemorrhagic, and fleshy because of focal infarction resulting from torsion of the stalk. Microscopically, these are of the mesenchymal or fibrotic type with metaplastic mesothelial cells that look like fibroblasts. Abundant hyalinized collagen is frequently present and there may be foci of calicification. Over the serous capsule, one can occasionally iden-

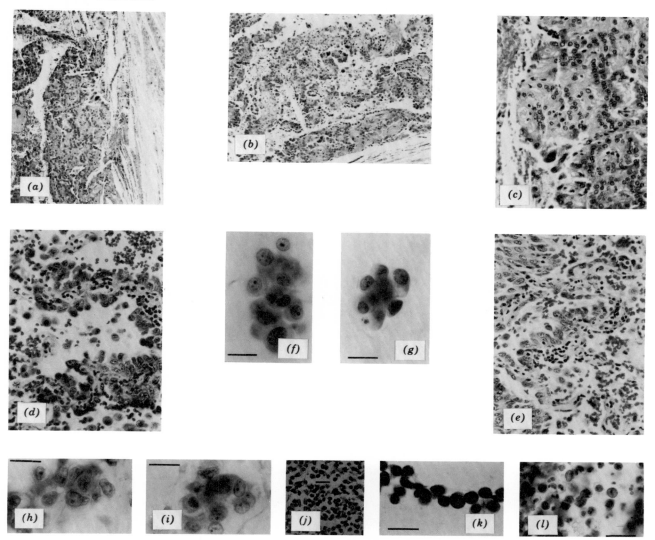

Fig. 15. (*a*) Proliferations of alveolar lining cells which line fibrous stalks containing vascular channels characterize scerosing hemangionas. Note cholesterol clefts at bottom. X80. (*b*) Vessels cut transversely occupy center of fibrous stalks. Some of the lining epithelial cells have desquamated into newly formed lumens. X80. (*c*) In some foci epithelial proliferations obscure vascular nature of the lesion, leading to misdiagnosis of bronchioloalveolar carcinoma. X200. (*d*) A bronchioloalveolar carcinoma lines preexisting alveolar septa. Note absence of thick central vessels, cholesterol clefts, and fibrous cores. X200. (*e*) Fingerlike tumor processes extend along alveolar septa without pushing margin. X200. (*f,g*) Exfoliated bronchioloalveolar carcinoma cells in a deep papillary cluster. Cells are similar and contain micronucleoli. X400. (*h,i*) Bronchogenic adenocarcinomas exfoliate more variable, slightly larger neoplastic cells. X400. (*j*) Small similar-sized hyperchromatic individual cells of lymphosarcoma with little cytoplasm. X250. (*k,l*) Molded hyperchromatic cells on a sputum (X500) and more variable cells with some vesicular nuclei and moderate cytoplasm of oat cell carcinoma contrast to Fig. 14*j*. X500.

tify hyperplastic cuboidal mesothelial cells with rare transitional forms to the underlying fibrous component. This variety of localized mesothelioma is sometimes referred to as pleural fibroma (Fig. 16*a,b,c*). They are not associated with asbestos exposure, do not metastasize, and are more common in individuals over 50 years of age, with no apparent sexual predominance. The pedunculated fibrous' type is not associated with ectopic hormonal or endocrinal syndromes or the characteristic stoop produced by the fibrous retraction of diffuse mesotheliomas within the thorax. Although cases of clubbing and pulmonary osteoarthopathy have been described, this form of mesothelioma is usually discovered incidentally on routine chest radiographs.

The diffuse form is the most common and is rarely discovered early as a small plaque of thickened visceral or parietal pleura often associated with larger hyalinized, almost acellular, calcified, fibrous plaques (Fig. 17*a,b*).

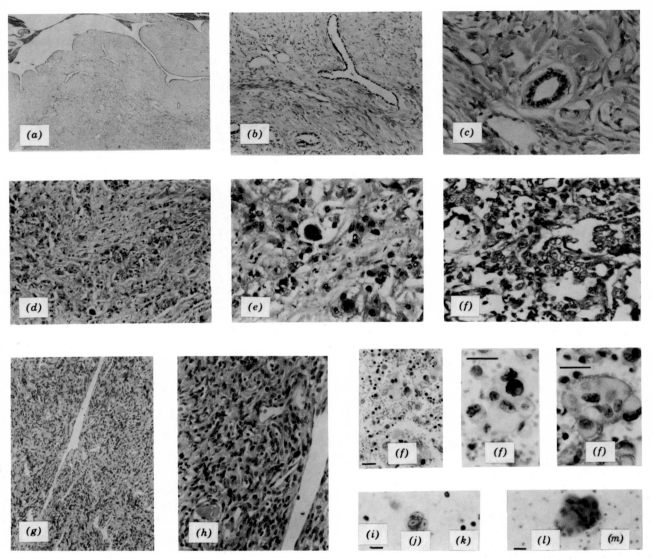

Fig. 16. (a) Histological appearance of a pedunculated mesothelioma sometimes referred to as a pleural fibroma. Nodules of fibrous tissue predominate, X80. (b) Small nests of cuboidal mesothelium are trapped, X100, and (c) hyalinized fibrocytes form an almost acellular growth. X200. (d) Epithelial mesotheliomas resemble metastatic adenocarcinoma. Plump epithelial mesothelial cell nests are enmeshed in a fibrous stroma. X80. (e) Transitional cells in between fibroblast-like cells and epithelial cells aid in determining origin of tumor, X200. (f) In less dense foci, papillary fronds of mesothelioma simulate adenocarcinoma. X200. (g) Fibrosarcomatous mesothelioma composed of plump fibroblastic cells in whorls, X80. (h) Transitions to more cuboidal epithelial cells, X200, aid in determining origin of tumor. (i) Multinucleated mesothelial cells with variable nuclei (bottom tier, l and m) are part of the cellular population, X400. (i) (upper left) shows abundant acceptable mesothelial cells with transitional forms to malignant cells. X200. (j) (center) depicts malignant nuclei, and (k) shows a multinucleated mesothelial cell with typical peripheral cytoplasmic vacuolization. X400.

These plaques are associated with asbestos exposure, although demonstration of asbestos bodies in this material is not very successful. When present, asbestos bodies are more easily identified in adjacent pulmonary parenchyma.

Many papers discuss the relationship between asbestos exposure and mesotheliomas.[133,140,186,195] The association of definite or probable asbestos exposure to mesothelioma ranges from 20% in 10-year studies to over 70% in smaller series specifically related to one type of industrial exposure.

Industrial and mining studies suggest that of the various forms of asbestos, chrysotile seems less related to the development of mesothelioma than crocidolite and

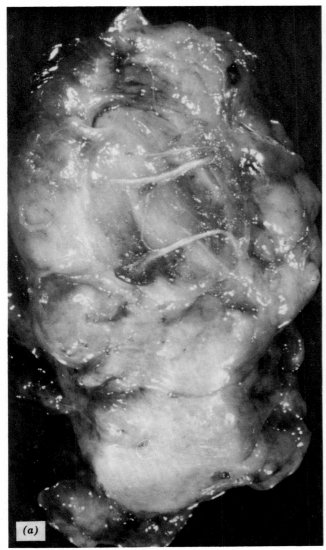

(a)

(b)

Fig. 17. (a) A shiny, nodular thickened plate of pleura showing portion of a fibrosarcomatous mesothelioma. (b) Small lobules with finely serrated margin typify the growth of an extensive epithelial mesothelioma.

amosite.[118] Pneumoconiotic involvement of the lung in individuals with mesothelioma is much more frequent than mesothelioma in individuals with asbestosis.

Diffuse mesothelioma affects men twice as often as women, and their exposure to asbestos can be confirmed to be three times that of women. Often asbestos exposure has been related to the commonest type of mesothelioma, the mixed histologic variety. Although some studies indicate that tubulopapillary or epithelial mesothelioma is most common, different histologic criteria may have been used for the inclusion of some tumors in the mixed type.

The fibrotic, mesenchymal or fibrosarcomatous variety is the rarest, and has seldom been associated with hypoglycemic syndromes, although the volume of the tumor may be the sole etiologic basis (Fig. 16a). Histologically, it is composed of large fusiform cells with elongated pleomorphic nuclei. Sheetlike, herringbone and whorled patterns mimic the usual fibrosarcoma (Fig. 16g,h). Electron micrographic studies show the epithelial nature of the cells in this form of mesotheliomatous growth.[89,188]

The mixed type represents a mixture of the fibrous and tubulopapillary or epithelial growth patterns. Zones of transition between tubulopapillary and fibromatous cells are the most helpful histological criteria in distinguishing mesothelioma from metastatic adenocarcinoma. Additional studies that aid in this distinction are the determination of acid mucopolysaccharide content in effusion material and the use of special stains such as mucicarmine and colloidal iron.[180] Cytologic study of effusion material may be particularly useful in mixed and epithelial mesotheliomas.[154]

The tubulopapillary form has papillary fronds with a central vascular stalk, lined by enlarged, variably sized squamoid mesothelial cells with pyramidal arrangement of the cells that constitute the frond (Fig. 16d,e). If present, the abundant epithelial component frequently obscures any fibromatous or fibrosarcomatous element (Fig. 16f). This may represent the converse of the small epithelial component, which is dominated in some tumors by abundant hyalinized, acellular, calcified material similar to that seen in hyaline plaques.

Grossly, the mixed and tubulopapillary forms grow as a thickened irregular, granular plaque that extends over the parietal pleura and into the endothoracic fascia to involve intercostal muscle and adipose tissue. It further coats the visceral pleura, lining all its invaginations, and produces irregular, frequently superficial nodular protrusions into the lung parenchyma. Often the fibrosarcomatous variant is less sheetlike and forms a larger more localized, invasive and compressed nodular mass. This macroscopic type may represent a transitional phase in biologic behavior between the diffuse and localized forms. Although some epithelial component is often present, this variety is relatively localized and only superficially involves the lung. With wide local excision of pleura and underlying lung, disease-free states have been recorded for almost a decade. With recurrence, reoperation may be successful but termination is frequently similar to that in the diffuse type.

The diffuse variant covers both parietal and pleural surfaces encrusting the lungs, and often forms a new cavity or preserves focally the original pleural space. Significant serosanguineous effusions accumulate here, decreasing lung volume and inducing protein catabolism. This growth lines fissures and, once it has permeated visceral pleura, involves lung parenchyma. Here it gains access to lymphatics and metastasis to ipsilateral and contralateral hilar lymph nodes ultimately results. Subsequent pleural involvement occurs and leads to constriction of the lung. In the majority of cases, mesotheliomas remain confined to the thoracic cavity. The peritoneal and pleural cavities are involved in 10% of cases and the peritoneal cavity in 30% of all cases of mesothelioma. Rare examples of cerebral metastases have been recorded.

REFERENCES

1. Abrahamson, J. R., and Friedman, N. D.: Intrapulmonary stromal mesothelioma. J. Thorac. Cardiovasc. Surg. 51:300, 1966.

2. Ackerman, L. V., and Rosai, J.: Respiratory tract/lung page 226. In Surgical Pathology, 5th ed., C. V. Mosby, St. Louis, 1974, p. 226.

3. Adamson, J. S., Senior, R. M., and Merrill, T.: Alveolar cell carcinoma: an electron microscopic study. Am. Rev. Respir. Dis. 100:550, 1969.

4. Allen, M. S., and Drash, E. C.: Primary melanoma of the lung. Cancer 21:154, 1968.

5. Al-Saleem, T., Peale, A. R., and Norris, C. M.: Multiple papillomatosis of the lower respiratory tract: clinical and pathologic study of eleven cases. Cancer 22:1173, 1968.

6. American Joint Committee for Cancer Staging and End Result Reporting: Clinical staging system for carcinoma of the lung. Ca 24:87 (March/April 1974).

7. Anthony, C. W., and Koneman, W. E.: Visceral Kaposi's sarcoma. Arch. Path. 70:740, 1960.

8. Auerbach, O.: Cancerous and precancerous lung changes: A slide review. Ca 19:138 (May/June 1969).

9. Auerbach, O., Gere, J. B., Pawlowski, J. M., Muehsam, G. E., Smolin, H. J., and Stout, A. P.: Carcinoma in situ and early invasive carcinoma occurring in tracheobronchial trees in cases of bronchial carcinoma. J. Thorac. Surg. 34:298, 1957.

10. Auerbach, O., Gere, J. B., Foreman, J. B., Petrick, T. G., Smolin, H. J., Muehsam, G. E., Kassouny, D. V., and Stout, A. P.: Changes in bronchial epithelium in relation to smoking and cancer of the lung—a report of progress. New Engl. J. Med. 256:97, 1957.

11. Auerbach, O., Stout, A. P., Hammond, E. C., and Garfinkle, L.: Changes in bronchial epithelium in relation to sex, age, residence, smoking, and pneumonia. New Engl. J. Med. 267:111, 1962.

12. Auerbach, O., Stout, A. P., Hammond, E. C., and Garfinkle, L.: Multiple primary bronchial carcinomas. Cancer 20:699, 1967.

13. Axelsson, C., Burcharth, F., and Johansen, A.: Mucoepidermoid lung tumors. J. Thorac. Cardiovasc. Surg. 65:902, 1973.

14. Ayella, R. J.: Hemangiopericytoma: Report of a case with arteriographic findings. Radiology 97:611, 1970.

15. Azzopardi, J. G., and Williams, E. D.: Pathology of "nonendocrine" tumors associated with Cushing's Syndrome. Cancer 22:274, 1968.

16. Babbayan, G. A., Woodruff, J. D., and Shelley, W. M.: Latent ectopic pulmonary choriocarcinoma associated with renal cell carcinoma. Am. J. Obstet. and Gynecol. 114:1009, 1972.

17. Backwinkel, K. D., and Diddams, J.: Hemangiopericytoma: Report of a case and comprehensive review of the literature. Cancer 24:896, 1970.

18. Bahadori, M., and Liebow, A. A.: Plasma cell granulomas of the lung. Cancer 31:191, 1973.

19. Barnard, W. G.: Embryoma of the lung. Thorax 7:299, 1952.

20. Batson, E. M.: So-called hamartoma of the lung—a true neoplasm of fibrous connective tissue of the bronchi. Cancer 31:1458, 1973.

21. Bauermeister, D. E., Jennings, E. R., Beland, A. H., and Judson, H. A.: Pulmonary blastoma, a form of carcinosarcoma. Am. J. Clin. Pathol. 46:322, 1966.

22. Bennett, D. E., and Sasser, W. F.: Bronchiolar carcinoma: a valid clinicopathologic entity. Cancer 24:876, 1969.

23. Bensch, K. G., Gordon, G. B., and Miller, L. R.: Electron microscopic and biochemical studies on bronchial carcinoid tumor. *Cancer* **18**:592, 1965.

24. Bensch, K. G., Gordon, G. B., and Miller, L. R.: Studies on the bronchial counterpart of the Kulchitsky (argentaffin) cell and innervation of bronchial glands. *J. Ultrastruct. Res.* **12**:668, 1965.

25. Bensch, K. G., Corrin, B., Pariente, R., and Spencer, H.: Oat-cell carcinoma of the lung—its origin and relationship to bronchial carcinoid. *Cancer* **22**:1163, 1968.

26. Bensch, Klaus G.: (Editorial) What is the function of the bronchial counterpart of the intestinal argentaffin (Kulchitsky) cell? *Ann. Thorac. Surg.* **14**:568 (November 1972).

27. Berkheiser, S. W.: Significance of bronchiolar atypia and lung cancer. *Cancer* **18**:516, 1965.

28. Boylen, C. T., et al: High-speed trephine lung biopsy: methods and results. *Chest* **63**:59 (January 1973).

29. Broders, A. S.: Epithelioma of the genito-urinary organs. *Ann. Surg.* **75**:577, 1922.

30. Buell, P. E.: Importance of tumor size in prognosis for resected bronchogenic carcinoma. *J. Surg. Oncol.* **3**:559, 1971.

31. Bull, J. C., and Grimes, O.: Pulmonary carcinosarcoma. *Chest* **65**:9, 1974.

32. Burcharth, F., and Axelsson, C.: Lung carcinoids. *Scand. J. Thorac. Cardiovasc. Surg.* **7**:72, 1973.

33. Carstens, P. H. B.: Ultrastructure of granular cell myoblastoma. *Acta Pathol. Microbiol. Scand.* **78A**:685, 1970.

34. Chaudhuri, M. R.: Independent bilateral primary bronchial carcinomas. *Thorax* **26**:476 (July) 1971.

35. Chaudhuri, M. R., Eastham, W. N., and Fredriksz, P. A.: Pulmonary blastoma with diverse mesenchymal proliferation. *Thorax* **27**:487, 1972.

36. Coalson, J. M., Mohr, J. A., Pirtle, J. K., Dee, A. L., and Rhoades, E. R.: Electron microscopy of neoplasms in the lung with special emphasis on the alveolar cell carcinoma *Am. Rev. Respir. Dis.* **101**:181, 1970.

37. Cox, F. H., and Helwig, E. B: Kaposi's sarcoma. *Cancer* **12**:289, 1959.

38. Danziger, H.: Pulmonary blastoma. *Can. Med. Assoc. J.* **102**:146, 1970.

39. Davis, P. W., Briggs, J. C., Seal, R. M. E., and Storring, F. K.: Benign and malignant mixed tumors of the lung. *Thorax* **27**:657, 1972.

40. Delarue, J., Abelanet, R., and Chomette, G.: Vascularization of malignant tumors. *Presse Med.* **73**:1517 (May 1965).

41. Delarue, N. C., Anderson, W., Sanders, D., and Starr, J.: Bronchio-alveolar carcinoma; a reappraisal after 24 years. *Cancer* **29**:90, 1972.

42. Dines, D. E., et al.: Malignant pulmonary neoplasms predisposing to spontaneous pneumothorax. *Mayo Clin. Proc.* **48**:541 (August 1973).

43. Dixon, D. S., and Breslow, A.: Pulmonary blastoma. *Am. Rev. Respir. Dis.* **108**:968, 1973.

44. Doyle, W. F.: Lung cancer: pathological cell types. Classification and frequency. *Present Concepts* **7**(1):1, 1974.

45. Eggleston, J. and Carter, D.: Reported at International Academy of Pathology, short course on lung, San Francisco (February 1974).

46. Emory, W. B., Mitchell, W. T., and Batch, H. B.: Mucous gland adenoma of the bronchus. *Am. Rev. Respir. Dis.* **108**:1407, 1973.

47. Etherton, J. E., Conning, D. M., and Corrin, B.: Autoradiographical and morphological evidence for apocrine secretion of dipalmitoyl lecithin in the terminal bronchiole of mouse lung. *Am. J. Anat.* **138**:11.

48. Farinacci, C. J., Blauw, A. S., and Jennings, E. M.: Multifocal pulmonary lesions of possible decidual origin (so-called pulmonary deciduosis): report of a case. *Am. J. Clin. Pathol.* **59**:509, 1973.

49. Fechner, R. E., Bentinck, B. R., and Askew, J. B., Jr.: Acinic cell tumor of the lung. A histologic and ultrastructural study. *Cancer* **29**:501, 1972.

50. Feinstein, A. R., Gelfman, N. A., and Yesner, R.: Observer variability in the histopathologic diagnosis of lung cancer. *Am. Rev. Respir. Dis.* **101**:671, 1970.

51. Feldman, F., and Seaman, W. B.: Primary thoracic hemangiopericytoma. *Radiology* **82**:998, 1964.

52. Felton, W. L., Liebow, A. A., and Lindskog, G. F.: Peripheral and multiple bronchial adenomas. *Cancer* **6**:555, 1953.

53. Feyrter, F.: Uber die peripheren endokrinen (parakrinen) Druesen des Menschen. W. Maudrich Press, Vienne, Dusseldorf, 1953.

54. Friedman, P. J., and Tisi, G. M.: "Alveolarization" of tantalum powder in experimental bronchography and the clearance of inhaled particles from the lung. *Radiology* **104**:523–535 (September 1972).

55. Frost, J. K.: An evaluation of cellular morphologic expression of biologic behavior. *Monographs in Clinical Cytology: The Cell in Health and Disease*, Vol. 2, Williams and Wilkins, Baltimore, 1969.

56. Fusco, F. D., and Rosen, S. W.: Gonadotropin—producing anaplastic large cell carcinomas of the lung. *New Engl. J. Med.* **275**:507, 1966.

57. Gallivan, G. J., Dolan, C. T., Stam, R. E., Eggertsen, B. S., and Tovey, J. D.: Granular cell myoblastoma of the bronchus; report of a case. *Am. Rev. Respir. Dis.* **96**:923, 1968.

58. Gamsu, G., et al.: Clearance of tantalum from airways of different caliber in man evaluated by roentgenographic method. *Am. Rev. Respir. Dis.* **107**:214 (February 1973).

59. Garancis, J. C., Komorowski, R. A., and Kuzma, J. F.: Granular cell myoblastoma. *Cancer* **25**:542, 1970.

60. Garland, L. H., et al.: The apparent sites of carcinomas of the lung. *Radiology* **78**:1, 1962.

61. Gmelich, J. T., Bensch, K. G., and Liebow, A. A.: Cells of Kulchitsky type in bronchioles and their relation to the origin of peripheral carcinoid tumors. *Lab. Invest.* **17**:88, 1967.

62. Gmelich, J. T., Huvos, A. G., and Turnbull, A. D.: Carcinoid tumors of the lungs—prognostic significance of pathologic features. *Am. J. Clin. Pathol.* **1**:143 (January 1973).

63. Goodner, J. T., Berg, J. W., and Watson, W. L.: The non-benign nature of bronchial carcinoids and cylindromas. *Cancer* **14**:539, 1961.

64. Greenberg, S. D., Smith, M. N., and Spjut, H. J.: Bronchoalveolar carcinoma—cell of origin? (electron microscopy study of five cases). *Lab. Invest.* **30**:376 (March 1974).

65. Greenberg, S. D., Smith, M. N., and Spjut, J. J.: The nonciliated bronchiolar epithelial (Clara) cell: comparative ultrastructure in mouse, rat, rabbit, calf and man. *Am. J. Pathol.* (Abstr.) **106**:48a (January/March 1974).

66. Greenberg, S. D., Heisler, J. G., Gyorkey, F., and Jenkins, D. E.: Pulmonary lymphomas versus pseudolymphomas: A perplexing problem. *South. Med. J.* **65**:775, 1972.

67. Guccion, J. G., and Rosen, S. H.: Bronchopulmonary leiomyosarcomas and fibrosarcoma. *Cancer* **30**:1972.

68. Haas, J. E., Yunis, E. J., and Totten, R. S.: Ultrastructure of a sclerosing hemangioma of the lung. *Cancer* **30**:512, 1972.

69. Haddad, R., and Massaro, D.: Idiopathic diffuse interstitial pulmonary fibrosis (fibrosing alveolitis), atypical epithelial proliferaton and lung cancer. *Am. J. Med.* **45**:211, 1968.

70. Hadley, G. G., and Bullock, W. K.: Autopsy reports of pulmonary carcinomas: survey of Los Angeles County Hospital for 1951. *Calif. Med.* **79**:431, 1953.

71. Hajdu, S. I., Winawer, S. J. and Meyers, W. P. L.: Carcinoid tumors. A study of 204 cases. *Am. J. Clin. Pathol.* **6**:521, 1974.

72. Hammond, E. C., Auerbach, O., Kirman, D., and Garfinkle, L.: Effects of cigarette smoking on dogs. *Am. Cancer Soc.* **21**:78, 1971.

73. Hartmann, W. H.: Peculiar proliferation of bronchial cartilage. *Arch. Pathol.* **84**:422–424 (October 1967).

74. Hathaway, B. M., Copeland, K., and Gurley, J.: Giant cell adenocarcinoma of the lung. *Arch. Surg.* **98**:24 (January 1969).

75. Hattori, S., Matsuda, M. Tateishi, R., Nushihara, H., and Horai, T.: Oat cell carcinoma of the lung. *Cancer* **30**:1014, 1972.

76. Hayashi, H., et al.: Chemotactic factor associated with invasion of cancer cells. *Nature* **226**:174 (April 11, 1970).

77. Heilbrunn, A., and Crosby, I. K.: Adenocystic carcinoma and mucoepidermoid carcinoma of the tracheobronchial tree. *Chest* **61**:145, 1972.

78. Herman, D. L., Bullock, W. K., and Waken, J. K.: Giant cell adenocarcinoma of the lung. *Cancer* **19**:1337, 1966.

79. Hill, G. S., and Eggleston, J. C.: Electron microscope study of so-called "pulmonary sclerosing hemangioma." Report of a case suggesting epithelial origin. *Cancer* **30**:1092, 1972.

80. Hoch, W. S., Patchefsky, A. S., Takeda, M., and Gordon, G.: Benign clear cell tumor of the lung (an ultrastructural study). *Cancer* **33**:1328, 1974.

81. Hochberg, L. A., and Schacter, B.: Benign tumors of the bronchus and lung. *Am. J. Surg.* **89**:425, 1955.

82. Hukill, P. B., and Stern, H.: Adenocarcinoma of the lung: Histological factors affecting prognosis. *Cancer* **15**:504 (May/June 1962).

83. Iverson, L.: Bronchopulmonary sarcoma. *J. Thorac. Surg.* **27**:130, 1954.

84. Iverson, R. E., and Straehley, C. J.: Pulmonary blastoma; long-term survival of juvenile patients. *Chest* **63**:436, 1973.

85. Jonas, A. M., and Hukill, P. B.: Histogenesis of a pulmonary adenocarcinoma in the cat. *Arch. Path.* **85**:573 (June 1968).

86. Kakos, G. S., Williams, T. E., Assor, D., and Vasko, J. S.: pulmonary carcinosarcoma. Etiologic, therapeutic, and prognostic considerations. *J. Thorac. Cardiovasc. Surg.* **61**:777, 1971.

87. Kalus, M., Rahman, F., Jenkins, D. E., and Beall, A. C.: Malignant mesenchymoma of the lung. *Arch. Pathol.* **95**:199, 1973.

88. Katz, A., and Lattes, R.: Granulomatous thymoma or Hodgkin's disease of thymus? A clinical and histologic study and a reevaluation. *Cancer* **23**:1, 1969.

89. Kay, S., and Silverberg, S. G.: Ultrastructural studies of a malignant fibrous mesothelioma of the pleura. *Arch. Pathol.* **92**:499, 1971.

90. Keith, R. G., and Taylor, G. A.: Use of flexible fiberoptic bronchoscope in diagnosis of malignant tumors of lung. *Cancer J. Surg.* **16**:118 (March 1973).

91. Kennedy, A.: Pathology and survival in operable cases of giant cell carcinoma of the lung. *J. Clin. Pathol.* **22**:354, 1969.

92. Kennedy, W. R., and Jimenez-Pabon, E.: The myasthenic syndrome associated with small cell carcinoma of the lung (Eaton-Lambert Syndrome). *Neurology* **18**:757, 1968.

93. Kern, W. H., Crepeau, A. G., and Jones, J. C.: Primary Hodgkin's disease of the lung. *Cancer* **14**:1151, 1961.

94. Kinloch, J. D., Webb, J. N., Eccleston, P., and Zeitlin, J.: Carcinoid syndrome associated with oat cell carcinoma of the bronchus. *Br. Med. J.* **12**:1533, 1965.

95. Kirchner, J. A.: Papilloma of the larynx with extensive lung involvement. *Laryngoscope* **61**:1022, 1963.

96. Klein, H. Z.: Mucinous carcinoid tumor of the vermiform appendix. *Cancer* **33**:770 (March 1974).

97. Korbitz, B. C.: Massive cavitation of the lung in Hodgkin's disease. *Chest* **58**:542, 1970.

98. Korn, D., Bensch, K., Liebow, A. A., and Castleman, B.: Multiple minute pulmonary tumors resembling chemodectoma. *Am. J. Pathol.* **37**:641, 1960.

99. Kreyberg, L.: *Histological lung cancer types: a morphological and biological correlation*, Norwegian Universities Press, Oslo, 1962.

100. Kreyberg, L., Liebow, A. A., and Uehlinger, E. A.: *Histological Typing of Lung Tumors*, International Histological Classification of Tumors, No. 1, WHO, Geneva, 1967.

101. Kyriakos, M., and Webber, B.: Cancer of the lung in young men. *J. Thorac. Cardiovasc. Surg.* **67**:634 (April 1974).

102. Lambert, M. W.: Accessory bronchiole-alveolar communications. *J. Pathol. Bacteriol.* **70**:311, 1955.

103. LeLarve, N. O., Anderson, W., Sanders, D., et al.: Bronchioloalveolar carcinoma. *Cancer* **29**:90, 1972.

104. Lerner, H. J.: Giant cell carcinoma of the lung. *Arch. Surg.* **94**:891 (June 1967).

105. LeRoux, B. R., Williams, M. A., and Kallichurum, S.: Squamous papillomatosis of the trachea and bronchi. *Thorax* **24**:673, 1969.

106. Lichtiger, B., Mackay, B., and Tessmer, C. F.: Spindle cell variant of squamous carcinoma. *Cancer* **26**:1311 (December 1970).

107. Lieberman, P. H., et al.: Reappraisal of eosinophilic granuloma of bone, Hand-Schuller-Christian syndrome, and Lettered-Siew syndrome. *Medicine* **48**:375–399 (September 1969).

108. Liebow, A. A.: Tumors of the lower respiratory tract. In *Atlas of Tumor Pathology*, Sect. V, Fasc. 17, National Research Council, AFIP, Washington, D.C., 1952.

109. Liebow, A. A., and Hubbell, D. S.: Sclerosing hemangioma (histiocytoma, xanthoma of the lung). *Cancer* **9**:53, 1956.

110. Liebow, A. A.: Bronchiolo-alveolar carcinoma. *Adv. Intern Med.* **10**:329, 1960.

111. Liebow, A. A., and Castleman, B.: Benign clear cell ("sugar") tumors of the lung. *Yale J. Biol. Med.* **43**:214 (February/April 1971).

112. Liebow, A. A.: Neoplastic and Non-Neoplastic Lesions of the

to 8 months. Chahinian[14] analyzed volume doubling times in primary lung cancer in 30 patients. Among small cell carcinomas, the range was ½ to 2½ months with a mean of 1.3 months, whereas epidermoid carcinoma had a range of 7 days to 9 months, with a mean of 3 months, and adenocarcinoma a range of 1½ to 2½ months, with an average of 2 months.

Straus[48] summarized information from the English-language literature and compiled the following data: 91 epidermoid carcinomas, range of volume doubling times 7 days to 13 months, mean 3½ months; 41 adeno-carcinomas, range ½ to 20 months, mean 6.2 months; 33 undifferentiated carcinomas, range 1.1 to 16 months, mean 3.3 months; 5 small cell carcinomas, range ½ to 2½ months, mean 1.1 month; 3 large cell carcinomas, range 1½ to 3.7 months, mean 3 months. The mean doubling time for adenocarcinoma was significantly longer than the mean of each of the other cell types. Weiss[54] was able to show that although certain tumors follow a consistent discernible pattern of growth, others have irregular spurts that cannot be fitted to a constant pattern of tumor growth.

Nathan et al.[40] related the tumor volume doubling time to the histologic diagnosis. Of 10 lesions with a tumor doubling time of less than 7 days, all were due to a benign process such as pneumonia, pulmonary infarction, or abscess; 17 of 18 lesions with tumor doubling times over 500 days were usually due to granulomas or benign tumors.

The significance of the tumor volume doubling time observations lies in the possibility of estimating the length of growth of clinically discernible bronchogenic carcinomas with possible prognostic significance. If one assumes a cell content of 10^9 cells/cc of tumor tissue and a tumor volume doubling time of 4 months, according to the above mentioned studies, an estimate of growth can be arrived at as shown in Table 2. The clinical range and the potential salvage rate are indicated for patients treated effectively for lung cancer.

The relationship between doubling time and prognosis has been investigated by Meyer.[38] Meyer examined the growth rate of primary bronchogenic carcinomas in 22 patients and classified them into three categories. One category, with doubling times of about 80 days, showed no survivors among 4 patients undergoing resection; 7 patients with doubling times of 80 to 150 days underwent resection, and 4 survived 5 years. Of 5 patients with doubling times of over 150 days, 1 died of

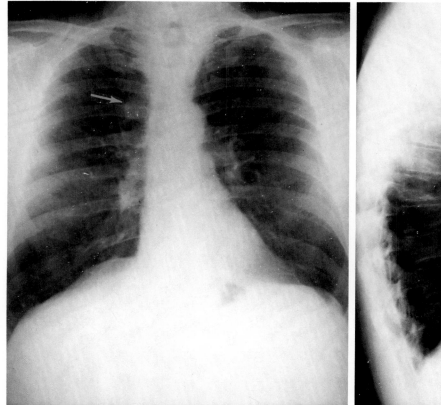
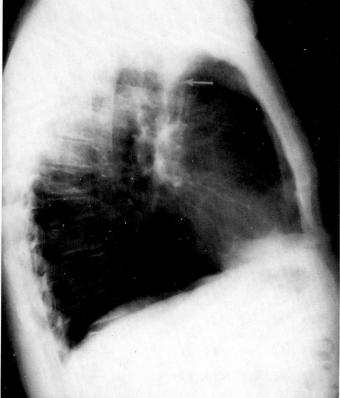

Fig. 1. Patient C. D. Postero-anterior and left lateral chest x-ray, 4/27/68. A coin lesion of the right upper lobe of the lung can be seen.

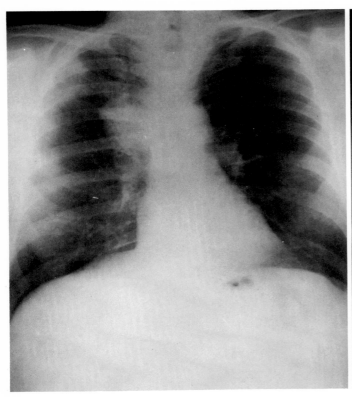

Fig. 2. X-rays of the same patient obtained on 12/30/68. This lesion showed a volume doubling time of 50 days, calculated on the basis of these two examinations and assuming a constant growth rate. The tumor was an epidermoid carcinoma.

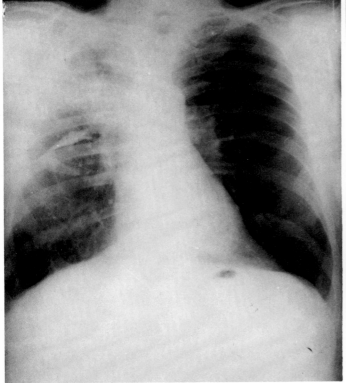

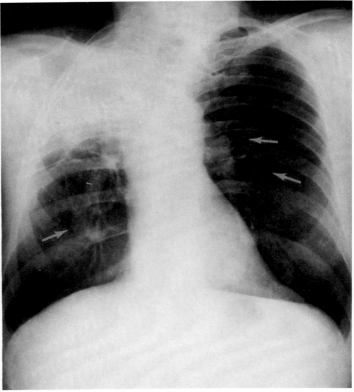

Fig. 3. Same patient, following radiation therapy to the right upper lobe. On 4/10/69 a suspicion of lung metastasis was raised, and on 7/29/69 multiple bilateral pulmonary metastatic nodules are clearly visible. Estimated volume doubling time is 17 days.

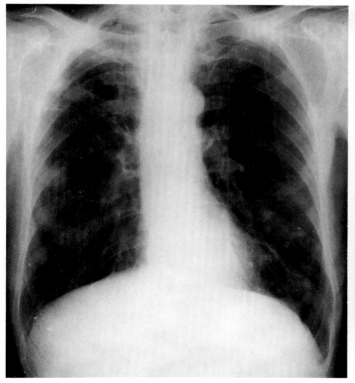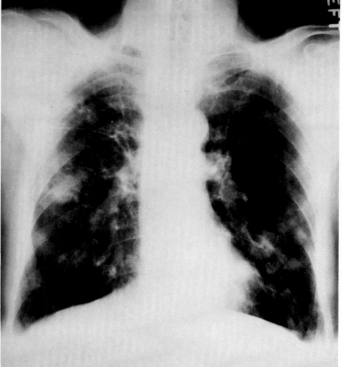

Fig. 4. Patient J. W. Metastatic carcinoma, primary site: adeno-carcinoma of the left submandibular salivary gland. Figure on left obtained on 2/19/71, figure on right on 2/8/74. Volume doubling time on the basis of these two films is 34 months. No treatment for the lung metastasis was administered.

recurrence at 56 months, 2 died of intercurrent disease, and the remainder are doing well.

Joseph et al.[26] also reviewed the experience in 113 patients with nonpulmonary malignant tumors who had pulmonary metastasis, and were able to correlate improvement of survival after resection to long doubling times. It is noteworthy that they encountered a significant number of patients in whom the tumor doubling times varied by at least 100% of the time determined for the slowest growing lesion, when comparing several lesions in the same patients.

The mitotic activity of a tumor is related to the volume doubling time. Weiss[52] examined this relationship, but was unable to correlate the mitotic activity with survival from the time of tumor detection. There were differences in mitotic activity between histologic types of tumor, with an increase in mitotic rate from adenocarcinoma to low-grade epidermoid carcinoma to high-grade epidermoid to oat cell carcinoma.

Malaise et al.[32] examined the relationship between labeling indices from radioactive tracer studies and tumor volume doubling times. They found a fair relationship between increasing doubling time and decreasing labeling index, the latter showing 8.3% of the cells

TABLE 2.   ESTIMATE OF TUMOR GROWTH (VOLUME DOUBLING TIME: 4 MONTHS)

Year	Number of Volume Doublings	Number of Tumor cells	Diameter (cm)	Weight (g)	Clinical Range	Estimated Percentage of Patients Surviving after Treatment
0	0	1	$10\,\mu$			
7	20	10^6	0.1 cm	10^{-3}		
10	30	10^9	1.25 cm	1	Asymptomatic	90%
11	32	4×10^9	1.8 cm	4	Asymptomatic	60%
11.5	33.5	3×10^{10}	4.0 cm	32	Asymptomatic	30%
12	35	5×10^{11}	10.0 cm	500	Metastatic	0%

n epidermoid carcinomas and 2.1% in adeno-
ca..... .as. An increasing labeling index also was correlated with increasing cell loss. Muggia and De Vita[39]
determined the labeling index after intratumoral injection of radioactive thymidine in metastatic sites. Biopsies
from small cell carcinoma showed a labeling index of
24%, whereas those from anaplastic carcinoma showed
6%.

Volume doubling time and labeling indices are only
part of the information necessary to assess cell proliferation kinetics in cancer of the lung. It is likely that the
growth fraction of the tumor, that is, the fraction of
cells participating in active mitotic activity, varies between histologic types and that it may be responsible
for some of the wide ranges of tumor volume doubling
times found within histologic types. Further research is
required.

The difference in prognosis between rapidly progressive carcinomas of the small cell variety and the less
aggressive primary lung cancers of the bronchioloalveolar
or low-grade adenocarcinoma type makes the growth rate
of the tumor clinically significant. To evaluate the effectiveness of therapy, we should consider the present
available knowledge of volume doubling time instead of
merely assessing the decrease in tumor volume from an
x-ray. A 50% increase in diameter of the pulmonary
primary lesion as visualized on the x-ray represents a
volume increase of approximately 85%. This may occur
in a period of 3 weeks in a patient with small cell carcinoma, while it would take about 5 months in a patient
with adenocarcinoma. There is, therefore, much less
time available to assess the effectiveness of a treatment
regimen on a tumor when small cell carcinoma is treated
as compared to adenocarcinoma. It is also likely that
metastatic spread is related not only to the volume of
tumor at various times in the clinical management of a
patient, but also to the time span during which the
tumor undergoes active proliferation. This may explain
the relatively poor prognosis of patients with adenocarcinoma, as compared to those with epidermoid carcinoma, in spite of the evidence presented on the basis of
tumor volume doubling times.

CLINICAL FEATURES OF LUNG CANCER

Among the 1211 patients with epidermoid carcinoma in
the Connecticut series (1935–1959),[17] there were 83%
male and 17% female patients. The age incidence from
the Memorial Hospital series[51] is given in Table 3.
Cough was the first symptom in approximately 50% of
patients, usually productive and often associated with
hemoptysis and/or chest pain. Weight loss occurred in
approximately 30% of patients, dyspnea in about 33%,

TABLE 3. EPIDERMOID CANCER OF THE LUNG[51]

Age	Number	Percent
10–20 years	1	
20–30 years	2	
30–40 years	20	1.5
40–50 years	165	12
50–60 years	475	36
60–70 years	570	38
70–80 years	135	10
80–90 years	11	1
Total	1,318	

and chest pain in 33%. Less frequently, anorexia, hoarseness and pain from bone metastasis occurred. In this
series, only 4% of the patients were asymptomatic;
75% had symptoms for less than one year and 15% for
1 to 2 years. A summary of the symptoms occurring in
a number of other series is given in Table 4.

Among 380 patients with oat cell carcinoma at the
Memorial Hospital, only 1.3% were asymptomatic.
Hemoptysis occurred in 4.4% of patients; the remainder
of the symptoms were distributed among the patients
with epidermoid carcinoma. The male to female ratio
was 11:1 with ages ranging from 32 to 83 years; 72%
of the patients were between 50 and 70 years. Only 1%
of the patients with oat cell carcinoma reported by Kato
et al.[28] were asymptomatic; 80% developed symptoms
within 3 months of diagnosis, and only 4% had symptoms 1 to 2 years prior to diagnosis.

In the study by Bennett et al.,[5] the male to female
ratio for adenocarcinoma of the lung was 3:2. The
youngest patient reported in this series was 27 years old,
but 81% of the men were over 50. The incidence of the
various histologic groups at the Barnes Hospital is given
in Table 5. Among patients with adenocarcinoma, 28%
had no symptoms at the time of diagnosis, and an additional 28% had only cough; 17% had hemoptysis, 11%
pain, and 1% weight loss. If symptoms were present,
they occurred approximately 1 to 2 years later than in
epidermoid carcinoma of the lung.

In bronchioloalveolar carcinoma the male to female
ratio was 2:1 in the Memorial series.[50] One percent of
the patients were under 30 years of age, 4% were between 30 and 40 years, 87% were from 40 to 70 years
old, and 8% were over 70. Twelve percent of the patients were asymptomatic, 22% had chest pain, 33% had
cough, and 7% hemoptysis. Symptoms occurred later
than in epidermoid carcinoma, and 17% of the patients
had symptoms for 18 months or more.

The significance of the biological behavior, especially
with reference to growth rate and metastasis, depends
on the histologic type of lung cancer. Although the size

TABLE 4. INITIAL AND EVENTUAL SYMPTOMS OF PATIENTS WITH CARCINOMA OF THE LUNG

Symptoms	First Symptom (%) Bjork[6] (342 patients)	Eventual Symptoms (%) Ochsner et al.[42] (129 patients)	Rienhoff[44] (327 patients)
Cough	58	92	71
Thoracic pain	11	67	50
Respiratory infection	10	60	18
Dyspnea	7	59	23
Hemoptysis	5	61	63
Loss of weight	—	79	39
Asthenia	3	7	—
Wheezing	—	17	—
Fever	2	—	13
Hoarseness	1	—	—
Dysphagia	—	—	—
Tightness of Chest	1	—	3

TABLE 5. CARCINOMA OF THE LUNG BARNES HOSPITAL (1948–63)[5]

Histologic Type	Men (1165 cases) (%)	Women (139 cases) (%)
Epidermoid	60	14
Oat cell	13	12
Other undifferentiated	9	16
Adenocarcinoma	9	49
Bronchioloalveolar	2	9
Unclassified	7	—

of the lesion at the time of treatment may be related to the prognosis in patients with epidermoid carcinoma of the lung, this is not the case in patients with adenocarcinoma because the longer growth time also allows more time for dissemination of the tumor. Metastatic malignancy in lymph nodes in patients with adenocarcinoma carries a worse prognosis than in patients with squamous cell carcinoma of the same size.

On the other hand, patterns of rapid local spread are important in the prognosis of oat cell carcinoma because up to 88% of the lesions show early involvement of the lymph nodes, and resectability and operability in oat cell carcinoma are significantly lower than in patients with epidermoid carcinoma in whom the tumor remains localized for longer periods of time.[51]

THE SPREAD OF CANCER OF THE LUNG

Our knowledge of the spread of lung cancer is based on autopsies performed on patients who died from broncho-genic carcinoma. The survival of such patients without specific treatment for bronchogenic carcinoma has been described by Buchberg et al.[11] in a careful study of 443 patients. The data are listed in Table 6. Of these patients, only 1.3% survived 5 years. Although this forms the largest group of patients reported without specific treatment for bronchogenic carcinoma, one must realize that some of these patients did not have histologic confirmation of their cancer.

At present, the incidence of metastasis at death is the best available means of assessing the progression of lung cancer from a localized lesion to metastasis. Although only untreated patients should be considered for classification of the natural history of bronchogenic cancer, published studies often contain a mixture of untreated and treated patients and will be reported upon. The large series of Budinger[12] and of Spjut and Mateo[47] reflect the incidence of metastasis at various sites at the time of death, without breakdown into histologic groups. Table 7 summarizes their data.

TABLE 6. SURVIVAL OF PATIENTS WITH UNTREATED CANCER OF THE LUNG[11]

Histologic Type	Number of Patients	1-Year Survival from Diagnosis (%)	2-Year Survival (%)
Epidermoid carcinoma	122	24.6	5.7
Adenocarcinoma	126	9.8	4.8
Anaplastic carcinoma	72	9.7	4.2

TABLE 7. METASTASIS IN AUTOPSIES OF PATIENTS WHO DIED OF BRONCHOGENIC CARCINOMA[12,47]

Site	Untreated (%)	Treated Patients Surviving over 1 Month (%)
Local tumor only	6.5	3
Regional lymph node metastasis	88	59
Distant metastasis, no regional node metastasis	6	38
Distant lymph node metastasis	—	34
All distant metastasis	65	—
Brain metastasis	20	58
Liver metastasis	42	45
Bone metastasis	31	40
Adrenal gland metastasis	33	41
Kidney metastasis	19	28
Opposite lung metastasis	10–23	53

Although these two studies represent the most recent addition to our knowledge of spread of bronchogenic carcinoma on the basis of autopsy findings, some of the older series contain significant information. It is important to emphasize that distant metastases are more frequent among patients treated for bronchogenic carcinoma than among those not specifically treated, since control of local cancer in the lung and mediastinum leads to a prolongation of life and later death from distant metastasis rather than from local extension or regional metastasis of the tumor. The result of this selection of patients is reflected in Table 8. Among the older studies, Olson[43] reported 57% local extensions in 67 cases

of unselected bronchogenic carcinoma. In 6% these local extensions were without metastasis. Local extensions were present in 65% of the oat cell carcinomas, in 55% of the epidermoid carcinomas and in 46% of the adenocarcinomas. A remarkable aspect of this series was the association of pulmonary inflammatory conditions, which were present in 59% of the cases. Bronchopneumonia prevailed, as did bronchiectasis and atelectasis of a lobe or an entire lung. Active tuberculosis was present in only 1.6%, healed parenchymal tubercular lesions were found in 6%. Pneumoconiosis was present in 2.9% of the patients.

The study of Engelman and McNamara[18] includes 234 autopsies published in 1954. Of note among the data published by these authors is an 18% incidence of abdominal and retroperitoneal lymph node involvement. Cervical lymph nodes were involved in 8% of cases. The rate of metastatic involvement of lymph nodes was related to the histologic diagnosis, with oat cell carcinoma showing a higher incidence of lymph node involvement than in epidermoid carcinoma or adenocarcinoma. Liver involvement was present in 33% of the epidermoid carcinomas, 48% of the oat cell carcinomas, and 43% of the adenocarcinomas. Adrenal gland metastasis occurred in 34% of the epidermoid carcinomas, 41% of the oat cell carcinomas, and 52% of the adenocarcinomas. Their findings, shown in Table 8, emphasize the importance of histologic type in the frequency of metastasis at various sites.

A recent study by Matthews et al.[33] provides information on 202 patients who underwent presumably curative surgery and died within a 30-day postoperative period. Seventy-three (35%) of the 202 patients had evidence of persistent disease upon postmortem examination. Of 131

TABLE 8. TREATED CANCER OF THE LUNG AT AUTOPSY[18,30]

Site of Metastasis	Epidermoid Carcinoma (%)	Oat Cell Carcinoma (%)	Adenocarcinoma (%)
All lymph nodes	54	85	75
Peribronchial lymph nodes	38	65	57
Mediastinal lymph nodes	37	50	48
Abdominal lymph nodes	16	22	14
Cervical lymph nodes	9	4	10
Brain	8–17	8–17	14–39
Liver	23–33	48–64	43–47
Bone	18–23	13–39	29–41
Adrenal	21–34	41–44	30–52
Kidney	15–26	15–26	20–43
Lung	12–14	7–12	14–24
Heart and major vessels	12	12	
Pleura	7–10	11–12	5–14
Spleen	5	9	5

patients with epidermoid carcinoma, 44 (33%) had persistent disease on autopsy; 22 (16%) had local disease identified only as disease at the bronchial stump or in the hilar or mediastinal lymph nodes; and 22 (16.5%) had distant metastatic disease. The majority of these distant metastatic sites were in the lymph nodes, liver, and adrenal glands.

Among 30 patients with adenocarcinoma, 13 (43%) had persistent disease. Although only 1 patient had residual local disease, 12 had distant metastasis; the adrenal glands, brain, and lymph nodes were the prevalent sites. There were 22 patients with large cell carcinoma, 3 (14%) of whom had distant metastasis at autopsy; kidney, adrenal glands, liver, and contralateral lung were the prevalent sites. There were no patients with only residual local disease. Of 19 patients with small cell carcinoma, 13 (70%) had persistent disease on autopsy. While there was 1 patient with residual local disease only, 12 had distant metastatic sites. The prevalent sites were the lymph nodes, adrenal glands, and liver. Other frequent metastatic sites in all histologic groups were the brain and the kidney.

More than 50% of the patients had one focus of tumor identified at autopsy, and the remainder had multiple sites of involvement. Table 8 also reports the findings of Line and Deeley.[30] The authors indicated that brain metastasis was solitary in 20% of all brain metastasis. The incidence of solitary cerebral metastasis was 27%

in the epidermoid carcinomas, 19% in the oat cell carcinomas, and 14% in the adenocarcinomas expressed as a percentage of all brain metastases in the histologic type.

Lymph node metastases are a significant feature even in primary lung cancers that are believed to have relatively little malignant activity, as shown by McNamara et al.[35] They found that among 43 patients with resected bronchioloalveolar carcinoma, 28% had lymph node metastasis, and of 38 patients operated on for single peripheral nodules with the same histologic diagnosis, 7 revealed lymph node metastasis.

Luomanen and Watson[31] have reported the incidence of metastasis in unusual organs as shown in Table 9. In their study, 43% of the patients with epidermoid carcinoma had bone metastasis; the vertebrae were involved in 53% of patients with bone involvement. For oat cell carcinoma the respective figures were 55% and 45%, and for adenocarcinoma, 2% and 46%.

THE CAUSE OF DEATH FROM CANCER OF THE LUNG

The cause of death, that is, the immediate process leading to the cessation of life, is frequently difficult to establish in patients with advanced metastatic malignant disease. Among the untreated patients in the Boston City Hospital study of Budinger[12] "the overwhelming majority of individuals died of respiratory failure, the end stage of recurrent pneumonia, bronchial obstruc-

TABLE 9. UNUSUAL SITES OF METASTASIS[31]

Sites	Number of Cases				
	Epidermoid Carcinoma	Oat Cell Carcinoma	Adenocarcinoma	Sarcoma	Total
Pancreas	36	51	9	2	98
Heart	33	24	29	2	88
Pericardium	36	21	14	4	75
Thyroid	29	20	10	2	61
Spleen	26	18	7	2	53
Small bowel	30	4	6	2	42
Diaphragm	12	10	18	1	41
Peritoneum	11	6	13	2	32
Subcutaneous tissue	13	5	7		25
Skin	10	5	6	2	23
Stomach	12	5	4	1	22
Omentum	8	2	4	2	16
Large bowel	8	2	5		15
Mesentery	6	1			11
Gallbladder	2	6	2		10
Bladder (urinary)	2	3	3		8
Testis	3	5			8
Trachea	6	1	1		8
Prostate	1	6			7
Ovary	3	2	2		7

tion, atelectasis, pulmonary fibrosis and unremittedly excessive bronchial secretions. This failure was often superimposed either on congestive heart failure, frequently associated with intractable pleura effusions and pulmonary edema, or extensive emphysema with fibrosis." Other immediate causes of death were rare; however, massive hemoptysis was felt to be the cause in 5 of 250 patients, stroke in 4 patients, hepatic failure in 3 patients, cardiac failure in 2 patients, and myocardial infarction in 1 patient.

Of the 676 autopsies reported from Memorial Hospital in New York,[31] 43 patients had no determinable immediate cause of death; 1 patient died of chemotherapy toxicity, and there were 2 suicides. Among the remaining patients, the following data were recorded regarding the immediate cause of death: 34% (153 of 348) of patients with squamous cell carcinoma died of an infection distant to known areas of disease, especially in the lung; 6.3% died from brain metastasis, 21.8% from multiple widespread metastasis, 15.5% because of cardiac complications, 2.9% from congestive complications, 2.6% from pulmonary embolism, and 2.9% from peptic ulcer; 1.7% of patients died from pulmonary hemorrhage, 1.2% of renal failure, and 2 patients each died of pulmonary tuberculosis and extrapulmonary infections.

Among the patients with oat cell carcinoma, infection was the immediate cause of death in 41%, brain metastasis 10%, multiple widespread metastasis 24.4%, cardiac complications 18.9%, surgical complications 1.6%, and pulmonary hemorrhage 1.6%; single patients died of pulmonary embolism, peptic ulceration and renal failure. Of 147 patients with adenocarcinoma of various grades, the corresponding causes of death were pulmonary infection 31.5%, brain metastasis 9%, multiple widespread metastasis 27.2%, cardiac complications 16.3%, pulmonary hemorrhage 1.4%, pulmonary embolism 2.8%, and peptic ulcer 2.2%. It is appropriate here to draw attention to the high incidence of multiple malignancies seen in patients who have arrest or "cure" of bronchogenic carcinoma, as will be shown later. The remarkable feature of these statistics is the high incidence of pulmonary infection as an immediate cause of death. Although the matter of how aggressively one should attempt to prolong life in patients with known incurable disease such as diffuse metastatic cancer, remains an ethical decision that the individual physician must make, the relative ease of specific treatment of pulmonary infection following appropriate culture and sensitivity studies should lead to a high degree of awareness of pulmonary infection as a major complication in patients under treatment or follow-up for lung cancer.

The significance of more extensive studies regarding the extent of the patient's disease at the time of initial diagnosis is shown by the increased emphasis among oncologic physicians on staging before specific treatment regimens are instituted. This interest should lead to earlier detection of metastatic disease by new scanning techniques using radionuclides, or by methods not previously used for this purpose, such as bone marrow aspirations. Details of these studies will be discussed later. Staging of patients with bronchogenic carcinoma not only allows better delineation of the extent of the patient's disease, but will also result in more appropriate decisions regarding treatment based on a rational approach. In the end, such information should lead to improved management and an increase in treatment efficacy and survival for patients with bronchogenic carcinoma.

MULTIPLE MALIGNANCY IN PATIENTS WITH CANCER OF THE LUNG

Multiple cancers may be classified as synchronous or metachronous. Since the etiologic factors for the malignant degeneration of lung tissue are well established, it is not surprising that multiple synchronous invasive carcinomas, growing apparently independent from each other, were seen in as many as 14.5% of the specimens examined by Auerbach et al.[2] The autopsy series of Memorial Hospital[31] showed evidence of other coexisting primary cancer of various areas in 53 of 676 patients. The most common site was found in the larynx, where there were 8 coexisting carcinomas. In the entire series of 5000 patients, 85 coexisting or successive laryngeal cancers were found. There were 11 cases of triple coexisting cancers on autopsy, all but 1 in the squamous cell group. One patient had four coexisting cancers, one each in the lung, breast and sigmoid and a lymphosarcoma.

Metachronous carcinomas were reported by Mersheimer et al.[37] who found carcinoma of the larynx in 3.2% of patients previously diagnosed as having lung cancer. Bronchogenic carcinoma followed arrest of carcinoma of the larynx in 8.9% of the patients. However, cancer of the larynx does not show the rapid increase in incidence that has been seen in bronchogenic carcinoma. In 1958 epidermoid carcinoma of the larynx was 1.4% of the total cancer incidence in Pennsylvania, and in 1970 it rose to 1.5%.[13] Corresponding figures for carcinoma of the trachea, bronchus, and lung were 7.7% and 10.6%.

Other primary sites associated with bronchogenic carcinoma in order of decreasing frequency are: carcinoma of the prostate gland, carcinoma of the skin, carcinoma of the large intestine, carcinoma of other digestive organs, and carcinoma of the bladder.[37] This order suggests that these malignancies occur in order of frequency in the general population.

SPONTANEOUS REGRESSION OF BRONCHOGENIC CARCINOMA

Apparent spontaneous regression of lung cancer has been reported in 3 patients.[4,8] One patient received 1200 rads postoperative radiation therapy through anterior and posterior portals following limited biopsy of an epidermoid carcinoma. The patient survived 6 years. The assumption of spontaneous regression was based on radiographic findings without further biopsy or postmortem examination in a second patient with epidermoid carcinoma who also survived 6 years with radiographic clearing of a lesion; a third patient died of a stroke 2 years after the diagnosis of adenocarcinoma of the lung without specific treatment. Here also, radiographic improvement was present before death. Only a few tumor cells were found at autopsy.

Bell[4] assumed that some form of immunological mechanism was responsible for the regression of the tumor in the first patient mentioned above. Examination of the peripheral lymphocytes for immunologic competence indicated a highly positive colony inhibition test.

IMMUNOLOGIC ALTERATIONS IN CANCER OF THE LUNG

The description of spontaneous regression of lung cancer and the recent interest in cancer immunology, usually with reference to hematologic neoplasms, has led to attempts to define the immunological status of patients harboring this tumor. Although tests of immune competence, such as lymphocyte transformation, may be altered by factors other than cancer cells, recent studies show that immune competence may play an important part in the prognostication of patients with lung cancer. The place of immune competence in the carcinogenesis of lung cancer is still unknown. The sparse reports in the literature must be analyzed with the awareness that heart disease, various drugs, and changes in the protein metabolism of the lung cancer patient may alter some of the tests of immune competence.

Krant et al.[29] examined the delayed hypersensitivity reaction in 73 patients with advanced bronchogenic carcinoma, using dinitrochlorobenzene (DNCB) sensitization and PPD reactions compared to age-matched controls as the test of immune competence. The PPD (purified protein derivative of tuberculin) reaction was negative in a much larger number of patients with bronchogenic carcinoma than among the controls. The DNCB challenge was also negative in a much larger number of cancer patients. Positive DNCB reactors were more frequent among patients with epidermoid carcinoma. Short survival times, more frequent among patients with oat cell carcinoma, were associated with negative DNCB tests.

Often, skin reactivity changed from positive to negative as the patient approached death. Circulating lymphocytes decreased greatly in number as the patients approached death, and in patients with bronchogenic cancer as compared to the control patients.

Braeman and Deeley[9] investigated lymphocyte transformation by phytohemagglutinine (PHA) in 32 patients with lung cancer. Although the authors found a lower average percentage of transformation in lung cancer patients as compared to a control population, neither the initial levels nor the tests after treatment could be related to prognosis. Han and Takita[22] found a greatly impaired lymphocyte response to PHA in operable patients with cancer of the lung, as did Ducos et al.[16] The authors felt that there might be some prognostic significance in this lymphocyte response to PHA. Similar results were reported by Jenkins et al.[25] A comparison of the various tests of immune competence in patients with cancer of the lung and their reliability in assessing immune deficiencies was reported by Brugarolas and coworkers.[10] There was a correlation of delayed hypersensitivity skin testing and lymphocyte stimulation testing with respect to the clinical state of the bronchogenic carcinoma patient. Two-thirds of the patients with cancer presented consistent skin tests and lymphocyte blastogenic indices of transformed cells in a stimulated culture and an unstimulated culture. Rosette formation after mixture with sheep red blood cells was much lower in the lymphocytes of lung cancer patients than in patients with breast cancer or control subjects. This occurred regardless of the stage of the disease, and may be important because thymus-derived lymphocytes (T-cells) rather than thymus-independent lymphocytes (B-cells) are presented in the rosette forming test, and it is believed that the T-cells play a major role in immunologic intervention at the target tumor cells of the host.

Israel and Halpern[24] reported improved survival in patients with tuberculin-positive skin reactions prior to chemotherapy compared to patients with negative skin tests.

Carcinoembryonic antigen (CEA) has been found in more than 50% of 19 lung cancers obtained at surgery or autopsy, as reported by Sizaret and Martin.[46] McIntire and Sizaret also reported tumor-associated human lung tumor antigens that are not tumor-specific in 30 examined cancers.[34] A specific antigen has been shown in bronchioloalveolar carcinoma.[41]

At present, the clinical significance for staging and diagnosis of the CEA level must be considered doubtful because of the high incidence of positive CEA levels in patients who are smokers (Concannon et al.,[15] Vincent and Chu,[49] Meeker et al.).[36] Approximately 50% of patients with benign lung disease had CEA values between

2.5 and 4.9 ng/ml.; 13%, most of them smokers, had CEA levels >5.0 ng/ml. Approximately 50% of patients with bronchogenic carcinoma, including advanced stages of the disease, had CEA values <5.0 ng/ml. Concannon and co-workers also pointed out that the initial CEA level was of little value in predicting patient survival after treatment.

SERUM STUDIES IN PATIENTS WITH CANCER OF THE LUNG

Biochemical studies involving serum level analysis of ubiquitous enzymes have been pursued by Bodansky.[7] Elevation of serum phosphohexose isomerase was found in 72% of 126 patients with lung cancer, elevated serum aldolase levels in 62% of patients, and in smaller percentages in the analysis of lactic acid dehydrogenase (53%), serum glutamic oxaloacetic transaminase (SGOT) (15%), malic acid dehydrogenase (25%), and serum glutamic pyruvic transaminase (SGPT) (7%). The elevation of these enzymes in the serum was attributed to one or more factors involving tissue damage by neoplastic growth or some other factor, the size of the organ or organs that were damaged, the concentration of enzyme in these organs, the rate of passage of enzyme from the tissue cells into the circulation, and the rate of disappearance from the circulation. Karcher[27] indicated that enzyme examination of the serum was more important in evaluating the response to treatment of bronchogenic cancer than in aiding diagnosis.

Metastatic cancer of the liver may be diagnosed using ubiquitous enzymes; reports by Bodansky[7] indicate that phosphohexose isomerase is elevated in 84% of patients, aldolase in 75%, lactic acid dehydrogenase in 69%, SGOT in 51%, and malic acid dehydrogenase in 62%. Karcher[27] has shown that not only absolute values, with elevations above the values found in a normal population group, but also relative changes are significant in the diagnosis of liver metastasis. If both SGOT and SGPT values are elevated, a quotient obtained by dividing the SGOT value by the SGPT value indicates a strong likelihood of metastasis if the quotient is above one.

Wieme et al.[55] examined serum lactic acid dehydrogenase (LDH) and its isoenzymes and found that elevation of the total serum LDH occurred in approximately 50% of the untreated cases and that cytostatic therapy produced a normalization of the total LDH levels and of the LDH isoenzyme levels, if the tumor responded.

Shaw and Kellermann[45] have described tests of lymphocytes in culture in 50 patients that correlate high levels of aryl hydrocarbon hydroxylase concentrations (AHH) with the high probability of lung cancer in cigarette smokers. Cigarette smokers with high AHH activity in their lymphocytes ran 36 times the risk of lung cancer compared to patients with low AHH inducibility. Patients with moderate levels ran 16 times the risk of those with low levels. About 9% of the American white population has a high AHH induction; the rest of the population is roughly divided between low and moderate levels. Although cancers in general are not necessarily associated with high AHH inducibility, there was a distinct pattern with lung cancer and smokers. There was a remarkable lack of lung cancer cases in the low inducibility group. Ninety-one percent of the healthy controls were in the low or moderate AHH inducibility group; 96% of the lung cancer group who were cigarette smokers had moderately or highly inducible AHH in their lymphocytes. Only 4% of those with cancer had poorly inducible AHH in their lymphocytes, which contrasted with poor inducibility of AHH in 45% of the control population.

Although profiles of serum chemistries and other components of serum have not yielded specific findings in lung cancer, Ashley,[1] reported a significantly higher frequency of blood group A in patients with proximal cancer of the lung as compared to distal cancer and to blood group O. His findings have not been confirmed by other authors.

REFERENCES

1. Ashley, D. J. B.: Blood groups and lung cancer. *J. Med. Genet.* **6**:183–186, 1969.
2. Auerbach, O., Stout, A., Harmond, E., and Garfinkel, L.: Multiple primary bronchial carcinomas. *Cancer* **20**:699–705, 1969.
3. Auerbach, O.: Cancerous and precancerous lung changes: slide review. *Cancer* **19**:138–145, 1969.
4. Bell, J. W.: Possible immune factors in spontaneous regression of bronchogenic carcinoma. *Am. J. Surg.* **120**:804–806, 1970.
5. Bennett, D. E., Sasser, W. F., and Ferguson, T. B.: Adenocarcinoma of the lung in men. *Cancer* **23**:431–439, 1969.
6. Bjork, V.: Bronchial carcinoma. *Acta Chiv. Scandinav.* **95** Suppl. 123:1–113, 1947.
7. Bodansky, O.: Use of ubiquitous enzymes in cancer management. *Cancer* **23**:275–280, 1973.
8. Boyd, W.: *The Spontaneous Regression of Cancer.* Charles C. Thomas, Springfield, Illinois, 1966.
9. Braeman, J., and Deeley, T. J.: Immunological studies in irradiation. *Ann. Clin. Res.* **4**:355–360, 1972.
10. Brugarolas, A., Han, T., Takita, H., and Minowada, J.: Immunologic assays in lung cancer. *N.Y. State J. Med.* **73**:747–750, 1973.
11. Buchberg, A., Lubliner, R., and Rubin, E. H.: Carcinoma of the lung: duration of life of individuals not treated surgically. *Dis. Chest* **20**:257–275, 1951.

References

12. Budinger, J. M.: Untreated bronchogenic carcinoma. *Am. J. Cancer* **11**:106–116, 1958.

13. Cancer Mortality and Morbidity in Pennsylvania. Commonwealth of Pennsylvania, Department of Health, Cancer Control Section. Harrisburg, Pennsylvania, 1970.

14. Chahinian, P.: Relationship between tumor doubling time and anatomical clinical features in fifty measurable pulmonary cancers *Chest* **61**:340–345, 1972.

15. Concannon, J. P., Dalbow, M. H., Liebler, G. A., Blake, K. E., and Cooper, J. W.: The carcinoembryonic antigen (CEA) assay in bronchogenic carcinoma. *Cancer*. In preparation.

16. Ducos, J., Migueres, J., Colomics, P., Kessous, A., and Poujoulet, N.: Lymphocyte response to PHA in patients with lung cancer. *Lancet* **1**:1111–1112, 1970.

17. Eisenberg, H., Shames, J. M., Holloway, W., and Barrett, H.: Cancer of the bronchus and lung. Connecticut 1935–1959, *J. Chronic Dis.* **17**:1033–1054, 1964.

18. Engelman, R., and McNamara, W.: Bronchiogenic carcinoma, statistical review of 234 autopsies. *J. Thorac. Surg.* **27**:227–237, 1954.

19. Falor, W. H., Gordon, M., and Kaczala, O. A.: Chromosomes in bronchoscopic biopsies. *Cancer* **24**:198–209, 1969.

20. Garland, L. H, Beier, R. L., Coulson, W., Heald, J. H., and Stein, R. L.: The apparent sites of origin of carcinoma of the lung. *Radiology* **78**:1–11, 1962.

21. Garland, L. H., Coulson, W., and Wollin, E.: The rate of growth and apparent duration of untreated primary bronchial carcinoma. *Cancer* **16**:694–707, 1963.

22. Han, T., and Takita, H.: Immunologic impairment in bronchogenic carcinoma: a study of lymphocyte response to phytohemagglutinin. *Cancer* **30**:616–620, 1972.

23. Herman, D. L., and Crittenden, M.: Distribution of primary lung carcinoma in relation to tissue as determined by histochemical techniques. *J. Natl. Cancer Inst.* **27**:1227–1271, 1961.

24. Israel, L., and Halpern, B.: Le corynebacterium parvum dans les cancers avances. *Nouv. Presse Med.* **1**:19–23, 1972.

25. Jenkins, V. K., Olson, M. H., and Ellis, H. N.: In vitro methods of assessing lymphocyte transformation in patients undergoing radiotherapy for bronchogenic cancer. *Cancer* **31**:19–28, 1973.

26. Joseph, W. L., Morton, D. L., and Adkins, P. C.: Variation in tumor doubling time in patients with pulmonary metastatic disease. *J. Surg. Oncol.* **3**(2):143–249, 1971.

27. Karcher, K.: Fermentuntersuchungen in Serum and Gewebe in: Einfuehrung in die Klinisch -experimentelle Radiologie, Urban and Schwarzenberg, Munich, 1964.

28. Kato, Y., Ferguson, T. B., Bennett, D. E., and Burford, T. H.: Oat Cell carcinoma of the lung. A review of 138 cases. *Cancer* **23**:517–524, 1969.

29. Krant, M. J., Manskopf, G., Brandrup, C. S., and Madoff, M. A.: Immunologic alterations in bronchogenic cancer. *Cancer* **21**: 623–631, 1968.

30. Line, D., and Deeley, T.: Palliative therapy. In *Modern Radiotherapy, Carcinoma of the Bronchus,* Appleton-Century, London, 1971.

31. Luomanen, R. K. J., and Watson, W. L.: Autopsy findings. In *Lung Cancer, A Study of Five Thousand Memorial Hospital Cases,* William L. Watson, Ed., C. V. Mosby, St. Louis, 1968.

32. Malaise, E. P., Chavaudra, N., and Tubiana, M.: The relationship between growth rate labeling index and histological type of human solid tumors. *Eur. J. Cancer* **9**:305–312, 1973.

33. Matthews, M. J., Kanhouwa, S., Pickren, J., and Robinette, D.: Frequency of residual and metastatic tumor in patients undergoing curative surgical resection for lung cancer. *Cancer Chemother. Rep.,* Part 3, **4**:63–68, 1973.

34. McIntire, K, and Sizaret, P.: Detection of antigens associated with carcinoma of the lung. Presented at the XIth International Cancer Congress, Florence, 1974.

35. McNamara, J., Kuigsley, W., Paulson, D., Arndt, J., Salines-Izaquine, S., and Upschel, H.: Alveolar cell carcinoma of the lung. *J. Thorac. Cardiovasc. Surg.* **57**:648–656, 1969.

36. Meeker, R. W., Kashmiri, R., Hunter, L., Clapp, W., and Griffen, W. O.: Clinical evaluation of carcinembryonic antigen. *Arch. Surg.* **107**:266–273, 1973.

37. Mersheimer, W. L., Ringel, A., and Eisenberg, H.: Some characteristics of multiple primary cancers. *Ann. N.Y. Acad. Sci.* **114**:896–921, 1964.

38. Meyer, J. A.: Growth rate versus prognosis in resected primary bronchogenic carcinomas. *Cancer* **31**:1468–1472, 1973.

39. Muggia, F. M., and DeVita, V.: In vivo tumor cell kinetics studies. Use of local thymidine injections followed by fine needle aspiration. *J. Lab. Clin. Med.* **80**:297–301, 1972..

40. Nathan, M. H., Collins, V. P., and Adams, R. A.: Differentiation of benign and malignant pulmonary nodules by growth rate. *Radiology* **79**:221–231, 1962.

41. Nordquist, R. E.: Specific antigens in human alveolar cell carcinoma. *Cancer Res.* **33**:1790–1795, 1973.

42. Ochsner, A., et al.: Primary pulmonary malignancy. *J. Thorac. Surg.* **5**:641–672, 1936.

43. Olson, K. B.: Primary carcinoma of the lung. *Am. J. Pathol.* **11**:449–468, 1935.

44. Rienhoff, W. F., Jr.: A clinical analysis and follow-up study of 502 cases of carcinoma of the lung. *Dis. Chest* **17**:33–53, 1950.

45. Shaw, C. H., and Kellermann, G.: Hydroxylase variation and susceptibility to bronchogenic carcinoma in Man. Presented at the XIth International Cancer Congress, Florence, 1974.

46. Sizaret, P., and Martin, F.: Brief communication: carcinoembryonic antigen in extracts of pulmonary cancers. *J. Natl. Cancer Inst.* **50**:807–809, 1973.

47. Spjut, H. J., and Mateo, L. E.: Recurrent and metastatic carcinoma in surgically treated carcinoma of lung, an autopsy survey. *Cancer* **18**:1462–1466, 1965.

48. Straus, Marc J.: The gross characteristics of lung cancer and its application to treatment designed. *Semin. Oncol.* **1**:167–174, 1974.

49. Vincent, R. G., and Chu, T. M.: Carcinomembryonic antigen in patients with carcinoma of the lung. *J. Thorac. Cardiovasc. Surg.* **66**:320–328, 1973.

50. Watson, W. L., and Farpour, A.: Terminal bronchiolar or "alveolar cell" cancer of the lung. *Cancer* **19**:776–780, 1966.

51. Watson, W.: *Lung Cancer.* C. V. Mosby, St. Louis, 1968.

52. Weiss, W.: Mitotic index in bronchogenic carcinoma. *Am. Rev. Respir. Dis.* **104**:536–543, 1971.

53. Weiss, W., Boucot, K. R., and Cooper, D. A.: The Philadelphia pulmonary neoplasm research project. Survival factors in bronchogenic carcinoma. *J. A. M. A.* **216**:2119–2123, 1971.

54. Weiss, W.: The growth rate of bronchogenic carcinoma. Is it constant? *Cancer* **32**:167–171, 1973.

55. Wieme, R. J., VanHove, W. Z., and VanDerStraeten, M. E.: The influence of cytostatic treatment on serum LDH patterns of patients with bronchial carcinoma and its relation to tumor regression. *Ann. N.Y. Acad. Sci.* **151**:213–221, 1968.

Chapter Six

The Role of the Lymphatics in Metastasis from Cancer of the Lung

The pulmonary lymph capillaries are closely associated with the alveolar walls, the pulmonary blood vessels, and the bronchial walls. Collecting trunks accompany blood vessels and bronchial branches to their termination in lymph nodes. Lymphatic capillaries are also present in the layers of the bronchi surrounding the bronchial musculature and cartilage. They continue on the outer surface of the bronchial walls in collecting vessels that are located on the outer surface of the major bronchi and pulmonary blood vessels with localized collections of lymphoid cells. Intrapulmonary lymph nodes are located at major branching angles of the bronchi. They conform to the different lobar arrangement in the right and left lungs. In the hilar areas, the nodes have a close relationship with the veins.

In the periphery of the lung, subpleural lymphatics underlie the visceral pleura and form large vessels that empty into the regional lymph nodes. These vessels are mainly responsible for the direction of outflow of lymph from the lungs. The collecting vessels of the lung periphery contain lymph which is flowing toward the pleura, while the vessels of the deep and central portions convey lymph toward the hilum. The peripheral portions of the lower lobes of the lung carry the lymph to lymph nodes in the immediate diaphragmatic region through an anterior node located in the pulmonary ligament.

In the anatomic classification of Gardner et al.,[4] the group of lymph nodes clinically described as "hilar" consists of the bronchopulmonary and pulmonary nodes that are located along the main stem bronchi. These nodes in turn drain into the mediastinal nodes, which are conveniently divided into the inferior and superior tracheobronchial nodes according to their relationship to the main stem bronchus (Fig. 1). The paratracheal and paraesophageal lymph nodes form the craniad part of the mediastinal lymph nodes. They leave the thorax through the bronchomediastinal lymph trunks which drain into the thoracic duct on the left and into the junction of the internal jugular and subclavian veins on the right, although anatomic variants are common. These lymph ducts relate closely to the supraclavicular lymph nodes.

Other mediastinal nodes include the anterior mediastinal nodes in the superior mediastinum, the posterior mediastinal nodes around the lower part of the thoracic esophagus, and subcarinal nodes which form part of the aforementioned inferior tracheobronchial nodes. The azygos node forms part of the right superior tracheobronchial nodes.

Operative specimens from pneumonectomies and lobectomies provide the best source of information about the incidence of lymph node metastasis from various primary sites of lung cancers. Table 1 contains data from

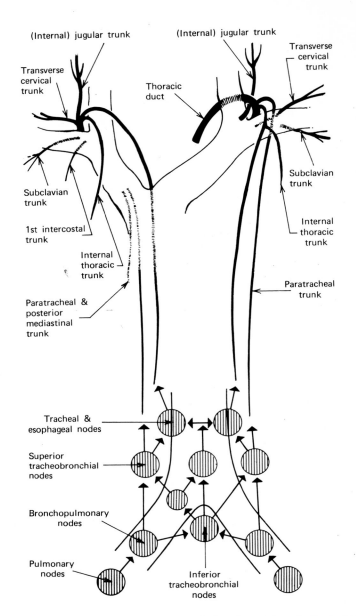

Fig. 1. Schematic representation of the visceral lymphatic nodes and collecting trunks of the thorax. (Courtesy of W. B. Saunders.[4])

such a study reported by Baird.[1] In this series, metastases were found in 77% of the patients, regardless of whether right- or left-sided lesions were present. The left lung may frequently metastasize to the right supraclavicular node through the communications between the left hilar and mediastinal nodes and the azygos node on the right. Involvement of the left supraclavicular nodes from a right-sided lesion is rare[1,2,5] (see Table 2).

Although the lymph nodes form one pathway for dissemination of lung cancer, hematogenous spread via the bronchial veins is another significant factor. Reports on studies of injection of blood vessels supplying pulmonary

TABLE 1. LYMPH NODE METASTASIS IN OPERATIVE SPECIMENS[1]

Primary Site	Frequency (% of all patients)	No Node Metastasis	Hilar Node Metastasis	Mediastinal Node Metastasis	Supraclavicular Right	Left
Right upper lobe and right hilum	41%	40.5%	59.5%	40.5%	30%	0%
Right middle lobe	5%	36%	64%	19%	30%	0%
Right lower lobe	11%	23%	77%	54%	3%	0%
Left upper lobe and left hilum	32%	27%	73%	46%	9%	31%
Left lower lobe	9%	24%	76%	40%	8%	0%

TABLE 2. SCALENE NODE METASTASIS[1,2,5a]

Primary Site	Right Upper Lobe	Right Middle Lobe	Right Lower Lobe	Left Upper Lobe	Lingula	Left Lower Lobe
Right scalene nodes	11–(31)–37.5	2–(2)–9	0.4–(7)–7	0–(1.7)–9	0–7	0–(2)–5
Left scalene nodes	0–(8.5)–10	0–(1)–7	0–(0.5)–3.5	12–(17)–32	0–3.5	0–(4.5)–7

[a] In percent of all positive biopsies: lowest–(median)–highest.

carcinomas following the patient's death indicate that involvement of the veins was present in 66% of the patients with oat cell carcinoma, compared to 28% in patients with epidermoid carcinoma.[5] The relationship of venous involvement to stage of tumor and lymph node involvement given in Table 3 indicates the progressive involvement of the vascular system as the tumor invades adjacent structures. The relationship between lymph node metastasis and distant metastasis was established by Croxatto and Barcat,[3] who found lymph node metastasis in 90% of patients with metastasis in distant organs, whereas lymph node metastasis occurred in only 17% of patients who did not have distant organ metastasis.

In summary, hilar node metastasis with lung cancer occur in about 60% of right upper lobe and middle lobe lesions and in approximately 75% of primary tumors arising in the remaining portions of both lungs. Mediastinal adenopathy occurs in 40 to 50% of operative specimens, with the exception of the right middle lobe where it is less common. Supraclavicular node metastasis predominate on the ipsilateral side, with an incidence up to 30% in the right upper, right middle, and left upper lobes. Left lower lobe lesions may metastasize to the contralateral, right scalene lymph nodes in about one-third of all scalene node metastases from this site.

Although it is likely that distant metastases usually occur following involvement of regional lymph nodes, the relative importance of other factors such as aggressiveness of tumor growth and vascular invasion is not known at this time.

TABLE 3. EXTENT OF PRIMARY TUMOR RELATED TO LYMPH NODE METASTASIS AND VENOUS INVOLVEMENT IN 211 CASES[5]

Description	Total	Node Metastasis Number	Node Metastasis Percent	Venous Involvement Number	Venous Involvement Percent
Tumor limited to the lung	77	51	66	15	19
Tumor invading the pleura	83	56	67	26	31
Tumor invading the mediastinum or chest wall	51	42	82	32	63
Oat cell carcinoma					66
Undifferentiated carcinoma					41.4
Squamous cell carcinoma					28.5

REFERENCES

1. Baird, J. A.: The pathways of lymphatic spread of carcinoma of the lung. *Br. J. Surg.* **52**:868–875, 1965.

2. Brantigan, O. C., and Moszkowski, E.: Bilateral biopsy of non-palpable cervical lymph nodes. Diagnosis and prognosis in carcinoma of the lung. *Dis. Chest* **50**:464–469, 1966.

3. Croxatto, O. C., and Barcat, J. A.: Lymph node metastasis in bronchogenic carcinoma. Study on its role in dissemination. *Johns Hopkins Med. J.* **126**:121–129, 1970.

4. Gardner, E., Gray, D., and O'Rahilly, R.: *Anatomy*. W. B. Saunders, Philadelphia, 1960.

5. Nohl, H.: *The Spread of Carcinoma of the Bronchus*. Year Book Publishers, Chicago, 1962.

Chapter Seven

Detection and Treatment of Early Bronchogenic Carcinoma

itely 50% of bronchioloalveolar carcinomas, f epidermoid and adenocarcinomas, and 96% of oat cell carcinomas are diagnosed initially when either locally advanced or metastatic. The lack of early symptoms, the inaccessibility of the primary tumor to clinical examination, and the uncertainties of radiographic examination as a diagnostic test contribute to the difficulties in the early diagnosis of bronchogenic carcinoma. Although some of the changes in the peripheral blood such as the carcinoembryonic antigen and serum enzymes show promise for the future, major recent efforts toward early diagnosis have been based on radiographic examination and cytologic studies. These two methods supplement each other in that peripheral lesions may be seen on x-rays when they reach approximately 1 cm in diameter, but they rarely show early malignant cells in the sputum. On the other hand, since small tumors near the hilum are difficult to detect radiographically because they blend with the mediastinum, early diagnosis through exfoliation of malignant cells and their finding in the sputum shows promise.

Early diagnosis of bronchogenic carcinoma by x-ray examination involves the detection and differential diagnosis of solitary pulmonary nodules. A combined study of the Veterans Administration and the Armed Forces[17] in 217 male patients with solitary pulmonary nodules revealed that 34% were due to bronchogenic carcinoma, 4.5% were benign tumors, 55% granulomas, 4.5% miscellaneous other conditions, and 2% metastatic tumors. There were 23% epidermoid carcinomas, 3.5% adenocarcinomas, 5% oat cell carcinomas, and 1.5% bronchioloalveolar carcinomas. In 130 lesions reported by Pellett and Gale,[14] 25% were primary bronchogenic cancers, 12% metastatic malignancies, 14% benign tumors, 45% granulomas, and 4% miscellaneous other conditions. In patients who were 50 years or older, 51% of the lesions were malignant.

Prospective studies regarding the value of periodic radiographic screening of high-risk populations have been carried out in Great Britain and in this country. Brett[3] offered 29,723 English men aged 40 and over six monthly chest x-rays over a 3-year period and compared the survival rate with that of a control group of 25,311 men of the same age and with similar smoking habits who were x-rayed at the beginning and end of the study. Among the test group, 65 bronchogenic carcinomas were discovered by routine x-ray examination and 36 in between surveys because of symptoms requiring radiographic examination. Among the control group, 76 developed bronchogenic carcinoma diagnosed on the basis of symptoms. The 5-year survival rate of the patients in the test group was 15%, usually following surgical treatment, and in the control group it was 6%. If the patients whose malignancy was detected on routine examination were analyzed separately, the 5-year survival was 23%. The overall annual incidence of bronchogenic carcinoma in the groups of patients under consideration was approximately 1/1000.

In a similar study, Nash et al.[12] reported on six monthly chest x-rays performed on male volunteers over 45 years of age. A total of 67,400 patients had at least one x-ray examination, and 197,500 follow-up x-rays were obtained. On the basis of the radiographic examinations, 147 cases of primary lung cancer were discovered. Of these, 83 patients came to resection and 39 survived 4 years. This 4-year survival rate of 27% among the group screened and found to have lung cancer is very similar to the previously mentioned study. The authors also followed carefully those patients who did not appear for reexamination. All patients could be followed except for 202 who could not be traced: 40 had left Great Britain, and the remaining 162 nonemigrants were known not to have been registered as dead in the National Registry. An additional 87 cases of primary lung cancer were traced among the group which did not undergo reexamination. Of these 87 only 5 (6%) lived 4 years or more. The group that benefited most from the routine surveys and detection of asymptomatic lung cancer were patients over 55 years of age who had epidermoid carcinoma or adenocarcinoma.

A large study carried out under the auspices of the Subcommittee on Lung Cancer of the Philadelphia County Medical Society by the Philadelphia Pulmonary Neoplasm Research Project has been evaluated by Boucot and Weiss.[2] A population of 6,136 male volunteers 45 years or older were screened every 6 months by chest fluoroscopy and questionnaires about symptoms. During a 10-year period of follow-up, 121 bronchogenic carcinomas were found; 94 cases of lung cancer were proven histologically and the remaining 27 were believed to have lung cancer on the basis of x-rays and clinical findings. Only 8% of the 121 patients survived 5 years following treatment. The 5-year survival rate in 67 men whose tumors were detected within 6 months of a negative x-ray was 12%, whereas there were 54 patients with intervals between examinations exceeding 6 months. Only 4% of these patients survived 5 years. Although the 5-year survival results as a group were disappointing, only 2 of the 10-year survivors were not detected by the screen and diagnosed on the basis of symptoms requiring medical attention. As in the previous studies, patients over 55 years of age who had epidermoid or adenocarcinoma fared better than younger patients or those who had poorly differentiated carcinoma. No patients under 55 or over 65 years of age survived. It was also shown that patients who smoked less than one pack of cigarettes a day, who did not have chronic cough, who were asymptomatic at the time of detection of lung cancer, and who had a peripheral roentgenographic lesion showed better 5-year survival rates than their counterparts.

A critique of the disappointing results of the Philadelphia project has been presented by Fontana[7] with reference to patient selection, a high postoperative mortality rate, and a lack of dual reading of the x-rays. It is noteworthy that while Boucot and Weiss[2] estimated the cost of a lung cancer "cure" to be $83,000, the British studies projected a cost between $500 and $2,500 in equivalent British pounds.

The disappointing results of radiographic diagnosis in early lung cancer were pointed out by Cooley,[5] who also indicated the need for a strong suspicion of cancer on the part of the radiologist to offer the patient the best chance for curative resection. Approximately one-third of lung cancers are partly or completely hidden by other structures until they become symptomatic and/or nonresectable. Only 20 to 30% of lung cancers begin as solitary peripheral nodules. On the other hand, the common nonnodular signs of asymptomatic peripheral pulmonary cancer such as scars, thickened caps, pleural plaques or nonspecific infiltrative processes are frequently associated with pulmonary fibrosis, pleural scarring, or emphysema and make accurate radiographic diagnosis difficult.

Remarkable progress has been made during recent years in the cytologic diagnosis of asymptomatic lung cancer. A review of the early experience was presented by Clerf and Herbut[4] in 1946. They showed that the value of cytology in the early diagnosis of lung cancer had been emphasized since about 1926. A large series of cytologically diagnosed lung cancer was reported by Kirsh et al.[9] in 1970. They presented an 86% rate of accuracy in the cytological typing of 104 primary bronchogenic carcinomas regardless of the histological type of the cancer. If ambiguous cases with a strong suspicion of malignancy are included, the overall accuracy of diagnosis is 95%. The location of the lesions diagnosed by cytology was analyzed by Rosa et al.,[15] who found that at least three sputum specimens, central location of the cancer, and absence of atelectasis yielded the most accurate results. The diagnosis of cancer was established by one sputum in 49% of the patients, by two in 55%, and by three sputum examinations in 65%. The overall sensitivity was 71% of all cancers. Peripheral tumors were diagnosed in 48% of lesions, metastasis in 62%, and central carcinoma in 82.5%. Positive cytologies were recorded in 84.5% of all epidermoid cancers, 70% in oat cell carcinomas, and 57% in adenocarcinomas. Lilienfeld[10] showed that single cytologic screening was

positive in only 33%. Multiple cytologic studies sometimes made with sputum inducers in the form of aerosol inhalants often eliminate false-negative reports (Fig. 1). He also emphasized the possibility that cells from malignant lesions of the larynx, pharynx, and oral cavity might appear in the expectorated sputum.

The encouraging results with sputum cytology have led to prospective studies using this technique in the early diagnosis of lung cancer. In 1967, Pearson et al.[13] reported 41 patients with malignant cells in the sputum but without visible tumor on chest x-rays; 25 patients underwent sputum examination because of findings that suggested bronchial carcinoma; 5 patients had radiographic lesions which were later shown to be benign and unrelated to the coexisting bronchogenic carcinoma.

In this survey restricted to male cigarette smokers over 40 years of age, sputum examination of 1586 patients with an average of 1.4 sputum samples per patient showed approximately 10% with moderate or severe dyskaryosis. In addition to x-ray examination, bronchoscopy, bronchography, and tomography were used to localize the tumor. Eleven patients showed evidence of malignant cells as the only sign of a malignant tumor, and only 3 of the 11 tumors had been located at the time of the report; 8 patients were still being followed. Thirty-seven cytologies indicated the presence of epidermoid carcinoma. Two-thirds were early invasive and one-third were *in situ* carcinomas. Of the 19 living pa-

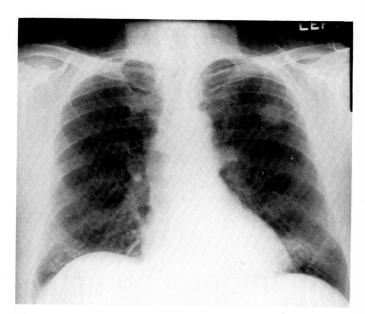

Fig. 1. Patient W. W. Coin lesion. Multiple examinations of sputa did not reveal the histologic nature of this left upper lobe carcinoma of the lung. No malignant cells were obtained after stimulation of the sputum by aerosol inhalation. Mediastinal biopsy revealed evidence of anaplastic carcinoma.

tients in whom a tumor was located, there were 14 resections and 5 patients were treated by radiation therapy only. To date none of the 14 patients treated by resection has died of recurrent cancer. One patient died of a coronary thrombosis during operation. One of the 5 patients treated by radiotherapy died of unrelated disease 12 months after treatment and there was no sign of residual tumor at autopsy. Another patient died of unrelated disease following radiotherapy without autopsy. The remaining 3 patients showed progression of their tumor and they died at 22, 32, and 38 months respectively after radiation therapy. At present, follow-up is 2 to 6 years after surgery. Follow-up cytologic tests have remained negative in all patients who have been examined postoperatively.

The difficulty in identifying the tumor site in patients with positive cytology without radiographic findings of lung cancer has been confirmed by Bell.[1] Only 6 of 12 patients in whom positive sputum was obtained had identification of the tumor site. Saksena et al.[16] found bronchoscopy the most valuable study in the workup of patients with positive cytology for lung cancer without radiographic findings. They found 11 malignant lesions in 8 patients with lung cancer detected by sputum cytology. One of the patients was treated by radiation therapy only and died eight months after radiation therapy without residual carcinoma at autopsy. The remaining 7 patients underwent various forms of surgery; 4 have survived 20 to 96 months free of tumor and an additional 3 died 24 to 48 months postoperatively. The authors pointed out the importance of follow-up by repeat cytology.

The localization of early bronchogenic carcinoma has been greatly advanced by the use of flexible fiberoptic equipment instead of the conventional straight Jackson bronchoscope (Figs. 6 and 7, chapter 11). The presence of unexpected large areas of carcinoma *in situ* surrounding small areas of invasive carcinoma have been reported by Marsh et al.[11]

Simultaneous screening for lung cancer using chest x-ray and sputum cytology has been advanced by Grzybowski and Coy.[8] A group of 2112 male cigarette smokers over the age of 40 who suffered from chronic bronchitis and showed long-standing radiologic abnormalities or had recently recovered from pneumonia were screened by sputum cytology and chest x-ray. In the study, 17 lung cancers were detected, an incidence of 0.8%; 8 of these cases were detected by x-ray alone, 7 by cytology alone and 2 by both methods. Of the 17 patients, 13 died of lung cancer, 1 died of another cause, and 3 are alive and well. The 3 survivors were among 6 patients exposed to a thoracotomy and the remaining 11 patients had contraindications to surgery.

A prospective study regarding the value, acceptance, and effectiveness of a combined screening by cytology and x-ray examination for lung cancer is being carried out by the Mayo Lung Project.[6] Smokers 45 years or older are the subjects under study. Chest x-rays and lung health questionnaires are used, as well as a 3-day pooled sputum specimen for cytologic examination. A control group receives care and advice according to current standards at the Mayo Clinic. Participants in the study will undergo extensive bronchogenic carcinoma screening every 4 months. Although patient acceptance of this program has been good, results of the study are not yet available.

An estimate of the best results to be expected by earlier diagnosis of cancer of the lung may be based on reports of treatment of *in situ* and early invasive lung cancer by Woolner et al.[18] Surgery performed in 28 patients resulted in only 3 failures, 2 of them were due to multiple lesions.

It is not likely that radiographic diagnosis of early bronchogenic carcinoma will be improved significantly at reasonable cost in the future. Therefore, our hopes for improvements of early diagnosis rest upon the use of screening by sputum cytology in association with the other established methods of diagnosing lung cancer. Although it is not widely used at present, and the dilemma of locating a small lesion which is shedding malignant cells into the sputum remains serious, the results of treatment are encouraging. One must remember that cytologic screening was first employed in carcinoma of the cervix, for which diagnosis and treatment have advanced so far that, theoretically at least, invasive carcinoma need no longer occur.

REFERENCES

1. Bell, J. W.: Positive sputum cytology and negative chest roentgenograms. A surgeon's dilemma. *Ann. Thorac. Surg.* 9:149–157, 1970.

2. Boucot, K. R., and Weiss, W.: Is curable lung cancer detected by semiannual screening? *J. A. M. A.* 224:1361–1365, 1973.

3. Brett, G. Z.: Earlier diagnosis and survival in lung cancer. *Br. Med. J.* 4:260–262, 1969.

4. Clerf, L. H., and Herbut, P. A.: Diagnosis of bronchogenic carcinoma by examination of bronchial secretions. *Ann. Otol. Rhinol. Laryngol.* 55:646–655, 1946.

5. Cooley, R. N.: Radiographic detection of preclinical and asymptomatic cancer of the lung. *Am. J. Roentgenol. Radium Ther. Nucl. Med.* 107:440–442, 1969.

6. Fontana, R. S., Sanderson, D. R., Miller, W. E., Woolner, L. B., Taylor, W. F., and Uhlenhopp, M. A.: The Mayo Lung Project: preliminary report of "early cancer detection" phase. *Cancer* 30:1373–1382, 1972.

References

7. Fontana, R. S.: Editorial. *J. A. M. A.* **225**:1373, 1973.

8. Grzybowski, S., and Coy, P.: Early diagnosis of carcinoma of the lung. Simultaneous screening with chest x-ray and sputum cytology. *Cancer* **25**:113–120, 1970.

9. Kirsh, M. M., Orvald, T., Naylor, B., Kahn, D. R., and Sloan, H.: Diagnostic accuracy of exfoliative pulmonary cytology. *Ann. Thorac. Surg.* **9**:335–338, 1970.

10. Lilienfeld, A.: An evaluation of radiologic and cytologic screening for the early diagnosis of lung cancer. *Cancer Res.* **26**:2083–2121, 1966.

11. Marsh, B. R., Frost, J. K., Erozan, Y. S., and Carter, D.: Occult bronchogenic carcinoma. Endoscopic localization and television documentation. *Cancer* **30**:1348–1352, 1972.

12. Nash, F. A., Morgan, J. M., and Tomkins, J. G.: South London lung cancer study. *Br. Med. J.* **2**:715–721, 1968.

13. Pearson, F. G., Thompson, D. W., and Delarue, N. C.: Experience with the cytologic detection, localization, and treatment of radiographically undemonstrable bronchial carcinoma. *J. Thorac. Cardiovasc. Surg.* **54**:371–382, 1967.

14. Pellett, J. R., and Gale, J. W.: The solitary pulmonary lesion. What is it? What is the treatment? *Arch. Surg.* **83**:97–108, 1961.

15. Rosa, U. W., Prolla, J. C., and da Silva Gastal, E.: Cytology in diagnosis of cancer affecting the lung. Results in 1,000 consecutive patients. *Chest* **63**:203–207, 1973.

16. Saksena, D. S., Parrish, C. M., Hughes, R. K., and Fullmer, C. D.: Sputum cytology in occult lung cancer. *Rocky Mt. Med. J.* **70**:33–36, 1973.

17. Walske, B. R.: The solitary pulmonary nodule. A review of 217 cases. *Dis. Chest* **49**:302–304, 1966.

18. Woolner, L. B., David, E., Fontana, R. S., Andersen, H. A., and Bernatz, P. E.: In situ and early invasive bronchogenic carcinoma: Report of 28 cases with postoperative survival data. *J. Thorac. Cardiovasc. Surg.* **60**:275–290, 1970.

Chapter Eight

Diagnostic Radiology in Cancer of the Lung

Arnold Chait, M.D.

Radiology is an indispensable tool in the study of bronchogenic carcinoma and plays a role in three stages of the investigation of this disease: detection, differential diagnosis, and evaluation of spread and operability.

Of all the organs of the body, the lung would appear to be the one most readily accessible to radiologic investigation, particularly in the diagnosis of solid tumors. The air content of the lung should serve as a perfect backdrop against which to detect the soft tissue densities of new growths. It is therefore disappointing that the early detection of pulmonary neoplasms at a stage when such early detection might be translated into better prognosis has not had greater success, although there has been some enthusiasm for mass screening procedures and some indication that they may prove useful. For example, in a study of mass screening of over 1,800,000 persons in Los Angeles, 244 were found to have bronchogenic carcinoma. Three times as many asymptomatic as symptomatic patients with cancer of the lung were found to be alive and well 7 years after surgery, and resectability was found to be twice as great before the onset of symptoms as it was after they appeared.[8]

In a Finnish study[29] radical surgery was carried out in 34% of the group of carcinomas discovered by compulsory mass screening, whereas such surgery was possible in only 13% of cases discovered after they became symptomatic. Three-year survival was 28% in the first group but only 12% in the second.

The fact remains, however, that a lung mass must reach a relatively large size, perhaps 1 cm in diameter, before it can be detected radiographically. The reasons for this are many and include reader error as well as the inherent limitations of the resolving power of the radiographic imaging system. It should be further emphasized that fluoroscopy of the lungs, even with image intensification, for the purpose of detecting or evaluating lung masses, should be roundly condemned. The resolution of the fluoroscopic system is far inferior to that of radiography, and the possibility of permanent record keeping is lost.

Radiography, too, is a far from perfect tool. Yerushalmy[42] reports that in a study of 1256 14×17 chest films interpreted by five competent readers, the number of positive diagnoses ranged from 56 to 100! Perhaps even more important, each reader in this study frequently disagreed with his own interpretation when he examined the same film a second time. Dual reading will reduce this potential error but at great cost, and while minimizing the number of false-negative readings it will increase the number of false-positives. The same author reports poor correlation in the interpretation of serial chest films, with two of the readers disagreeing with each other in about one-third of cases as regards changes of regression, progression, or of stability of disease. Thomas,[34] in a study of search patterns made by radiologists reading chest films, found that all investigators failed to explore some areas in detail.

In addition to the problems mentioned, it is evident that abnormal mediastinal nodes must grow beyond the normal contours of the mediastinal silhouette before they can be seen at all, and must reach a fairly large size, often several centimeters,[6] before they are considered to represent something other than normal anatomy or an anatomic variant. Even when a mediastinal lesion is large enough to be seen, it may be mistaken for benign (Fig. 1) or malignant (Fig. 2) disease other than bronchogenic carcinoma. Peripheral lesions may be concealed by overlying ribs, clavicles, or scapulae. Nodular densities, while still small, may be mistaken for pulmonary arteries or veins seen end-on. Bronchogenic carcinoma in the apices of the lungs is frequently mistaken for scar-

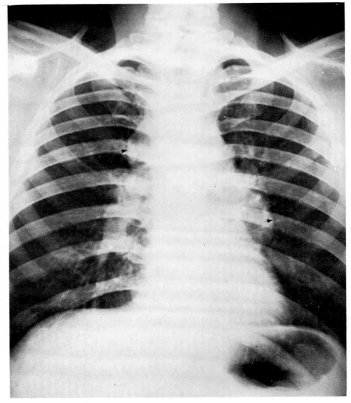

Fig. 1. Mimicking of a benign lesion. Mediastinal lesions of bronchogenic tumor may mimic other mediastinal lesions such as sarcoidosis. This 34-year-old man was thought to have sarcoidosis because of the x-ray findings shown here. This adenopathy, closely mimicking sarcoidosis, was demonstrated on mediastinoscopy to be a poorly differentiated oat cell carcinoma.

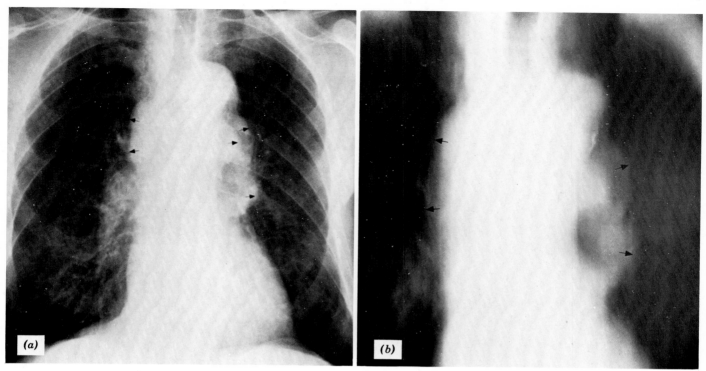

Fig. 2. Hilar adenopathy. This 76-year-old man presented with a history of anorexia, weight loss, nausea, and vomiting for 3 weeks. (a) His chest x-ray shows bilateral extensive hilar adenopathy (arrows) resembling mediastinal lymphoma. (b) The body section x-ray (arrows) shows these lesions and their relationships to normal mediastinal structures more clearly. At autopsy, this was found to be a poorly differentiated carcinoma of the lung with involvement of mediastinal and hilar nodes.

ring due to chronic inflammatory disease (Fig. 3), particularly tuberculosis.

To help resolve some of these problems, multiple special techniques have been devised to more clearly visualize concealed areas in the thorax, and to more accurately delineate poorly seen lesions and regions. Of course, a lesion must first be suspected before these additional views and techniques can be applied. In addition to the usual posteroanterior and lateral films of the chest, the following simple techniques can readily be added to the standard study on suspicion or discovery of a lesion while the patient is still in the x-ray department on his initial visit.

A. Oblique chest films. These views are often helpful in displacing shadows under investigation from mediastinal structures and from overlying or underlying ribs. They help to localize lesions in an anteroposterior orientation.

B. Apical lordotic view of the chest (Figs. 3,4). This view serves to displace the clavicles and the anterior ribs from the apical portions of the lungs, resulting in a more or less bonefree look at the apices. Very large lesions that have been overlooked on standard roentgenograms may be seen with this technique.

C. Body section radiography (tomography, laminography). With this technique, body parts in front or in back of the area of interest are obscured by an intentional blurring motion during filming and the area of interest is sharply visualized. This technique is particularly applicable to the study of:

1. "Coin lesions" (Figs. 5,6). These are nodular densities, usually single and well circumscribed, although no universal definition has been accepted. One of the many definitions of a coin lesion is that of any solitary circular mass of 6 cm in diameter or less situated within the lung substance with or without cavitation.[21] The presence or absence of calcium within such a lesion can be very important in deciding whether the lesion is benign or malignant. The presence of calcium may be clearly shown on laminography, and strongly suggests that the lesion is benign, either the result of chronic inflammation or of benign tumor. It should be clearly understood, however, that a bronchogenic tumor may engulf a benign calcification resulting from chronic inflamma-

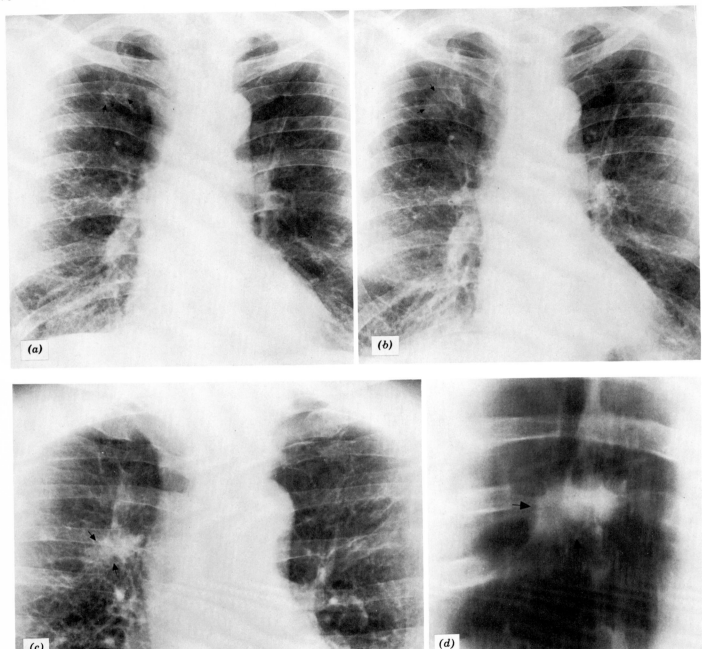

Fig. 3. Three-year observation of an upper lobe lesion. (a) This 64-year-old male physician had a long history of chronic obstructive lung disease and was known to have had a right upper lobe "density" for 8 years (arrows, 1965). (b) Although it grew during this period of time (arrows, 1967), it was thought to be of an inflammatory nature and related to patient's known bronchiectasis. (c)

Apical lordotic films (arrows) and (d) laminography (arrows) showed a "shaggy" and poorly marginated lesion, but did not help in reaching a diagnosis. Bronchoscopy was negative. At autopsy, the lesion was found to be an adenocarcinoma of the lung with lymphagitic spread and metastases to the left lower lobe of the liver, and several vertebral bodies.

tory disease and that, more rarely, calcification may occur in a necrotic area of tumor. The presence of calcification therefore does not entirely rule out the possibility of carcinoma, but does make it unlikely. Solitary

densities in the lung that are ill-defined or "shaggy" are probably malignant.

2. Cavitation. It is not unusual for a bronchogenic carcinoma to cavitate. This occurs in from 2 to 10% of

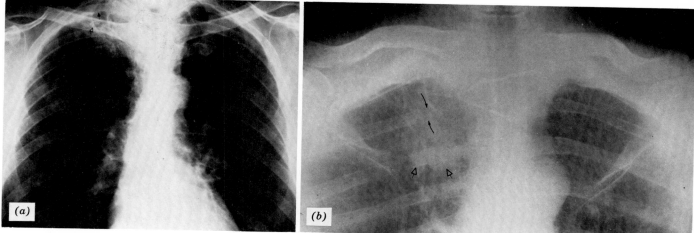

Fig. 4. Value of apical lordotic view. This 56-year-old man complained of pain in the right posterior and lateral upper chest over a period of 6 months. (a) His initial chest x-ray showed right apical pleural thickening (solid arrow), and an associated area of calcification (open arrow). Partly because of this calcification, the lesion was considered inflammatory, probably secondary to old tuberculosis. (b) Three months later, an apical lordotic film showed the mass character of this lesion (open arrows) with partial destruction of the posterior portion of the second right rib (slender arrows). This lesion between the open arrows is well visualized, and its poor margination is frequently seen in bronchogenic tumor. The presence of calcification, common in benign lesions, does not exclude the existence of a coincidental tumor or tumor with calcification.

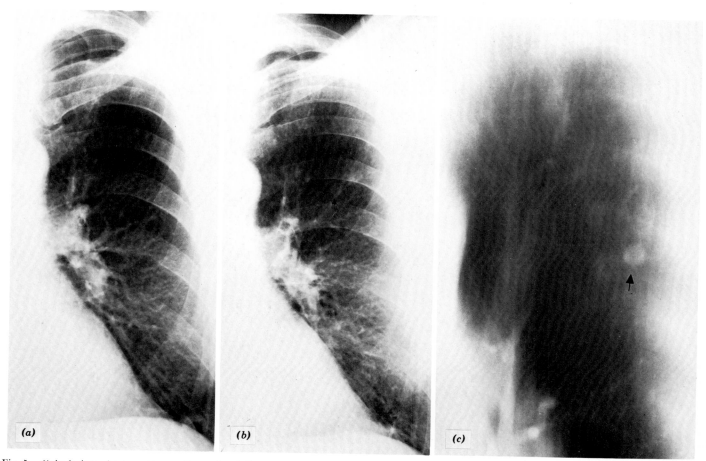

Fig. 5. Coin lesion—body section radiography. When a small lesion is found on x-ray, a review of previous films of the same patient may reveal that the lesion existed unrecognized at an earlier stage, or may give no hint of such a lesion. (a) Film made in September, 1967 during admission for benign prostatic hypertrophy. Even in retrospect, no lung lesion is appreciated. (b) 13 months later in a well-defined, uncalcified lesion, approximately 7 mm in diameter was seen in the left upper lobe (arrow). (c) Laminography shows the lesion to better advantage (arrow). At surgery, this was a poorly differentiated carcinoma.

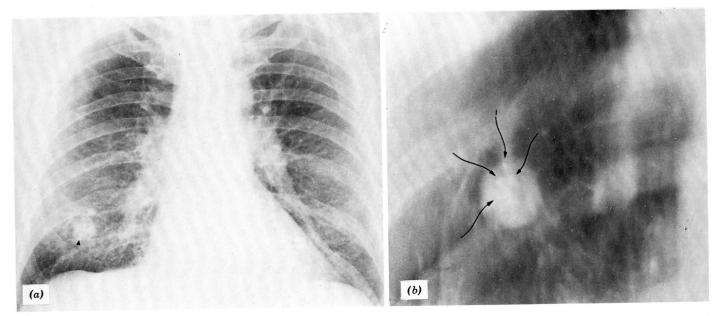

Fig. 6. Calcified Coin Lesion—tomography. Body section radiography demonstrates calcium in lung nodules. (a) This 66-year-old man was asymptomatic, but a 15 mm nodule was present in his right lower lobe (arrow). (b) Laminography shows multiple flecks of calcium (arrows) within this nodule. This lesion was observed over a period of several years and did not change in size or appearance. It is felt to represent a benign granuloma.

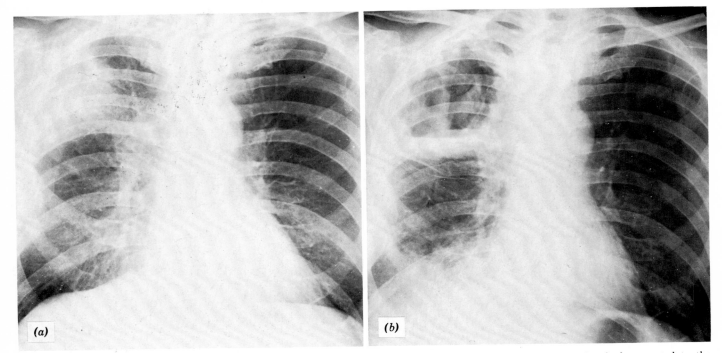

Fig. 7. Cavitation. This 60-year-old man was admitted 5 months before these films were made with an episode of pleuritic pain in the right chest that increased in severity until a right upper lobe was shown. (b) Two months later the lesion had excavated to the extent seen here. Rapid cavitation is not unusual in bronchogenic carcinoma, and is most commonly seen in epidermoid carcinoma.

cases, most frequently in the upper lobes and with epidermoid carcinomas.[14] This excavation can occur with surprising rapidity (Fig. 7). Although tomography is not usually required for the diagnosis of the presence of a cavity, it can demonstrate the character of a cavity clearly and, based upon the nodularity or smoothness of the cavity wall and upon wall thickness, a judgment as to the benign or malignant nature of the lesion can be made. The inner borders of malignant cavities are often quite irregular with fingerlike projections extending into them from the periphery (Fig. 8), whereas benign cavitations tend to be smooth-walled.

3. Bronchial stenosis. Particularly centrally located bronchial lesions may be clearly defined with laminography, and amputation or stenosis of a bronchus may be visualized (Fig. 9).

4. Mediastinal masses. On standard roentgenograms, mediastinal masses due to bronchogenic carcinoma frequently blend imperceptibly with adjacent normal struc-

tures, and may mimic mediastinal masses types of lesions (Figs. 1,2). With lamino normal can often be differentiated from the

5. Apical lesions. The pulmonary apex is always at least partially obscured by the ribs and the clavicle. Often it is also frequently the site of old fibrotic lesions, the result of chronic inflammation. Tomography is useful in helping to differentiate tumor from fibrosis (Figs. 3,10).

6. Extent of tumor. It is often possible, with the use of tomography, to demonstrate that a lesion discovered on plain film involves contiguous structures. Such a demonstration may obviate the need for a more involved investigation (Fig. 11).

Alveolar cell carcinoma. Alveolar cell carcinoma (Figs. 12,13) deserves special mention. It originates in bronchiolar epithelium, probably as a single primary focus, although it is often radiographically visualized as a multi-

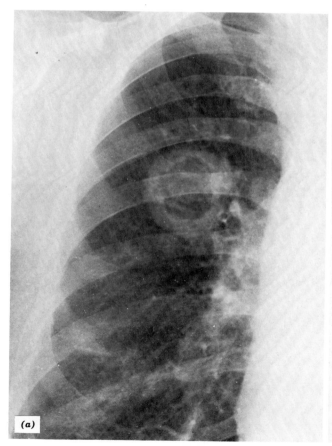

(a)

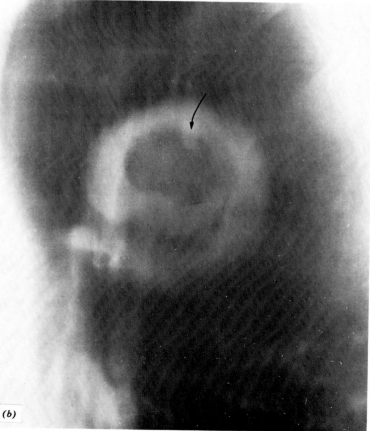

(b)

Fig. 8. Excavating lesion. On x-ray an excavating lesion may be benign or malignant. (*a*) The thick-walled lesion seen here can be better evaluated on a laminographic section. (*b*) The irregular wall of this lesion with areas of intraluminal projection (arrow) suggests malignancy. This was demonstrated surgically to be an epidermoid carcinoma.

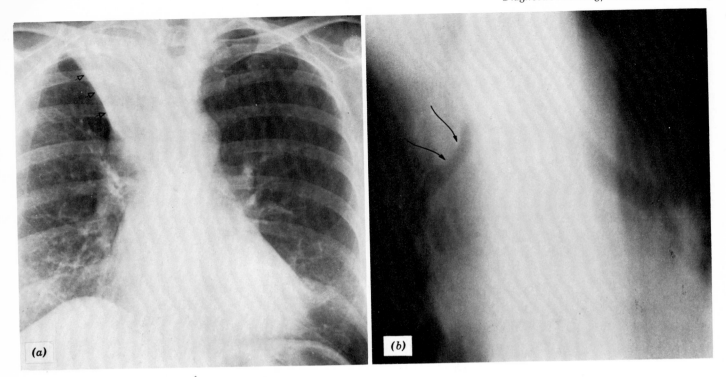

Fig. 9. Tomography with endobronchial lesion: atelectasis. This 47-year-old woman noted pain and fullness in her right upper chest for a period of several months. She had smoked 2 packs of cigarettes a day for over 20 years. (a) A posteroanterior film of the chest shows total collapse of the right upper lobe (arrows). (b) A tomographic section demonstrates total occlusion of the right upper lobe bronchus and involvement with narrowing of the bronchus intermedius (arrows).

centric lesion. On serial roentgenograms, some of the diffuse bilateral lesions have been shown to have begun as localized nodules.[20] The lesions are usually well circumscribed and peripheral, and classifications of nodular, infiltrative, and segmental forms have been described. The lymph nodes are usually involved late. Although single lesions as large as 10 cm in diameter have been described, the lesions may be radiographically invisible when symptoms start.[17] These may enlarge and spread locally or generally. Cavitation and collapse are rare.

Scar carcinoma. There appears to be a positive correlation between the presence of tuberculosis and bronchogenic carcinoma. This may be related to the occasional carcinoma that arises in an area of scarring and which appears to be unrelated to bronchi. Presumably, it originated in epithelial metaplasia with ultimate carcinoma (Fig. 14).

An endobronchial tumor often makes its presence known not by virtue of its soft tissue density, but by its effect on local or distant structures. Stenosis of a bronchus may lead to accumulation of secretions in the segments normally drained by it with resultant pneumonia and/or abscess formation. Usually, the pneumonia so produced does not subside entirely with appropriate chemotherapeutic management. Such a nonresolving pneumonia should always be suspect for the presence of underlying tumor (Fig. 15).

In cases of complete bronchial obstruction (Figs. 9,16), atelectasis of the corresponding lung segment may give the first clue to the nature of the underlying problem. In a Mayo Clinic series[14] 16.7% of patients with squamous cell carcinoma showed atelectasis as the only roentgenographic sign. Atelectasis was present in this series in 36.4% of squamous cell carcinomas.

Involvement of the phrenic nerve, usually by metastatic disease rather than by the primary tumor, will lead to paralysis of the corresponding diaphragm. This can sometimes be appreciated on a standard posteroanterior chest film as poor descent of the diaphragm on inspiration (to be differentiated from diaphragmatic elevation due to atelectasis [Fig. 17a]; fluoroscopy and cineradiography are helpful in differentiating a high but normally innervated diaphragm from a paralyzed one. Static films made on inspiration and expiration would also be useful in making this diagnosis.

The esophagus (Fig. 18a) is a valuable indicator of mass lesions in the mediastinum. Thus it is often useful

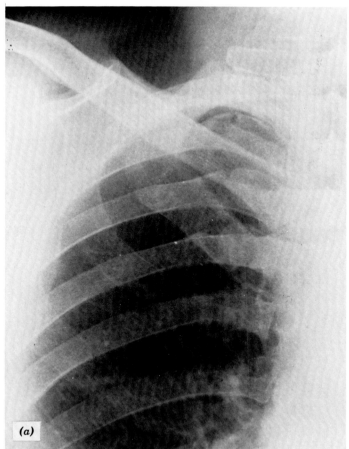

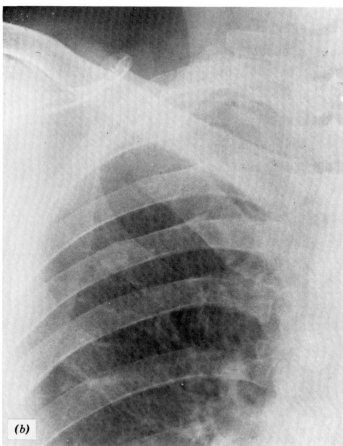

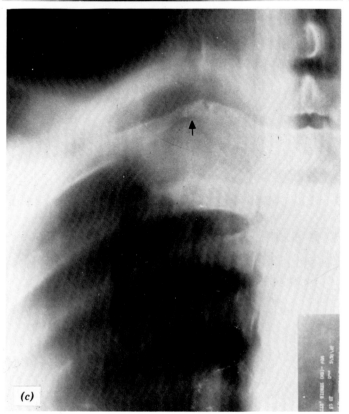

Fig. 10. Superior sulcus tumor: tomography. Apical cancers are often difficult to differentiate from apical scarring resulting from old inflammatory disease. (*a*) This 49-year-old man was first seen in 1953 with pain in the neck and back, and a persistent cough associated with an upper respiratory tract infection. This film shows minimal scarring in the right upper lobe. (*b*) In 1966, the right upper lobe apical scarring was much more evident but still not ominous. (*c*) Body section radiography demonstrates the soft tissue apical mass more clearly and also shows partial destruction of the third rib posteriorly. Exploratory thoracotomy showed tumor involving the right superior pulmonary sulcus, invading the chest wall, the body of the third thoracic vertebra, and the third rib. Autopsy diagnosis was bronchioloalveolar carcinoma.

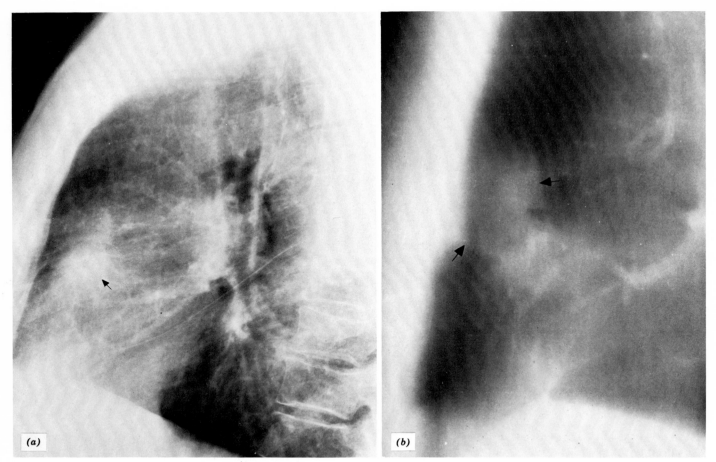

Fig. 11. Body section radiography. Body section x-rays often show densities that are obscure on standard films. (a) This 70-year-old man had epidermoid carcinoma of the right middle lobe bronchus. However the nature of the poorly defined density seen on the lateral film of the chest (arrow) was not well appreciated until body section radiographs were made. (b) These show the density to be a well-defined mass (arrows) contiguous with the anterior chest wall, and thought to be tumor extension through the anterior mediastinum involving the anterior chest wall. Autopsy confirmed the diagnosis.

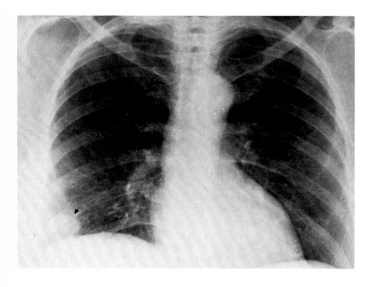

Fig. 12. Bronchioloalveolar carcinoma—single lesion. This 59-year-old woman has bronchioloalveolar carcinoma, represented by a single mass (arrow) on chest x-ray.

to opacify the esophagus with barium to evaluate the displacement or invasion of this structure. When invasion of the esophagus occurs, it may be impossible to differentiate a primary esophageal carcinoma from an invading bronchogenic carcinoma. The trachea may also be displaced by mediastinal mass (Fig. 18b), and this may be appreciated on the standard chest film as a dislocation of the tracheal air shadow.

When a pulmonary lesion is visualized, it is valuable to compare the current examination with whatever previous films are available (Figs. 5,19). A coin lesion that has been present for many years and has not changed in size can be ignored with relative safety. If there has been enlargement, however, more intensive diagnostic efforts are warranted.

BRONCHOGRAPHY (Fig. 17)

Although opacification of the bronchial tree appears to be an ideal method for localization and characterization

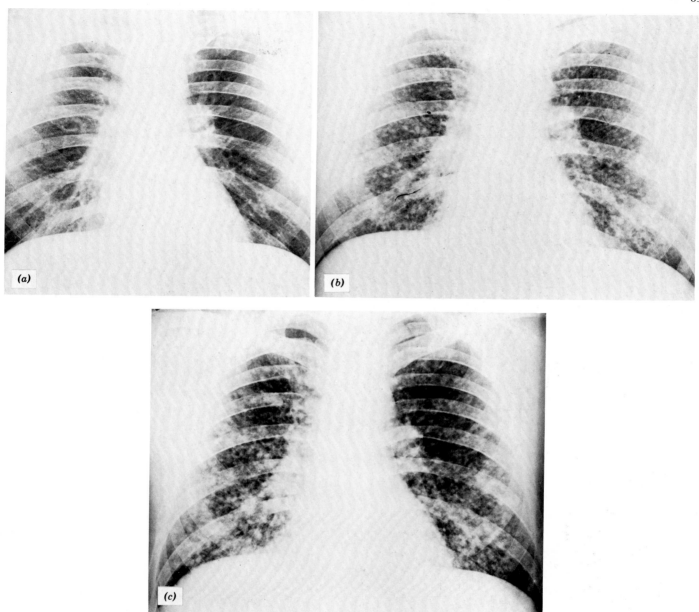

Fig. 13. Bronchioloalveolar carcinoma—multiple lesions. Three chest films made in March, October, and December of the same year show the rapid progression of these myriad small, ill-defined bilateral densities in a 29-year-old man with progressive dyspnea and productive cough. At autopsy, diffuse bronchioloalveolar carcinoma was found.

of tumors of the bronchus, there has been less and less enthusiasm for this technique in recent years, partly because of the advent of rapid and safe mediastinoscopy. Nevertheless, Nelson and Christoforidis[24] in 1973 were able to list seven indications for the performance of bronchography: hemoptysis, cough, repeated pneumonias, localized emphysema, unilateral hilar adenopathy, persistent unilateral infiltrates, and the differential diagnosis of persistent cavities or cysts. They consider the signs of tumor to be obstruction, indentation and displacement of bronchi, localized narrowing, cavitation, and bronchial relocation. Rinker et al.[27] claimed an accuracy in diagnosing carcinoma with bronchography ranging from 94.2% to 97.3%. Charpin et al.[5] performed bronchography with cineradiography and attached great significance to the sign of bronchial rigidity on cine films as an indication of tumor. Bronchography probably retains its greatest application in segmental and

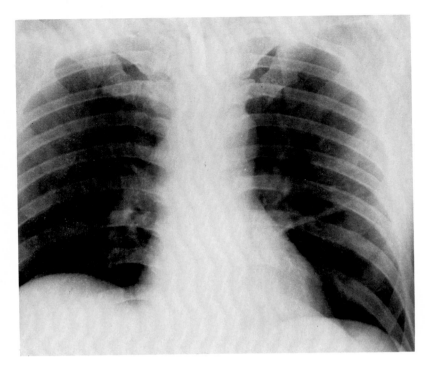

Fig. 14. Scar carcinoma. This 41-year-old man died with a peripheral mucin-producing, poorly differentiated carcinoma with intrapulmonary metastases as well as metastases to bone and the central nervous system. The arrow indicates the pulmonary scar in which a focus of carcinoma was found at autopsy.

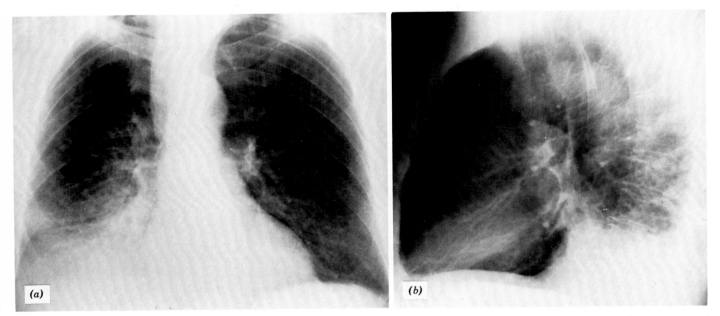

(a)

(b)

Fig. 15. Drowned lung. Often the only roentgenographic sign of endobronchial tumor may be pneumonia and abscess behind it, caused by poor drainage. This 59-year-old man was treated for pneumonia for 4 months before these films were made, but clearing was never radiographically complete despite several courses of antibiotics. The patient was asymptomatic except for a low grade fever. This right lower lobe pneumonia was caused by a partially occluding, lower lobe bronchogenic carcinoma.

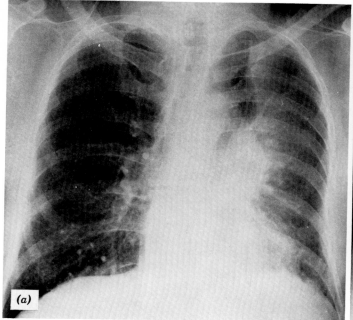 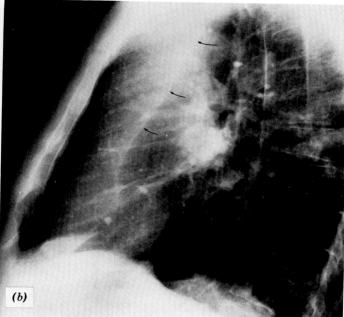

Fig. 16. Atelectasis. Bronchogenic carcinoma frequently presents as collapse of an obstructed segment without the obstructing mass itself being visualized. This patient had epidermoid carcinoma of the left upper lobe bronchus with resultant atelectasis. (a) The atelectasis is seen as a diffuse haziness on the posteroanterior film, and as an anteriorly collapsing density on the lateral view (b, arrows). The lesion itself is not visualized as is often the case.

subsegmental lesions that are difficult or impossible to reach with a bronchoscope, and in patients in whom a cytologic examination has been positive for tumor but in whom no lesion has otherwise been detectable.

BRONCHIAL ARTERIOGRAPHY

Since pulmonary neoplasms obtain their blood supply from bronchial arteries, there was, in the early 1960s, some enthusiasm for using bronchial arteriograms in the diagnosis of bronchogenic carcinoma, particularly in the differentiation of tumor from inflammatory lesions.[36] Unfortunately, bronchial arteriography has not been particularly helpful in making this differentiation, since there is a paucity of bronchial arteries supplying bronchogenic cancer, and tumor blush is infrequent. Even when abnormal vasculature is seen in the suspected mass, it is difficult to differentiate benign from malignant tumors.[22] Furthermore, inflammatory lesions often demonstrate increased or abnormal vascularity. Thus because of its failure to produce results, this procedure has been largely abandoned. There is also some hazard in performing bronchial arteriography, and transverse myelitis has been reported as a complication of the study.[11]

HYPERTROPHIC PULMONARY OSTEOARTHROPATHY (Figs. 20,21)[15,16]

Despite the fact that hypertrophic pulmonary osteoarthropathy was known in Hippocrates' day, the mechanism by which it is produced remains as much a mystery today as it was then. It occurs in a variety of chronic pulmonary diseases including bronchogenic carcinoma. The full-blown picture consists of periostitis of tubular bones, arthralgia, and clubbing of the digits. These findings may occur independently of one another. The periostitis is most marked at the diaphyses. The synovia may be inflamed, and there is sometimes joint effusion. The extremity is painful, there may be nonpitting edema of tissues over the ends of the long bones, and these are usually warm and tender. The primary change seems to be an overgrowth of vascular connective tissue and increased blood flow to the involved part.

There have been two theories about the nature of this entity, one humoral and the other neurogenic. There is good experimental evidence based on cross-circulation models that tends to rule out a humorally mediated cause. The fact that vagotomy may lead to prompt regression of swelling and pain supports the neurogenic theory. Following resection of the primary pulmonary

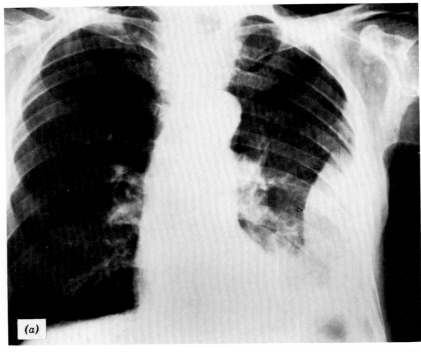

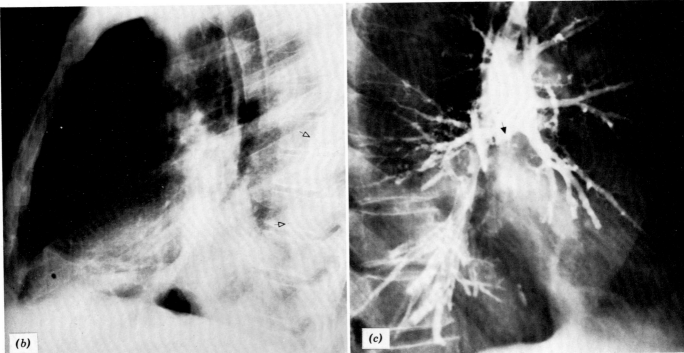

Fig. 17. Bronchogram. This 70-year-old man presented with a history of hoarseness and cough. (a) His posteroanterior and (b) lateral chest films show left lower lobe collapse with resultant elevation of the left dome of the diaphragm. A posteriorly loculated pleural effusion is also present (open arrows a and b). (c) A lateral bronchogram shows complete occlusion of the left lower lobe bronchus (closed arrow). Note the abrupt and ragged termination of this bronchus, typical of a malignant lesion.

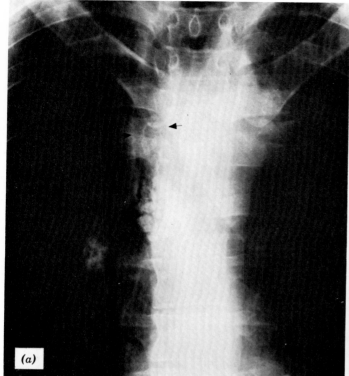

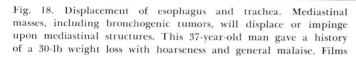

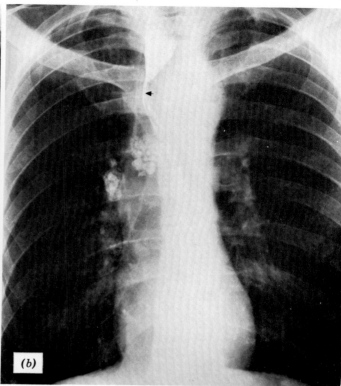

Fig. 18. Displacement of esophagus and trachea. Mediastinal masses, including bronchogenic tumors, will displace or impinge upon mediastinal structures. This 37-year-old man gave a history of a 30-lb weight loss with hoarseness and general malaise. Films of the chest show displacement of the barium-filled esophagus (b) and of the trachea (a, arrows) to the right. There was no evidence of invasion of either structure, although invasion of the esophagus is not unusual in patients with bronchogenic carcinoma.

tumor, the changes of hypertrophic pulmonary osteo-arthropathy may disappear.

Much of the emphasis in radiologic examination of patients with bronchogenic carcinoma has been on the determination of spread of disease and operability. The plain film of the chest is often sufficient to establish, or at least strongly suggest that the disease may be inoperable. The presence of a pleural effusion (Fig. 17), while not conclusive evidence of inoperability, does suggest this to be the case. Pericardial effusion (Fig. 22) is more convincing evidence of metastatic spread. It is sometimes possible, on the basis of the plain film of the chest, to suggest that there has been lymphagitic spread of tumor through the same lung (Fig. 23) or to the contralateral lung. This also suggests inoperability.

SUPERIOR VENACAVOGRAPHY (Fig. 24)

Involvement of the superior vena cava is usually readily manifest clinically as superior vena cava syndrome, but may be demonstrated angiographically by the simple technique of transvenous injection of contrast ma-terial. Although the superior vena cava may be completely occluded in patients with superior vena cava syndrome, this occlusion is generally due to extrinsic compression rather than direct tumor invasion of the vena cava which is rare. This occlusion does, however, indicate inoperability.[1]

AZYGOGRAPHY (Figs. 25,26)

The posterior mediastinum is one of the most difficult areas to approach radiographically, but it must often be evaluated in determining the operability or non-operability of bronchial cancer. One-third of explored tumors turn out to be unresectable.[19] Thus preoperative determination of this unresectability would obviate much unnecessary surgery. Although standard lymph-angiography performed from the feet is a convenient method of visualizing retroperitoneal lymph nodes, the mediastinal and hilar nodes do not regularly opacify with this technique. The azygous vein, in the posterior mediastinum, can be visualized radiographically and has been used as an indicator of mass lesions in this location. It may be opacified directly via a catheter passed through

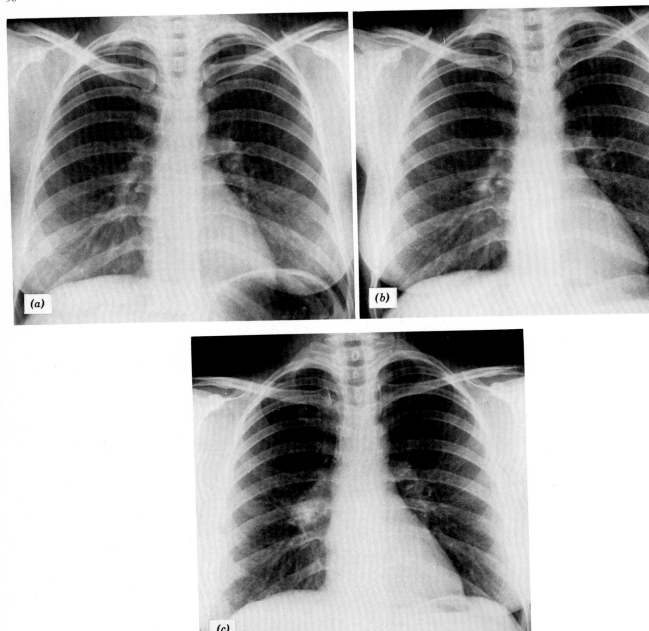

Fig. 19. Value of old films. The availability of previous films is important in the evaluation of minor changes. (*a*) This patient was 27 years old when this film was made in 1954. Even in retrospect, no abnormalities are seen. (*b*) In 1963, this film was interpreted as normal, and without the previous film for comparison it does appear unremarkable. However, when the right hilum in the second film is compared with that in the first, considerable enlargement is seen. (*c*) By 1965, the right hilar mass is obvious. A thoracotomy was performed revealing adenocarcinoma, and the patient died about 1 year later with widespread metastases.

the superior vena cava and then, selectively, into the azygous vein. This approach has been used with some success particularly in the study of lymphomas.[26] A more physiologic look at the azygous vein is obtained via the intraosseous route. Injection of contrast material into the medulla of the posterior portion of a rib will result in drainage through a subcostal vein into the azygous vein on the right or the hemiazygous vein on the left. Theoretically, an obstructed, displaced, or indented azygous vein indicates a posterior mediastinal mass and makes operability unlikely. Wolfel et al.[40] performed azyography on 35 patients with histologically proven

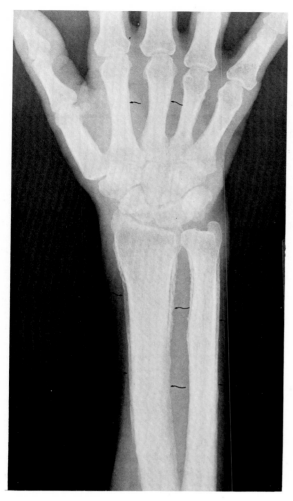

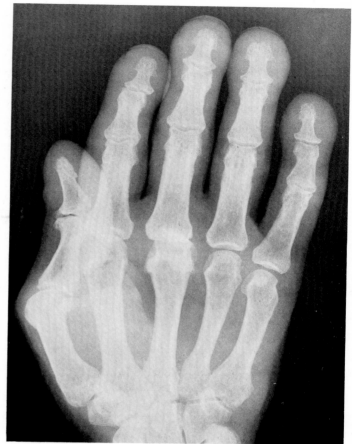

Fig. 20. Hypertrophic pulmonary osteoarthropathy. The long bones of this 40-year-old man show the marked periosteal new bone found in hypertrophic pulmonary osteoarthropathy. Here it is shown in the radius, ulna, and metacarpal bones, but also involves virtually all the other long bones. Note the irregularity of this periosteal new bone and its predilection for the diaphyses with relative sparing of the metaphyses. It may regress following lung surgery.

Fig. 21. Clubbing of the fingers. This 61-year-old man with epidermoid carcinoma of the lung had prominent soft tissue on the terminal digits of his hands. These spoon-shaped clubbing deformities are associated with bronchogenic carcinoma, or sometimes with the periosteal new bone growth of hypertrophic pulmonary osteoarthropathy. This patient did not show periosteal changes.

carcinoma of the lung, all of whom subsequently underwent thoracotomy. There were 4 false-negatives of the 25 azygograms read as normal, and 1 false-positive in the group of 10 read as positive. They conclude that azygography adds little to what is known by other means, but that an abnormal azygogram indicates inoperability. They also feel that a normal azygogram is of no value in predicting resectability. Rinker et al.[28] tend to confirm this evaluation of azygography. They had 1 false positive azygogram in 63 patients, and this error was due to postoperative fibrosis. They also suggest that the reopening of a previously blocked azygous vein following radiation therapy indicates that an unresectable lesion may have been converted into a resectable one.

Janower et al.[19] found that 20 of 65 patients thought operable on the basis of other criteria were in fact inoperable, and 50% of these had positive azygograms.

Possibly because of the large number of false-negative studies but probably due to the painful nature of the procedure, azygography has never found great favor as a routine part of the workup of bronchogenic cancer. Janower and co-workers[19] indicate that their patients suffered only slight discomfort during the study; our own patients have reported considerably more pain. The sporadic appearance of reports of good correlation of azygography with surgical findings, however, suggests that this procedure warrants a closer look.

PULMONARY ARTERIOGRAPHY AND LUNG SCANNING
(Figs. 27,28,29)

It is sometimes helpful to perform pulmonary arteriography in the evaluation of patients with bronchogenic

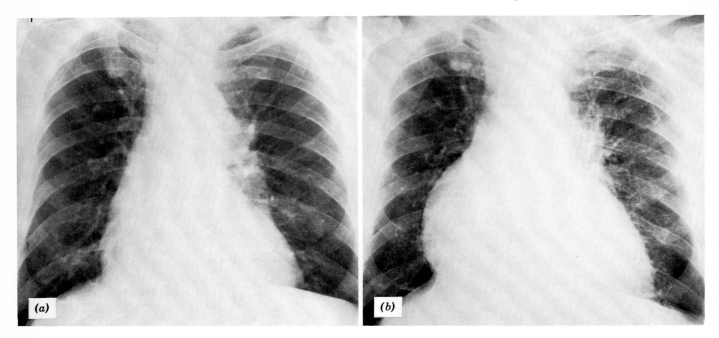

Fig. 22. Pericardial effusion. Pericardial effusion due to pericardial metastases can occur very rapidly, as is shown on the x-rays of this 61-year-old man who died of bronchogenic carcinoma of the left main stem bronchus with metastases to pleura, pericardium, heart, aorta, liver, regional lymph nodes, and diaphragm. (a) At the time of this film, the cardiac silhouette was only slightly enlarged. (b) A film made 19 days later shows a massive pericardial effusion. The immediate cause of death was cardiac tamponade.

cancer. Although actual invasion of the pulmonary arteries by mediastinal tumor is rare, it does occur. What happens more frequently, however, is a decrease in flow to the involved lung either because of extrinsic compression of a pulmonary artery branch, pulmonary venous compromise, or diminished perfusion of a large volume of lung for reasons that are still poorly understood. In some cases, hyperinflation of tumor-containing lung may be due to a check-valve mechanism caused by endobronchial cancer (Fig. 27). Whatever the cause, angiographic observation of diminished perfusion is frequently made in the presence of intact pulmonary arteries, and the area of underperfused lung is often much greater than would be thought probable on the basis of size or location of the tumor present (Fig. 28). It should be emphasized, however, that there is no specific arteriographic sign of bronchial cancer.[35] The phenomenon of air-trapping in these cases can often be better appreciated on films made on deep expiration. Sanders et al.[30] found that pulmonary angiography correctly predicted resectability in 81% of their patients. Combining angiography with mediastinoscopy raised their accuracy to 97%. Angiography is less sensitive to anterior mediastinal nodes than is mediastinoscopy.

Perfusion scanning of the lung with Tc 99m-labeled albumin microspheres, for example, is a noninvasive alternative to pulmonary arteriography. Secker-Walker et al. emphasize that the scanning defect (as the angiographic defect) due to bronchogenic cancer is often larger than the size of the tumor seen on x-ray and may involve the entire lung. Absence of perfusion is said to be more common in hilar and inoperable carcinomas, and the magnitude of the perfusion abnormality correlates well with resectability.[37] When the relative perfusion of the affected lung is less than one-third of the total, the tumor is probably inoperable.[32] Preoperative lung scanning is also used in the evaluation of the contralateral (normal) lung.

[67]Ga has been used as a tumor-seeking radiopharmaceutical (Fig. 29). When administered intravenously, it localizes in a variety of malignant tumors. Ito et al.[18] studied 21 patients with lung cancer with this material. They found the Ga scans were positive in 11 cases, and in 2 of these the scan became negative after radiation therapy. This suggests that Ga scanning may be useful in assessing the results of therapy. They also claim a great advantage for Ga scanning over routine radiography because the former clearly shows infraclavicular nodes and hilar and mediastinal lesions that may not be visible on x-ray. Edwards and Hayes[9] claim the greatest localization of ^{67}Ga in viable tumor, less in fibrotic or necrotic tumor, and diminished following radiation

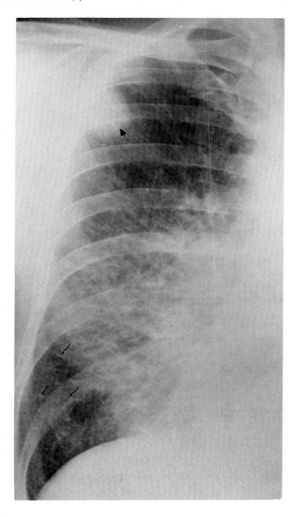

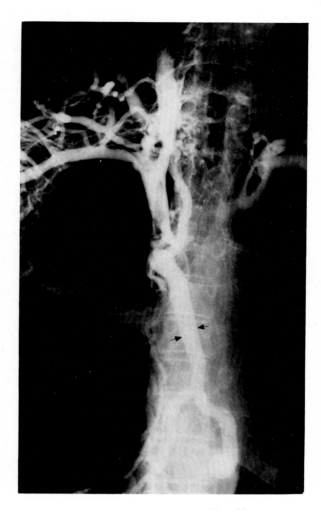

Fig. 23. Lymphangitic spread. This 44-year-old man presented with severe dyspnea of 2 to 3 months' duration. At autopsy, the large mass in the right upper lobe (solid arrow) was an adenocarcinoma. Extensive lymphangitic spread of tumor was found throughout both lungs. Although the fine linear streaks in the patient's right lung base (slender arrows) and elsewhere cannot be distinguished radiographically from the lines of Kerley seen in congestive failure and may be confused with pulmonary fibrosis, they are consistent with x-ray findings of lymphangitic spread of tumor. The patient was not in congestive failure at the time this film was made.

Fig. 24. Superior vena cava syndrome. This 57-year-old woman with lung cancer presented with swelling of the upper extremities and neck. A superior vena cavogram performed by injection of a right antecubital vein shows total occlusion of the superior vena cava below the entrance of the azygous vein. There is extensive retrograde filling of the neck and thoracic veins. The drainage of the upper extremities and head is mainly through the azygous (arrows) and lumbar venous system into the inferior vena cava.

and chemotherapy. They found tumor localization of Ga in 75% of patients with bronchogenic carcinoma. This localization appears to be best in epidermoid carcinoma. They claim two levels of potential application in clinical tumor scanning: the search for metastases in patients with known primary tumors, and the search for primary neoplasm in patients suspected of having cancer. Unfortunately, Ga localization is by no means specific for tumor, and this agent tends to localize well in areas

of inflammation. For this reason, it seems to be useful in outlining the walls of abscess cavities.

GAS MEDIASTINOSCOPY

Gas has been used as a contrast agent in outlining mediastinal structures. Either carbon dioxide or oxygen or a combination of the two is used to dissect the subfascial planes of the mediastinum. When this technique is combined with tomography, the mediastinal structures can often be seen with great clarity. Berne et al.[3] report no morbidity or mortality in 64 patients with 87.5%

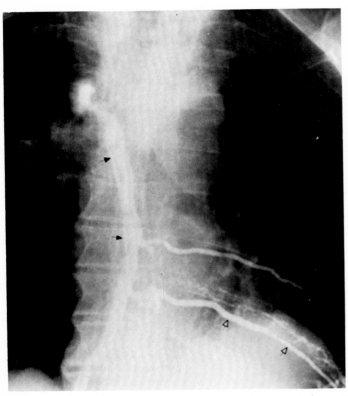

Fig. 25. Azygography—normal. This 66-year-old man presented with a superior mediastinal mass. Azygography was performed by injection into the left tenth rib and contrast is seen draining through the tenth subcostal vein (open arrows). Flow is predominately into the azygous vein (solid arrows) in a forward direction into the superior vena cava. By this criterion the lesion is operable. (Photograph courtesy Dr. Renate Soulen, Temple University Hospital, Philadelphia, Pa.)

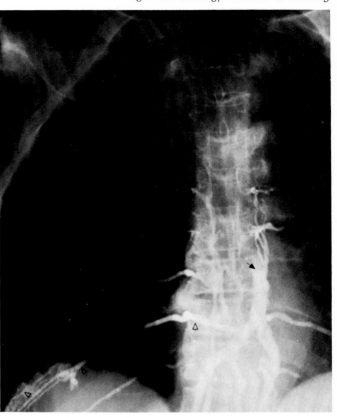

Fig. 26. Azygography—abnormal. Injection of contrast material has been made into the medullary space of the right ninth rib posteriorly, and the draining subcostal vein (open arrows) is opacified. Flow is into the azygous vein which occludes abruptly at the level of the eighth thoracic vertebral body (solid arrow). The bulk of the flow is in a retrograde direction into the ascending lumbar veins. This is a reliable sign of mediastinal mass, probably inoperable. (Photograph courtesy Dr. Renate Soulen, Temple University Hospital, Philadelphia, Pa.)

technically successful studies. They claim that the technique defines the extent of disease and helps in planning radiation therapy; that with this technique the diagnosis of occult lymph node disease is improved and subcarinal and paratracheal lymph nodes are well displayed. The azygous nodes are not well seen. Bariety et al.[2] found a 6.4% incidence of temporary clinical "incidents." They emphasize that with this technique, the exact nature of the mediastinal tumor cannot be determined, but when combined with tomography the diagnosis was facilitated in 250 cases of primary bronchogenic carcinoma. Easy dissection of the gas correlates with probable operability, whereas mediastinal impermeability to gas indicates probable inoperability. In 61 of their cases, surgery was contraindicated on the basis of gas mediastinoscopy alone. Nevertheless, 9 of these patients had surgery, and excision was possible in only 1.

METASTASES TO BONE (Figs. 30,31)

Metastases to bone from bronchogenic carcinoma are almost always lytic in nature, and may occur in any bone. Charkes and Sklaroff[4] claim that up to 85% of terminal patients with cancer of the breast, prostate, and lung have metastases at the time of death. Conventional roentgenograms fail to visualize 50% of bone lesions and, possibly, show none smaller than 1 to 1½ cm in diameter. One-half of the density of a vertebra must be lost before this change can be seen as an osteolytic lesion. Roentgen bone surveys made to detect occult metastases in evaluating the spread of cancer are expensive, time-consuming and, if the figures mentioned are to be believed, often unproductive. Even when the patient localizes bone pain to a specific area, the bone roentgenograms may not show the lesion, therefore bone scans seem to be a more sensitive alternative. Radio-strontium is deposited in growing

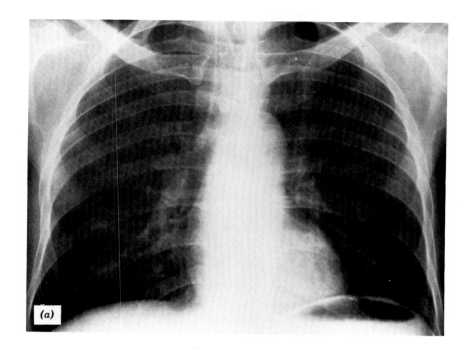

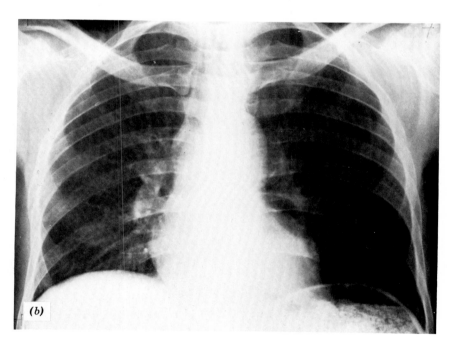

Fig. 27.   Hyperlucent lung with air-trapping. This 46-year-old man had a normal chest film in 1967. (a) In 1971, on inspiration, his chest film still appears normal. (b) On expiration, however, the mediastinum shifts to the right (the normal side), and the left lung appears hyperlucent. (c) A perfusion scan shows total lack of perfusion of the left lung. Courtesy of Dr. Abass Alavi, Hospital of the University of Pennsylvania. (d) On pulmonary arteriography, arterial flow to the left lung is greatly diminished, and (e) on the late phase of the arteriogram there is good demonstration of right-sided pulmonary veins (open arrows), but no sign of left-sided pulmonary veins. Even in this late venous phase the left pulmonary artery (solid arrows) has not yet emptied. There was no encroachment upon the main pulmonary artery angiographically, nor was there at autopsy. The pulmonary veins were also free of disease. An endobronchial carcinoma was found that was evidently responsible for the mediastinal shift on expiration as well as the hyperlucency seen in (b) and must have been responsible for the perfusion defect.

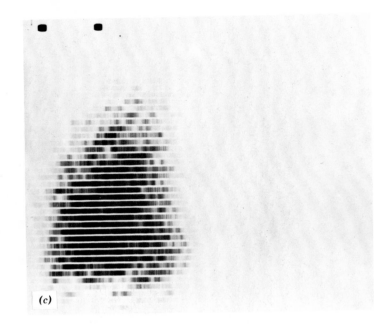

Fig. 27. (c)

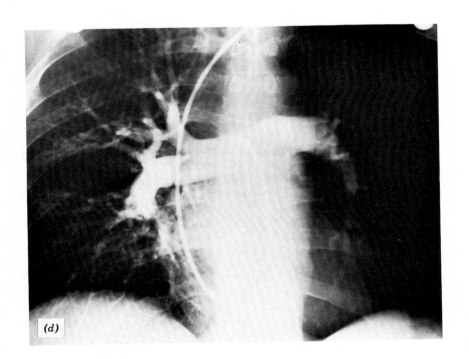

Fig. 27. (d)

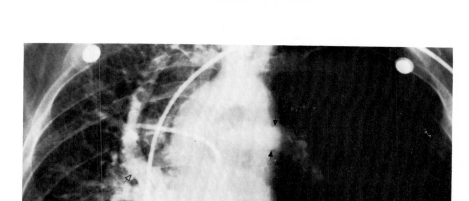

Fig. 27. (e)

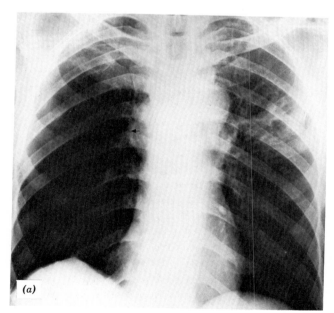

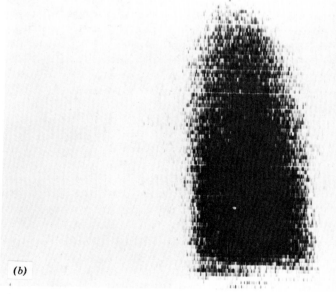

Fig. 28. Hyperlucent lung. (a) The right hilar mass (arrow) represents a bronchogenic tumor on this supine chest film. The right lung is hyperlucent and little of the vascular pattern can be discerned. (b) On a ^{99m}Tc albumin lung scan, the right lung appears entirely unperfused. The mechanism of this apparent nonperfusion is poorly understood, although in some cases it may be a check-valve mechanism (see Fig. 27), or arterial or venous occlusion by the primary tumor or by nodes. This phenomenon may also be seen in patients with bronchogenic carcinoma, with uninvolved major pulmonary vessels, and in whom there is no check-valve mechanism. Courtesy of Dr. Abass Alavi, Hospital of the University of Pennsylvania.

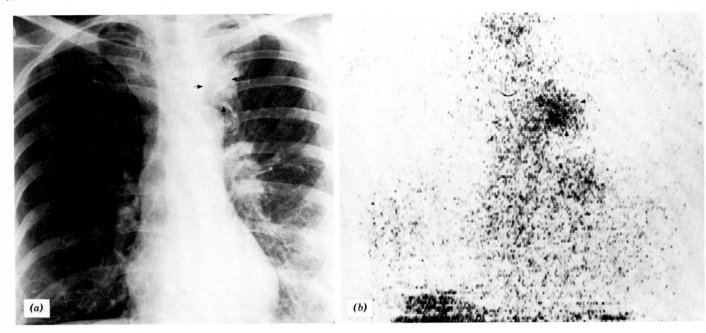

Fig. 29. ⁶⁷Gallium citrate scanning. (a) On the posteroanterior film of the chest, a superior mediastinal soft tissue density is apparent above the aortic knob (arrows). (b) ⁶⁷Ga citrate has localized in this area in what was eventually determined to be bronchial cancer (arrows). Of the bronchogenic carcinomas, epidermoid carcinoma appears to localize Ga best. Unfortunately, this localization is not specific for tumor and occurs in areas of inflammation and around abscess cavities. Courtesy of Dr. Abass Alavi, Hospital of the University of Pennsylvania.

bone as well as in new bone formed in reaction to the presence of tumor. Strontium is laid down in immature osteoid adjacent to invading malignant cells. Osteoid is not seen on standard radiography, but the deposited radio-strontium is detectable on scan. In 2% of cases, the scan will be negative despite the presence of lytic metastases. Bone biopsy in such cases shows no reactive bone, but simply destruction.

BRAIN SCANNING (Fig. 32)

Bronchogenic carcinoma frequently metastasizes to the brain. The brain scan represents an atraumatic, simple, and effective method of detecting these metastatic lesions and, when successful, obviates the necessity of performing the more expensive and uncomfortable carotid or vertebral arteriogram. The selective uptake of the isotope in the metastatic lesion depends upon local hypervascularity and increased vascular permeability of the lesion.[18]

In recent years, computer-assisted tomography of the brain has, to a great extent, displaced isotopic examination. The relative accuracy of these two techniques has yet to be established, but CAT scanning is totally noninvasive and has proven a most impressive tool.

VISCERAL ANGIOGRAPHY

Although angiography is an extremely sensitive tool in demonstrating metastatic disease from such vascular primary lesions as hypernephroma or leiomyosarcoma, it is less useful in the diagnosis of metastatic tumor secondary to bronchogenic carcinoma, an essentially avascular lesion seen angiographically. However, displacement and deformity of intrahepatic arteries can be seen when the defects are large enough[10] and Nebesar et al.[23] claim 86% accuracy in diagnosing liver metastases, stating that a lesion as small as 1 cm in diameter can be seen. Unfortunately, it has been the general experience that the liver may be diffusely infiltrated by metastases without these being evident angiographically. Confusion with the changes of cirrhosis or fatty liver is also possible. Although metastases to the kidney and pancreas have also been detected angiographically, this diagnosis is difficult and the procedure is unwarranted for this purpose because of its limited contribution to management.

LIVER SCANNING

Scanning of the liver after injection of radionuclides is of value in detecting metastases, although those smaller than 2 cm in diameter may not be visualized. Confusion

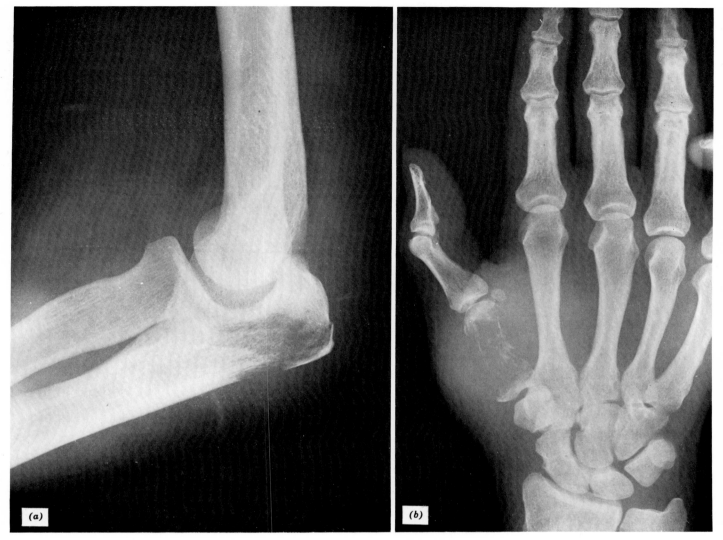

Fig. 30. Bone metastases. (a) Lesions in the long bones of the extremities are common. (b) Lesions in the digits are unusual but are of the same lytic nature as those found elsewhere.

with cirrhotic livers is possible since cirrhosis may also appear as filling defects. However, multiple filling defects without increased extrahepatic uptake are seen most frequently in tumor. Because of its noninvasive nature, this procedure is advisable where angiography may not be. Wilson et al.[39] found the scan to be 78% accurate in their 69 patients. The accuracy of liver function tests in predicting metastases was similar, but when the serum alkaline phosphatase determination was combined with radionuclide scanning, accuracy rose to 93%. In this same study, when both the scan and the serum alkaline phosphatase were normal, cancer was present in the liver in only 1 of 23 cases.

AORTOGRAPHY AND VENOGRAPHY (Figs. 33,34,35)

Variations in configuration of the mediastinal silhouette sometimes make it impossible to determine, with a plain roentgenogram whether a mediastinal prominence represents abnormal mass or a normal but atypical mediastinal structure. In Figure 33, an apparent mediastinal widening is seen on the right. Angiography showed that this widening was a prominent but otherwise unremarkable superior vena cava, and unnecessary thoracotomy was avoided. In Figure 34, a left-sided superior mediastinal mass was shown on aortography to represent a tortuous but otherwise unremarkable left subclavian artery

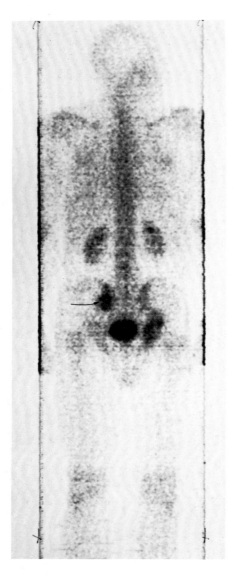

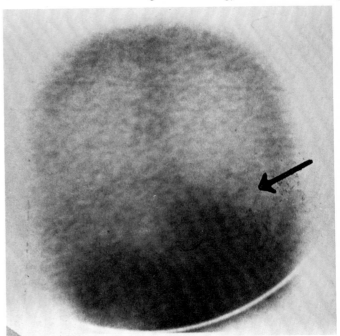

Fig. 32. Brain scan. This gamma camera scan with ^{99m}Tc pertechnetate demonstrates a posterior fossa lesion on the left. Courtesy of Dr. Abass Alavi, Hospital of the University of Pennsylvania.

Fig. 31. Bone scan (radiostrontium). This bone scan shows a "hot" area (arrow) in the right iliosacral region that represents a metastatic deposit from bronchogenic carcinoma. This painful lesion was undetectable by standard x-ray methods. Courtesy of Dr. Abass Alavi, Hospital of the University of Pennsylvania.

of no clinical significance. On the other hand, mediastinal tumors may masquerade as abnormal vascular masses. The appearance of the left-sided mass in Figure 35 is compatible with a thoracic aortic aneurysm. Aortography, however, showed that this lesion was extraaortic, and eventual thoracotomy proved that it was a solid tumor (neurolemmoma).

Although they are not strictly radiologic procedures, many of the newer methods of obtaining cytologic specimens from lung tumors require image-intensified fluoro-

scopy for their performance. Although the required skills for carrying out these procedures can be readily acquired by any interested physician, it seems appropriate that they remain the province of the radiologist:

PERCUTANEOUS TRANSTHORACIC BIOPSY

It is feasible for material from peripheral lung tumors to be aspirated through a needle passed percutaneously through the thorax. Although there is some morbidity associated with this technique in the nature of pneumothorax (35% in a series reported by Rabinov *et al.*[25]) as well as the potential for tumor transplantation,[41] it does provide an alternative to thoracotomy and has been reported to yield a correct diagnosis in 90% of patients with proved malignant lung lesions.

BRONCHIAL BRUSH BIOPSY (Fig. 36)

The technique of passing a "brush" into the bronchus under study and obtaining cells for microscopic examination is effective and safe. Fennessy[12] reported no significant complications in 100 patients and established a diagnosis in 62% of these. The accuracy of the technique is increased by preceding it with bronchography. The brush may be passed in conjunction with a fiberscope (as illustrated) or, as an alternative, through a transnasally

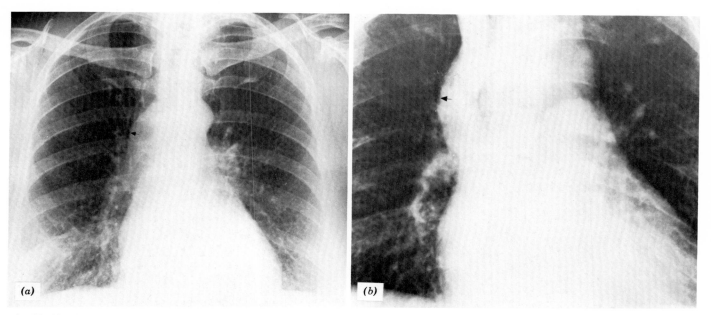

Fig. 33. Simulated mass. (a) It is sometimes difficult to determine whether a prominence on a chest x-ray represents an abnormal mass or normal structure (arrow). Angiography may be useful to outline the normal vasculature. (b) In this 56-year-old asymptomatic woman, the prominence seen on the chest x-ray was a tortuous superior vena cava (arrow). Thoracotomy was unnecessary.

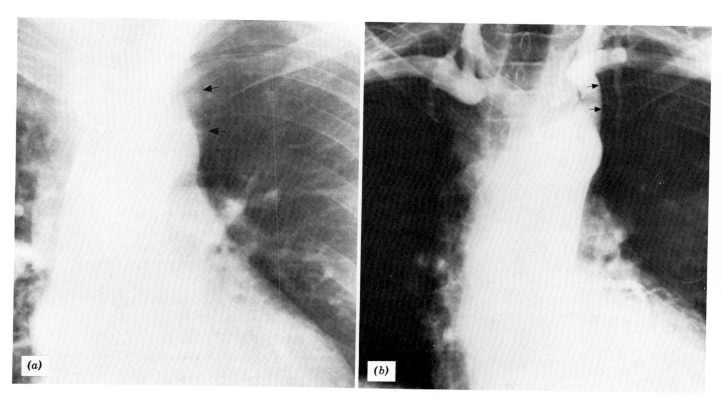

Fig. 34. Simulated mass (a) This 44-year-old man had a left superior mediastinal mass just above the aortic knob (arrows) on routine chest x-ray. (b) On aortography, this mass was shown to be a tortuous left subclavian artery (arrows).

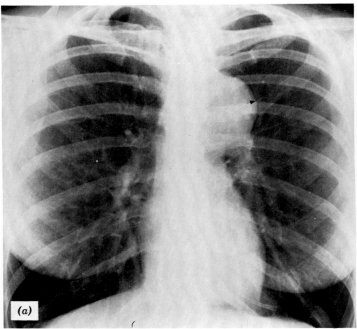

(a)

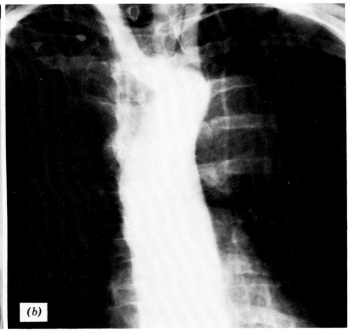

(b)

Fig. 35. Aortography. It is sometimes important to determine whether a mass adjacent to and silhouetting the mediastinum is vascular. (a) This 36-year-old woman was asymptomatic, having been admitted for a tubal ligation. She was found to have a mediastinal mass on routine chest x-ray (arrow). The appearance of this lesion on the posteroanterior film suggested aortic aneurysm. (b) However, on aortography the mass was shown to be extraaortic, and was eventually diagnosed as a mediastinal neurolemmoma.

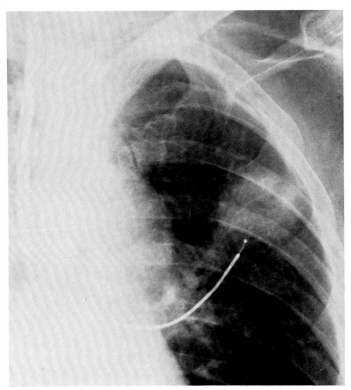

Fig. 36. Bronchial brush biopsy. The bronchial brush (arrow) has been passed with the aid of a fiberscope into the bronchus under investigation. Catheters of small diameter are also available for direction of the biopsy instrument. Localization in two planes is essential, and although simultaneous biplane fluoroscopy is useful, the procedure can be carried out in a standard fluoroscopic room.

or transorally introduced catheter, and followed fluoroscopically into the bronchus to be examined. "Steerable" catheter systems that are commercially available have been devised for use with this technique as an outgrowth of transarterial catheter systems.[38]

The more rapid method of transcricoid introduction of endobronchial catheters and brushes is an attractive alternative to the above procedure.[31] With this technique, however, there has been at least one instance of bronchogenic carcinoma transplanted to the puncture site in the cricoid region.[7] Thus this method of introduction should be approached cautiously.

REFERENCES

1. Amundsen, Per: Pulmonary angiography in lung and mediastinal tumors. In *Angiography*, Vol. 1, 2nd ed. Herbert L. Abrams, Ed. Little, Brown, Boston, 1971, pp. 539–565.

2. Bariety, Maurice, Coury, Charles, Monod, Olivier, Gimbert, Jean-Louis, and Wargon, Henri: Twelve years' experience with gas mediastinography (770 Cases). *Dis. Chest* **48**:449–454 (November 1965).

3. Berne, Alfred S., Ikins, Philip M., and Bugden, Walter F.: CO_2-O_2 Pneumomediastinography with polytomography for the preoperative evaluation of bronchogenic carcinoma. *Radiology* **88**:519–525 (March 1967).

4. Charkes, David N., and Sklaroff, David M.: The radioactive strontium and photoscan as a diagnostic aid in primary and metastatic cancer in bone. *Radiologic Clin. North America* **3**(3):449–509 (December 1965).

5. Charpin, J., Lallemand, M., Gayrard, P., and Chevrot, J.:

Cineradiography in bronchography of bronchogenic carcinoma. *J. Fr. Med. Chir. Thorac.* **20**:293–295 (April 1966).

6. Cooley, Robert N.: Radiographic detection of preclinical and asymptomatic cancer of the lung. *Am. J. Roentgenol.* **107**:440–442 (October 1969).

7. Curry, Joseph L.: Personal communication.

8. Davies, Dean F.: A review of Detection Methods for the early diagnosis of lung cancer. *J. Chron. Dis.* **19**:819–845, (August 1966).

9. Edwards, C. Lowell, and Hayes, Raymond L.: Scanning malignant neoplasms with gallium 67. *J.A.M.A.* **212**(7): 1182–1190 (May 18, 1970).

10. Evans, John A.: Techniques in the detection and diagnosis of malignant lesions of the liver, spleen and pancreas. *Radiol. Clin. North Am.* **3**(3): 567–582 (December 1965).

11. Feigelson, Howard H., and Ravin, Herbert A.: Transverse myelitis following selective bronchial arteriography. *Radiology* **85**:663–665 (October 1965).

12. Fennessy, John J.: Transbronchial biopsy of peripheral lung lesions. *Radiology* **88**:878–882 (May 1967).

13. Flipse, Robert C., Vuksanovic, Mario, and Fonts, Ernesto A.: Segmental brain scanning in radiation therapy of malignant tumors of the brain. *Am. J. Roentgenol.* **102**(1):93–96 (January 1968).

14. Fraser, Robert G., and Paré, J. A. Peter: Malignant neoplasms. In *Diagnosis of Diseases of the Chest*, Vol. 2, W. B. Saunders. Philadelphia, 1970, pp. 736–771.

15. Greenfield, George B., Schorsch, Hildegarde, A., and Shkolnik, Arnold: The various roentgen appearances of pulmonary hypertrophic osteoarthropathy. *Am. J. Roentgenol.* **101**:927–931 (December 1967).

16. Holling, H. Edward, Brodey, Robert S., and Boland, H. Christine: Pulmonary hypertrophic osteoarthropathy. *Lancet* **2**:1269–1274 (December 9, 1961).

17. Howells, J. B.: Alveolar cell carcinoma of the lung. *Clin. Radiol.* **15**:112–122, 1964.

18. Ito, Yasuhiko, Okuyama, Shinichi, Awano, Takayuki, Takahashi, Kunibumi, Sato, Tachio, and Kanno, Iwao: Diagnostic evaluation of the ⁶⁷Ga scanning of lung cancer and other diseases. *Radiology* **101**:355–362 (November 1971).

19. Janower, Murray L., Dreyfuss, Jack R., and Skinner, David B.: Azygography and lung cancer. *New Engl. J. Med.* **275**:803–808 (October 13, 1966).

20. Kittredge, Richard D., and Sherman Robert S.: Roentgen findings in terminal bronchiolar carcinoma. *Am. J. Roentgenol.* **87**: 875–883 (May 1962).

21. Levine, Arnold H., and Pais, M. Joyce: Enigma and dilemma of the pulmonary nodule. *Pa. Med.* **76**(12):50–55, (December 1973).

22. Milne, Eric N. C.: Bronchial arteriography. In *Angiography*, Vol. 1, 2nd ed., Herbert L. Abrams, Ed., Little, Brown, Boston. 1971, pp. 567–577.

23 Nebesar, R. A., Pollard, J. J., Edmunds, L. H., Jr., and McKhann, C. F.: Indications for selective celiac and superior mesenteric arteriography. *Am. J. Roentgenol.* **92**:1100–1109 (November 1964).

24. Nelson, Sidney W., and Christoforidis, Anthimos J.: Bron-

chography in diseases of the adult chest. *Radiol. Clin. North Am.* **11**(1): 125–152 (April 1973).

25. Rabinov, Keith, Goldman, Harvey, Rosbash, Hilde, and Simon, Morris: The role of aspiration biopsy of focal lesions in lung and bone by simple needle and fluoroscopy. *Am. J. Roentgenol.* **101**:932–938 (December 1967).

26. Ranninger, Klaus, and Collins, P. A.: Azygography: its value in the staging of lymphomas. Presented at the 59th Scientific Assembly and Annual Meeting of the Radiological Society of North America, Chicago, Ilinois, 1973.

27. Rinker, Carl T., Garrotto, Lewis J., Lee, Kyo Rak, and Templeton, Arch W.: Bronchography. Diagnostic signs and accuracy in pulmonary carcinoma. *Am. J. Roentgenol.* **104**:802–807 (December 1968).

28. Rinker, Carl T., Templeton, Arch W., MacKenzie, James, Ridings, G. Ray, Almond, Carl H., and Kiphart, Ridlon: Combined superior vena cavography and azygography in patients with suspected lung carcinoma. *Radiology* **88**:441–445 (March 1967).

29. Riska, Nils: Importance of compulsory mass x-rays for early diagnosis of lung cancer. *Geriatrics* **26**:172–182 (February 1971).

30. Sanders, D. E., Delarue, N. C., and Silverberg, S. A.: Combined angiography and mediastinography in bronchogenic carcinoma. *Radiology* **97**:331–339, (November 1970).

31. Sargent, E. Nicholas, and Turner, A. Franklin: Percutaneous transcricothyroid membrane selective bronchography. *Am. J. Roentgenol.* **104**(4): 792–801 (December 1968).

32. Secker-Walker, R. H., Provan, J. L., Jackson, J. A., and Goodwin, J.: Lung scanning in carcinoma of the bronchus. *Thorax* **26**:23–32 (January 1971).

33. Secker-Walker, Roger H., and Siegel, Barry A.: The use of nuclear medicine in the diagnosis of lung disease. *Radiol. Clin. North Am.* **11**(1):215–241 (April 1973).

34. Thomas, Edward Llewellyn: Search behavior. *Radiol. Clin. North Am.* **7**(3):403–417 (December 1969).

35. Viamonte, Manuel, Jr.: Angiographic evaluation of lung neoplasms. *Radiol. Clin. North Am.* **3**(3):529–542 (December 1965).

36. Viamonte, Manuel, Jr.: Selective bronchial arteriography in man. Preliminary report. *Radiology* **83**:830–839 (November 1964).

37. White, Robert I., Jr., James, A. Everette, Jr., and Wagner, Henry N., Jr.: The significance of unilateral absence of pulmonary artery perfusion by lung scanning. *Am. J. Roentgenol.* **111**(3):501–509 (March 1971).

38. Willson, James K. V., and Eskridge, Marshall: Bronchial brush biopsy with a controllable brush. *Am. J. Roentgenol.* **109**:471–477 (July 1970).

39. Wilson, Freddie E., Preston, David F., and Overholt, Edwin L.: Detection of hepatic neoplasm. Hepatic scanning combined with liver-function studies. *J.A.M.A.* **209**:676–679 (August 4, 1969).

40. Wolfel, Donald A., Linberg, Eugene J., and Light, John P.: The abnormal azygogram—an index of inoperability. *Am. J. Roentgenol.* **97**(4):933–938 (August 1966).

41. Wolinsky, Harvey, and Lischner, Mark W.: Needle tract implantation of tumor after percutaneous lung biopsy. *Ann. Intern. Med.* **71**:359–362 (August 1969).

42. Yerushalmy, J.: The statistical assessment of the variability in observer perception and description of roentgenographic pulmonary shadows. *Radiol. Clin. North Am.* **7**(3):381–392 (December 1969).

Chapter Nine

Medical Conditions Associated with Cancer of the Lung

TUBERCULOSIS

The relationship between chronic pulmonary tuberculosis and primary lung cancer appears to be accidental because of the frequency and possible coexistence of these conditions in any patient population. In a review of 54 cases with concurrent tuberculosis and bronchogenic carcinoma, Berroya et al.[2] found that this represented about 1% of the new cases seen in a state sanitarium in a 14-year period. Difficulties in diagnosing tuberculosis and cancer necessitate the evaluation of x-ray changes, with awareness that both conditions may be present in patients with chronic pulmonary disease who must be followed closely. Distribution of the cell type in the reported patients with tuberculosis followed the average distribution in patients with lung cancer, with epidermoid carcinoma predominating. Among the

54 patients studied, only 4 with coincidental cancer during a resection for residual cavitary tuberculosis survived 5 years. The authors felt that bronchogenic carcinoma may cause tuberculosis breakdown or reactivation because of a break into old tuberculous foci, and associated debility, cachexia, and loss of resistance. Of their patients, 83% had active tuberculosis when bronchogenic carcinoma was detected. If appropriate antibiotic treatment was begun for the tuberculosis, as reported by Fulkerson et al.,[12] it was controlled among 15 patients with coexisting lung cancer. Four patients had far advanced pulmonary tuberculosis, 7 moderately advanced, and the remainder had minimal tuberculosis; 7 patients each had active and inactive tuberculosis, and 1 patient had reactivation when bronchogenic carcinoma was diagnosed (Fig. 1). Similar results have been reported by Bobrowitz et al.[3] The difficulties in diagnosis make a

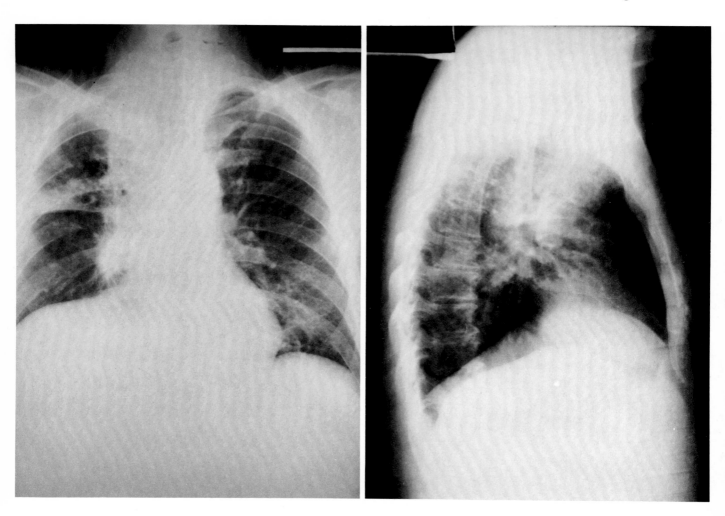

Fig. 1. Patient H. H. Epidermoid carcinoma of the upper lobe diagnosed by bronchoscopy and mediastinoscopy. Patient received radiation therapy and subsequently showed a clinical course with increasing septic temperatures. Although sputum studies were negative, a needle biopsy of the right upper lobe revealed caseating granulomas and produced m. tuberculosis in cultures.

high degree of suspicion necessary and may require multiple cancer and tuberculosis tests. In 2 of 28 patients with coexisting tuberculosis and lung cancer the tuberculin test reversed from positive to negative, according to Bonchek.[4] In Israel, Steinitz[28] found that death from lung cancer among tuberculous patients was higher than in the rest of the population, and the risk of lung cancer was comparable to that in a nontuberculous population of heavy smokers.

CHRONIC PULMONARY DISEASE

There is a complicated relationship between smoking, chronic bronchitis, and lung cancer, with a higher incidence of malignancy in smokers with chronic bronchitis.[24] Similarly silicosis, asbestosis, and other fibrotic lung diseases predispose to lung cancer. About half the adenocarcinomas and bronchioloalveolar carcinomas are associated with preexisting lung scars presumably because of malignant changes in the hyperplastic bronchiolar epithelium at the margin of such scars.[1]

Lung scars from tuberculosis, infarcts or bronchiectasis were associated with adenocarcinoma or bronchioloalveolar carcinoma in 17 of 20 patients reported by Ripstein et al.[25] Two patients had epidermoid carcinoma, and one had oat cell carcinoma. Although the etiological relationship between such fibrosis and cancer of the lung is not established beyond doubt, the significance of minor radiographic changes must be kept in mind even in patients with diffuse fibrosis, as has been stressed by Fraire and Greenberg[11] and Rigler.[23]

PNEUMOTHORAX

Among 1143 patients with spontaneous pneumothorax reported upon by Dines et al.,[9] 10 cases were attributed to malignant pulmonary neoplasm. In two cases a spontaneous pneumothorax occurred in patients who had not

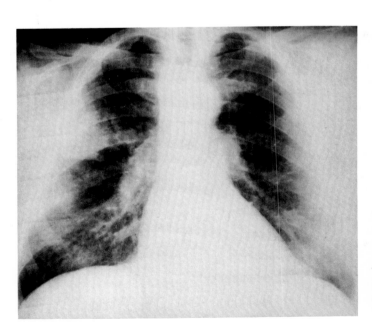

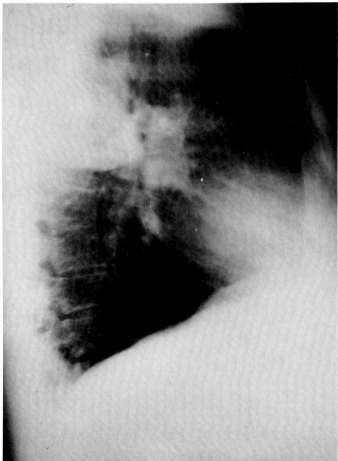

Fig. 2.   Patient C. D. Peripheral pneumonia in a patient with lung cancer. Bronchoscopy produced evidence of a squamous cell carcinoma of the right upper lobe bronchus.

shown roentgenographic evidence of pulmonary tumor. Six patients had multiple pulmonary metastasis from various types of sarcoma. Adenocarcinoma of the lung was diagnosed in 2 patients, and 1 had oat cell carcinoma and metastatic cells in the pleural fluid from a probable primary lung cancer; 3 of the ten patients had asymptomatic pneumothorax.

ENDOCRINE MANIFESTATIONS OF CANCER OF THE LUNG

The endocrine activity of bronchogenic cancer is important from a clinical point of view and because of the clues it provides to the biochemistry of cancer. Occasionally, metabolic consequences of endocrine abnormalities are the initial manifestation of bronchogenic carcinoma, and an alert examiner may suspect the underlying cancer. It has been estimated that extrapulmonary effects of bronchogenic carcinoma may be seen in up to 10% of patients.[8] Brown[6] was the first author to describe the association between oat cell carcinoma and Cushing's syndrome in 1928. In this cancer, Cushing's syndrome usually starts abruptly and pursues a rapid course, with weakness, pigmentation, and hypokalemic alkalosis. Elevated excretion of 17-hydroxycorticoids and 17-ketosteroids has been found in patients with lung cancer, especially in oat cell carcinoma.[18] Control of the tumor by surgery or radiation therapy may be associated with the clinical remission of Cushing's syndrome. It is likely that ACTH is produced by the malignant tumors.[14] Attempts at supressing urinary steroids with dexamethasone are usually unsuccessful, in contrast to classical Cushing's disease. A report by Bower and Gordon[5] indicates that very few epidermoid and adenocarcinomas produce this syndrome, the majority being oat cell carcinomas. In the series of Kato et al.,[15] 4 of 138 patients with oat cell carcinoma had signs and symptoms of hypercorticism. On the other hand, O'Neill et al.[21] reported that 6 of 15 patients studied had oat cell carcinoma of the lung as a source of ectopic corticotropin production.

Biochemical characteristics of hyperparathyroidism including hypercalcemia, hypercalciuria, and hyperphosphatemia have been shown to be present in patients with lung cancer and may improve after effective treatment of the cancer. It is believed that the cancers produce a substance similar to parathyroid hormone, and the clinical symptoms of lethargy, confusion, anorexia, nausea, vomiting, polydipsia, and polyuria should alert the examiner to this possibility. All histologic types of lung cancer are associated with this biochemical disturbance, but epidermoid carcinoma predominates.[19] In one study[26] of 4 patients with bronchogenic carcinoma who had parathyroid hormone in tumor tissue, 3 had epidermoid

carcinoma. The incidence of clinical symptoms that mimic hyperparathyroidism is less frequent than that in Cushing's syndrome. It is important to distinguish hyperparathyroidism from hypercalcemia secondary to metastatic bone disease. Metastatic involvement of the pituitary may also be confused with this syndrome due to diabetes insipidus.

Inappropriate excretion of antidiuretic hormone leads to hypernatremia and hypochloremia with the associated clinical symptoms of salt depletion. This has been described in patients with bronchogenic carcinoma of all histologic varieties. The tumor appears to be the site of hormone production, and treatment of the cancer is essential. The physician must be aware of this syndrome since the administration of salt will simply lead to the added excretion of salt. Water restriction may be the treatment until the tumor is controlled, although hypertonic saline may be used occasionally for temporary relief of acute symptoms of nausea, vomiting, and lethargy. The incidence of this syndrome is about half that in Cushing's syndrome.[20]

Gynecomastia is an occasional extrapulmonary manifestation of bronchogenic carcinoma, and gonadotropins were shown to be a major factor[10] in a number of patients with large cell carcinoma of the lung. A relationship to the clinical manifestations of pulmonary osteoarthropathy is suggested. Inappropriate secretion of other hormones such as insulin, serotonin, and others may occur in patients with tumor involving the lung.[5,13] Cutaneous flushing, diarrhea, and facial edema are associated with serotonin production of carcinoid tumors that metastasize to the lung and liver. A larger than normal amount of 5-hydroxy-indolacetic acid may be detected in the urine of these patients, occasionally without clinical manifestations of a carcinoid syndrome.

It is appropriate to add that the adrenal glands are frequently destroyed by metastasis from lung cancer, and the resulting defective indigenous production of corticosteroid hormones must be considered in the evaluating of a patient with bronchogenic carcinoma who presents with signs and symptoms of Addison's disease. This finding may explain the frequent beneficial effect of corticosteroids in terminal patients.

NEUROMUSCULAR AND SKELETAL EFFECTS OF CANCER OF THE LUNG

Clubbing of the terminal digits, (Fig. 3) occasionally associated with arthralgia, has been reported by Stenseth et al.[29] in 92% of 1879 malignant lung tumors. It occurred in 9% of the patients with epidermoid carcinoma of the lung, in 12% with adenocarcinoma, in 14% with large cell carcinoma, in 5% of oat cell carcinomas and

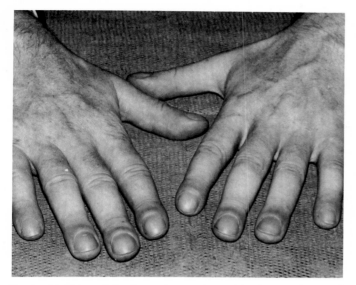

Fig. 3. Clubbing of the fingers in a patient with adenocarcinoma of the lung.

to varying degrees in other types of histologic tumors. There was a 3% incidence of clubbing among metastatic lung tumors. Among primary tumors, a larger tumor was more likely to be associated with hypertrophic pulmonary osteoarthropathy. There was no evidence of a prognostic significance in this syndrome. In 30% of the patients clubbing preceded the onset of pulmonary symptoms, but it disappeared immediately after operation in 37% of the patients, and by the end of the first month following operation in 84%. Sometimes up to 6 months elapsed before the arthralgia improved, and clubbing also regressed although more slowly. In at least 1 case clubbing improved but was still present 5 years postoperatively. Occasionally, x-ray therapy may lead to regression of symptoms in this syndrome that may be associated with ectopic growth hormone production. Clubbing is probably neurogenic in origin.

The symptoms of carcinomatous neuromyopathy are clinically significant because the affected patients are intolerant to muscle relaxants used during anesthesia. In a study by Trojaborg et al.,[30] 16% of patients with bronchogenic carcinoma had clinical manifestations of carcinomatous neuromyopathy; 6% of these patients had neurologic deficits, and up to 33% showed various abnormalities in electromyograms. Although polyneuropathy is the major clinical manifestation of this syndrome, a myasthenic picture may emerge. The neurologic symptoms may precede the diagnosis of bronchogenic carcinoma. Metastatic involvement of the spine or the spinal cord is an important differential diagnostic consideration. Nearly all patients reported with this syndrome in the literature had a diagnosis of epidermoid carcinoma. A number of patients showed improvement in clinical and laboratory findings following successful surgical treatment of the primary tumor.[16]

DERMATOLOGIC AND VASCULAR MANIFESTATIONS OF CANCER

In approximately 15% of patients with dermatomyositis there is an associated malignancy, occasionally bronchogenic carcinoma.[7] Other non-metastatic cutaneous manifestations of bronchogenic carcinoma are acanthosis nigricans and cutaneous manifestations of vascular changes, especially thrombophlebitis and fibrinolytic purpura. Lung cancer is the most frequent malignancy associated with thrombophlebitis in males.[17] Disseminated intravascular coagulation and coagulation defects have been described, and slow release of thromboplastin from tumor breakdown as well as infection have been implicated.[22] It is important to realize that in the treatment of cancer-related thrombophlebitis anticoagulants such as coumarin-type drugs are ineffective, therefore, heparin should be the treatment of choice.

REFERENCES

1. Bennett, D E., and Sasser, W. F.: Bronchiolar carcinoma: A valid clinicopathologic entity? *Cancer* **24**:876–886, 1969.

2. Berroya, R. B., Polk, J. W., Raju, P., and Bailey, A. H.: Concurrent pulmonary tuberculosis and primary carcinoma. *Thorax* **26**:384–387, 1971.

3. Bobrowitz, I. D., Elkin, M., Evans, J. C., and Lin, A.: Effect of direct irradiation on the course of pulmonary tuberculosis (using cancerocidal doses). *Dis. Chest* **40**:397–406, 1961.

4. Bonchek, L. I.: Diagnosis of lung cancer in tuberculous patients: use of tuberculin skin test and serum protein electrophoresis. *Chest* **60**:256–259, 1971.

5. Bower, B. F., and Gordon, G. S.: Hormonal effects of nonendocrine tumors. *Ann. Rev. Med.* **16**:83–118, 1965.

6. Brown, W. H.: A case of pleury glandular syndrome. Diabetes of bearded women. *Lancet* **2**:1022–1023, 1928.

7. Cormia, F. E., and Domokos, A. N.: Cutaneous reactions to internal malignancy. *Med. Clin. North Am.* **49**:655–680, 1965.

8. Croft, P. B., and Wilkinson, M.: The incidence of carcinomatous neuromyopathy in patients with various types of carcinoma. *Brain* **88**:427–434, 1965.

9. Dines, D. E., Cortese, D. A., Brennan, M. D., Hahn, R. G., and Payne, W. S.: Malignant pulmonary neoplasms predisposing to spontaneous pneumothorax. *Mayo Clin. Proc.* **48**:541–544, 1973.

10. Faiman, C., Colwell, J. A., Ryan, R. J., Hershman, J. M., and Shields, T. W.: Gonadotropin secretion from a bronchogenic carcinoma: Demonstration by radioimmunoassay. *N. Engl. J. Med.* **277**:1395–1399, 1967.

11. Fraire, A. E., and Greenberg, S. D.: Carcinoma and diffuse interstitial fibrosis of lung. *Cancer* **31**:1078–1086, 1973.

12. Fulkerson, L. L., Perlmutter, G. S., Zack, M. B., Davis, D. O., and Stein, E.: Radiotherapy in chest malignant tumors asso-

ciated with pulmonary tuberculosis. *Radiology* **106**:645–648, 1973.

13, Hattori, S., Matsuda, M., Tateishi, R., Tatsumi, N., and Terazawa, T.: Oat cell carcinoma of the lung containing serotonin granules. Gann **59**:123–129, 1968.

14. Jarett, L., Lacy, P. E., and Kipnis, D. M.: Characterization by immunofluorescence of ACTH-like substance in nonpituitary tumors from patients with hyperadrenocorticism. *J. Clin. Endocrinol. Metab.* **24**:543–549, 1964.

15. Kato, Y., Ferguson, T. B., Bennett, D. F., and Burford, T. H.: Oat cell carcinoma of the lung. *Cancer* **23**:517–524, 1969.

16. Kennedy, J. H., Coyne, N., and Khairallah, P.: Carcinomatous neuroendocrinopathy associated with cancer of the lung. *J. Thorac. Cardiovasc. Surg.* **57**:276–283, 1969.

17. Liberman, J. S.: Thrombophlebitis and cancer. *J. A. M. A.* **177**: 542–545, 1961.

18. Liddle, G. W., Island, D. P., Ney, R. L., Nicholson, W. E., and Shimizu, N.: Nonpituitary neoplasms and Cushing's syndrome. *Arch. Intern. Med.* **111**:129–133, 1963.

19. Myers, W. P. L.: Hormonal manifestations in lung cancer. C. V. Mosby, St. Louis, 1968, p. 488.

20. Omenn, G. S., and Wilkins, E. W., Jr.: Hormone syndromes associated with bronchogenic carcinoma: clues to histologic type. *J. Thorac. Cardiovasc. Surg.* **59**:877–881, 1970.

21. O'Neill, L. W., Kipins, D. M., Luse, S. A., Lacy, P. E., and Jarett, L.: Secretion of various endocrine substances by ACTH secreting tumors. *Cancer* **21**:1219–1232, 1968.

22. Peck, S. D., and Reiquam, C. W.: Disseminated intravascular coagulation in cancer patients: supportive evidence. *Cancer* **31**:1114–1119, 1973.

23. Rigler, L. G.: The natural history of untreated lung cancer. *Ann. N.Y. Acad. Sci.* **114**:755–768, 1964.

24. Rimington, J.: Smoking, chronic bronchitis and lung cancer. *Br. Med. J.* **2**:373–374, 1971.

25. Ripstein, C. B., Spain, D. M., Bluth, I.: Scar cancer of the lung. *J. Thorac. Cardiovasc. Surg.* **56**:362–370, 1968.

26. Sherwood, L., O'Riordan, M. J., Auerbach, G. D., and Potts, J. T.: Production of parathyroid hormones by non-parathyroid tumors. *J. Clin. Endocrinol. Metab.* **24**:140–146, 1967.

27. Sparagana, M.: Lung cancer associated with ectopic growth hormone production. Presented at the XIth International Cancer Congress, Florence, 1974.

28. Steinitz, R.: Pulmonary tuberculosis and carcinoma of the lung: a survey from two population-based disease registers. *Am. Rev. Respir. Dis.* **92**:758–766, 1965.

29. Stenseth, J. H., Clagett, O. T., and Woolner, L. B.: Hypertrophic pulmonary osteoarthropathy. *Dis. Chest* **52**:62–68, 1967.

30. Trojaborg, W., Frantzen, E., and Andersen, I.: Peripheral neuropathy and myopathy associated with carcinoma of the lung. *Brain* **92**:71:82, 1969.

Chapter Ten

Staging of
Carcinoma of the Lung

THE TNM SYSTEM OF STAGING

Anatomic and pathologic staging of lung cancer serves two purposes: first, it provides an accurate description of the disease in simplified terms and permits the exchange of information and comparison of data referring to results of treatment in a simple manner. Also, staging is usually closely related to the most effective treatment that may be available for a patient. Until recently there had been no commonly accepted staging system in cancer of the lung, until the American Joint Committee for Cancer Staging and End Results Reporting designed a TNM Classification, following the concepts initially introduced by the International Union Against Cancer (UICC). This complicated system is comprehensive and significantly related to treatment and prognosis.

Anatomic staging is done on the basis of clinical, laboratory, and radiographic information and surgical findings, including scalene node biopsy, mediastinoscopy, or exploratory thoracotomy. As a rule, patients should be staged by at least two physicians, usually a thoracic surgeon and a radiation therapist or a medical oncologist. Disagreement in opinion of the two examiners will place the patient in the lower, less advanced staging category, whereas treatment is permitted for the more advanced category.

The staging categories according to the TNM Classification are as follows:

T   Primary Tumor

T-0   No evidence of primary tumor

T-X   Tumor proven by the presence of malignant cells in secretions but not visualized roentgenographically or bronchoscopically.

T-1   Intrapulmonary, localized: a solitary tumor that is 3.0 cm or less in greatest diameter, surrounded by lung or visceral pleura and without evidence of invasion proximal to a lobar bronchus at bronchoscopy.

T-2   Intrapulmonary, extensive: a tumor more than 3.0 cm in greatest diameter or a tumor of any size which, with its associated atelectasis or obstructive pneumonitis, extends to the hilar region. At bronchoscopy, the proximal extent of demonstrable tumor must be at least 2.0 cm distal to the carina. Any associated atelectasis or obstructive pneumonitis must involve less than an entire lung and there must be no pleural effusion.

T-3   Extrapulmonary, intrathoracic, localized: this includes lesions which invade through the visceral pleura, into the pleural space or which are adherent to the parietal pleura; broncho-genic cancers within 2 cm of the carina; no visceral, vascular, neurologic, osseous or cardiac (including pericardial) invasion.

T-3.1   Lesions meeting such criteria limited to one lobe including associated atelectasis and infiltration.

T-3.2   Lesions as stated, limited to two lobes.

T-3.3A   Lesions as stated, limited to one main bronchus without atelectasis.

T-3.3B   Lesions with pleural effusion and negative cytology.

NB: It is important to recognize that T-3 lesions may require thoracic exploration to be determined. Such definition of T3.1, T3.2, and T3.3 represents T1 and T2 lesions clinically and radiographically assessed, which are beyond resection based upon location or evidence of extrapulmonary invasion at surgery.

T-4   Extrapulmonary, intrathoracic, extensive: a very extensive lesion involving nerves, major vessels, heart, vertebrae, and chest wall sites. It is beyond the parietal pleura and into the chest wall, viscera and/or deep mediastinal structures. Does not include patients with extrathoracic visceral metastasis.

T-4.1   Pleural effusion with positive cytology.

T-4.2   Superior vena caval obstruction associated with any lesion.

N   Regional Lymph Nodes

N-0   No demonstrable spread to lymph nodes.

N-1   Spread to lymph nodes in the ipsilateral hilar region (including direct extension).

N-2.1   Subcarinal and lower mediastinal lymph nodes.

N-2.2   High mediastinal lymph nodes.

N-2.3   Contralateral hilar nodes.

N-2.4   Posterior mediastinal, diaphragmatic and pericardial nodes.

N-3   Supraclavicular or biopsied scalene nodes.

M   Distant Metastasis

M-1   Solitary, isolated metastasis confined to one organ or anatomic site. This also applies to cervical, axillary or abdominal coeliac nodes.

M-2   Multiple metastatic foci confined to one organ system or one anatomic site, i.e., lungs, skeleton, liver, etc.

M-3   Multiple organs metastatic involvement.

Although this comprehensive staging system is well suited to departments that treat a large number of patients and are interested in detailed information based on a coding system, a stage grouping of the subclassifications is appropriate for individuals who are not interested in the amount of detail contained in the TNM

Classification. Such a stage grouping has been suggested by the Radiation Therapy Oncology Group of the National Cancer Institute and classifies patients as follows:

Stage Grouping of Carcinoma of the Lung

Stage O

| T-O, N-O, M-O | An occult carcinoma based upon positive cytology. |

Stage 1

| T-1, N-O, M-O | A tumor that can be classified T-1 without any spread to nodes or distant metastasis. |

Stage 2

| T-1, N-1, M-O | A pulmonary intrathoracic tumor classified as T-2, or spread to the lymph nodes in the ipsilateral hilar region only (N-1), or both T-2 and N-1. |
| T-2, N-O, M-O |
| T-2, N-1, M-O |

Stage 3

| T-3, N-O, or N-1 or N-2 with T-1, T-2, T-3, all M-O | Any extrapulmonary intrathoracic tumor or spread to the lymph nodes in the mediastinum. |

Stage 4

| T-4 with any N, N-3 with any T, M of any category | Extensive extrapulmonary invasion into viscera and bone or distant metastasis. |

The performance status of the patient may be coded as follows:

	%	
I. Able to carry on normal activity.	100	Normal; no complaints no evidence of disease.
	90	Able to carry on normal activity; minor signs or symptoms of disease.
	80	Normal activity with effort; some signs or symptoms of disease.
II. Unable to work; able to live at home, care for most personal needs; a varying amount of assistance is needed.	70	Cares for self, unable to carry on normal activity or to do active work.
	60	Requires occasional assistance, but is able to care for most personal needs.
	50	Requires considerable assistance and frequent medical care.
III. Unable to care for self; requires equivalent of institutional or hospital care; disease may be progressing rapidly.	40	Disabled; requires special care and assistance.
	40	Severely disabled; hospitalization is indicated, although death not imminent.
	20	Very sick; hospitalization necessary; active support treatment is necessary.
	10	Moribund; fetal process progressing rapidly.
	0	Dead.

SURGICAL CLASSIFICATION

For practical purposes, an obsolete staging system classifying patients as operable and inoperable has been used for many years. This classification involved a combination of historical, laboratory, and physical findings which were used to determine whether a patient would be eligible for an exploratory thoracotomy and possible resection. Although not universally agreed upon, contraindication to surgery was usually accepted if any of the following conditions were present:

The primary tumor is an oat cell carcinoma.
The primary tumor extends to within 1 cm of the carina, or a biopsy of the carina is positive for cancer.
There is involvement of the parietal pleural or chest wall, except in superior sulcus tumors.
There is atelectasis of an entire lung.
There is involvement of hilar or mediastinal lymph nodes.
There is malignant pleural effusion.
There is recurrent nerve paralysis.
There is phrenic nerve paralysis.
There is superior vena caval obstruction.
There are distant metastases, including metastasis in supraclavicular nodes.

THE PHYSICAL EXAMINATION AND STAGING OF PATIENTS WITH CANCER OF THE LUNG

There are certain findings on physical examination that indicate the need to investigate known regions of spread of bronchogenic carcinoma if present. Although the staging of patients with cancer of the lung uses history, physical examination and specific laboratory tests and surgical procedures, the physical examination is usually the first examination performed on which directed biopsies or tests should be based in addition to screening procedures. At the same time, the cardiovascular and pulmonary status of the patient must be considered, since a decision as to treatment should be made only after complete staging and medical evaluation. Significant findings on physical examination that direct attention to progression of the tumor include the following.

Vocal Cord Paralysis

Left vocal cord paralysis is an easily discernible feature of the physical examination if an indirect laryngoscopy is performed routinely in the physical examination of a patient suspected of having bronchogenic carcinoma. Among 100 consecutive cases of vocal cord paralysis without clinical evidence of tumor reported by Parnell and Brandenburg,[3] 32 were due to neoplasms in the mediastinum; 34 were traumatic, and the remainder were caused by mechanical factors, inflammatory or neurologic disorders, or were of unknown etiology. The left vocal cord was involved more often than the right, and 14% of the patients had bilateral cord involvement. Among the patients with trauma, vocal cord paralysis following thyroidectomy was the most common. Among those with neoplasm, 16 had lung cancer and 2 had Hodgkin's disease. In patients with proven bronchogenic carcinoma, recent onset of left vocal cord paralysis must be considered evidence for mediastinal involvement with metastatic malignancy, if prior causes of vocal cord paralysis are excluded. Current surgical opinion considers vocal cord paralysis to be one of the accepted contraindications for surgery. In rare cases, vocal cord paralysis may be secondary to involvement of cervical lymph nodes from a bronchogenic carcinoma.

Pleural Effusion

Although the presence of free pleural fluid is best determined by x-ray examination, physical examination by auscultation will show pleural fluid in nearly all cases with a large amount of fluid. If small effusions are suspected, a lateral decubitus chest x-ray is mandatory to distinguish old pleural changes from recent, free pleural fluid (Fig. 1).

Tandon[6] reported a large series of patients with pleural effusion associated with lung cancer. He found pleural effusion in 56 of 670 patients when primary carcinoma of the bronchus was first diagnosed. Among these 56 patients, 38 had small amounts of pleural fluid without significant symptoms due to the effusion. The distribution of histologic diagnosis among epidermoid carcinoma, undifferentiated carcinoma, adenocarcinoma, and oat cell carcinoma agreed with the incidence of these tumors in the entire series. Forty-three percent of the patients had bloody effusion, 43% serous effusion, and 14% had chylous effusion or empyema. Because of the high incidence of epidermoid carcinoma in the series, both serous and bloody effusions were usually associated with this type of cancer. The average survival time of patients with small effusions was 15.4 months; patients with

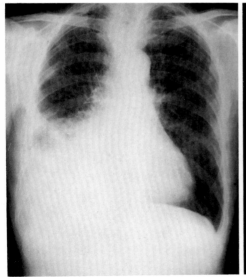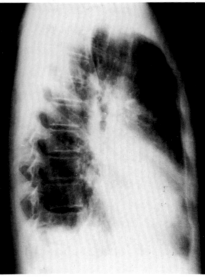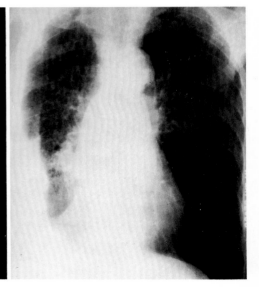

Fig. 1. Patient C. P. Squamous cell carcinoma of the right main stem bronchus diagnosed on bronchoscopy. The changes in the right lower lobe are shown to be due to free pleural fluid on the right lateral decubitus film. Aspiration revealed serosaguinous fluid with malignant cells on cytologic examination.

moderate effusions survived an average of 10.6 months. Patients with bloodstained pleural effusions failed to survive a year.

Although a bloody effusion is usually considered malignant, demonstration of malignant cells by appropriate cytologic studies is mandatory. Serous effusion, on the other hand, is not necessarily due to carcinoma and the usual diagnostic tests for tuberculosis and other infections should be carried out. Again, the demonstration of free malignant cells in the pleural fluid on cytologic examination is required to establish the malignant origin of the effusion. Although the diagnosis of empyema as part of initial diagnosis of cancer of the lung carries a poor prognosis, it should be emphasized that postoperative empyema after surgery for lung cancer has been associated with a better than average survival rate.[14] Empyema is a common complication, although it is less frequent now than in the early days of thoracic surgery mainly because of bronchopleural fistula after pneumonectomy. Ruckdeschel et al.[5] analyzed the fate of 489 patients who underwent lung resection between 1952 and 1966. Among the patients who suffered from primary lung cancer and survived at least 1 month after surgery, there were 18 patients with postoperative empyema. Among the resected patients in the general group, there were 22% who survived 5 years, whereas there were 50% in the empyema group. No other major differences were apparent between the two groups of patients.

The management of empyema should involve culture and sensitivity testing of the organism causing the effusion and specific antibiotic therapy should be started as early as possible. Definitive therapy by radiotherapy or surgery must usually be delayed until the acute manifestations of empyema are controlled.

Pericardial Effusion

The classical signs of pericardial effusion, venous distension, distant heart sounds, and paradoxical pulse are rare among patients with bronchogenic carcinoma at initial diagnosis. Later in the course of the disease, up to 35% of the patients with lung cancer may develop involvement of the pericardium, often because of secondary changes from involvement of the surrounding tissue with progressive growth into the pericardial sac. Localized progressive growth after unsuccessful treatment of lung cancer often produces a symptomatology of its own, so that pericardial involvement forms only a small part of the patient's clinical picture.

The treatment of pericardial effusion is part of the management of widespread metastatic disease. Chemotherapy can be used when pericardial metastasis is not life-threatening and when there is an effective chemotherapeutic agent for the tumor type. The treatment of choice for progressive pericardial effusion is radiation therapy (Fig. 2).

Superior Vena Caval Obstruction

The fully developed syndrome of superior vena caval obstruction with shortness of breath at rest, distended neck veins, suffusion of the head and neck, dilated collateral circulation of the anterior and lateral chest wall and upper abdomen, and cyanosis on reclining makes diagnosis easy. However, early stages may produce significant symptoms and are usually best determined by clinical examination in the upright and recumbent position which produces discernible changes even in the absence of distinctive symptoms.

On close examination, the patient frequently admits to slight shortness of breath upon reclining, and dilatation of the neck veins and bluish discoloration of the facial skin and neck while lying down are telltale signs of early superior vena caval obstruction (Figs. 3,4). In later stages, permanent edema of the neck structures is one of the outstanding symptoms. The majority of patients with superior vena caval syndrome have malignancy, usually bronchogenic carcinoma; in one large series, however, benign inflammatory lesions occurred in approximately one-third of the patients.[2] The superior vena caval syndrome is usually produced by compression of the superior vena cava because of adjacent lymph node involvement. Invasion of the wall of the vein by tumor occurs in only a small percentage of patients. In the series mentioned earlier, only 2 of 32 patients showed tumor invasion of the wall of the vein at postmortem examination. Superior vena caval syndrome indicates that there is metastatic disease in the mediastinum, and contraindicates curative surgery.

Staging of carcinoma of the lung has made great strides in recent years. Improvement in diagnostic techniques as well as increased awareness of the importance of detailed analysis of the extent of a patient's tumor before starting treatment has advanced our diagnostic acumen from a simple classification of operable or inoperable tumor to a complex system of disease description. Preliminary evidence suggests that the stage of disease relates significantly to prognosis if adequate treatment is administered. The staging of carcinoma of the lung has replaced the therapeutic nihilism which prevailed among physicians and surgeons with a rational approach to treatment that opened the door to a better understanding of the natural history of lung cancer and appropriate treatment that can significantly increase the survival of patients with bronchial carcinoma. Since

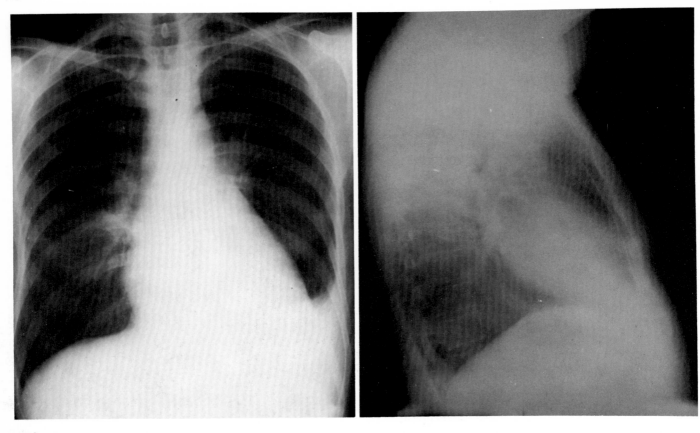

Fig. 2. Patient W. R. Posteroanterior and left lateral chest x-ray with evidence of cardiomegaly. This patient died, and epidermoid carcinoma of the left upper lobe of the lung with metastasis to the pericardium and to the left pleural and pericardial cavities were found on autopsy.

there is a close correlation between the staging of lung cancer and early diagnosis, more and more patients should be diagnosed at a time when effective curative treatment is available (Fig. 5). Although the long-term results of treatment of lung cancer are on the whole still disappointing, the meaning of the quality of life following treatment and improvement in the performance of treated patients is apparent to all with extensive experience in patient management.

The importance of staging is best demonstrated by its prognostic implications. Carr and Mountain[1] have published two-year survival data (Table 1) which show that for stage I disease epidermoid carcinoma has a 46.6% survival, adenocarcinoma 45.9%, large cell carcinoma 42.8%, and small cell carcinoma 6.0%. The respective figures for stage II disease were 39.8%, 14.3%, 12.9% and 5.0%, while in stage III, 11.5%, 7.9%, 12.9%, and 3.8% respectively survived 2 years.

TABLE 1. CARCINOMA OF THE LUNG: TWO-YEAR-SURVIVAL RATE

Cell Type	Stage I		Stage II		Stage III	
	Number	Percent	Number	Percent	Number	Percent
Epidermoid carcinoma	331	46.6%	66	39.8%	524	11.5%
Adenocarcinoma	151	45.9%	28	14.3%	334	7.9%
Large cell carcinoma	61	42.8%	17	12.9%	103	12.9%
Small cell carcinoma	38	6.0%	20	5.0%	302	3.8%

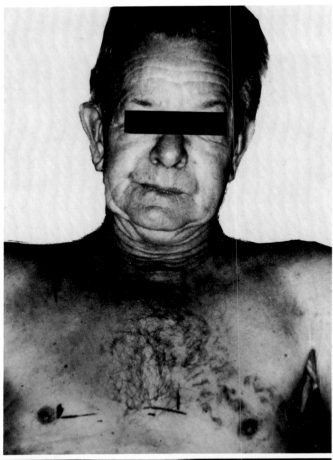

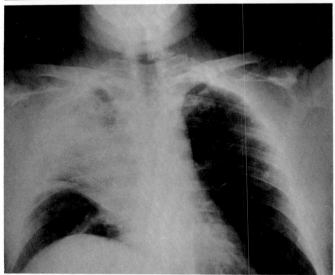

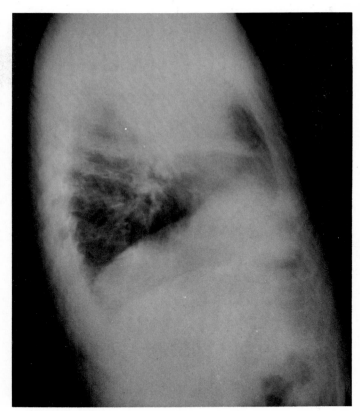

Fig. 3. Patient D. C. Superior vena caval syndrome with dilatation of neck veins and anterior thoracic veins, increase of circumference of the neck and suffusion of the face. The symptoms were aggravated by reclining and the patient was unable to lie flat because of shortness of breath. Diagnosis: epidermoid carcinoma.

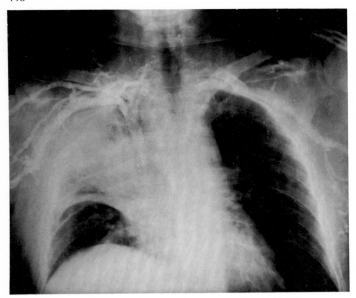

Fig. 4.   Same patient. Superior vena cavogram showing evidence of occlusion of the superior vena cava and collateral circulation.

REFERENCES

1. Carr, D. T., and Mountain, C. F.: The staging of lung cancer. *Semin. Oncol.* **1**:229–234, 1974.

2. Longacre, A. M., and Shockman, A. T.: The superior vena cava syndrome and radiation therapy, clinical response, survival, and postmortem findings. *Radiology* **91**:713–718, 1968.

3. Parnell, F. W., and Brandenburg, J. H.: Vocal cord paralysis. A review of 100 cases. *Laryngoscope* **80**:1036–1045, 1970.

4. Postoperative empyema and survival in lung cancer. Editorial. *Br. Med. J.* **1**:504, 1973.

5. Ruckdeschel, J. C., Codish, S. D., Stranahan, A , and McKneally, M. F.: Post-operative empyema improves survival in lung cancer. *N. Engl. J. Med.* **287**:1013–1017, 1972.

6. Tandon, R. K.: The significance of pleural effusions associated with bronchial carcinoma. *Br. J. Dis. Chest* **60**:49–53, 1966.

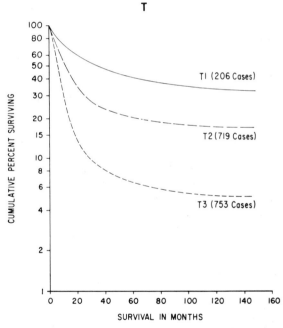

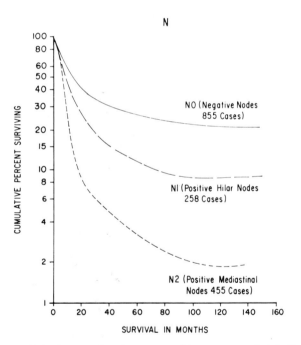

Fig. 5.   Survival in lung cancer stratified by the anatomic extent of the primary tumor (T factor) and of regional lymph node involvement (N factor), excluding undifferentiated small cell carcinoma. (From Mountain, C. F., Carr, D. T., and Anderson, W. A. D.: A clinical system for the staging of lung cancer. *Am. J. Roentgenol., Radium Ther. Nucl. Med.,* **120**:130–138, 1974. Courtesy of Charles C Thomas.)

Chapter Eleven

The Histologic Diagnosis of Cancer of the Lung

SPUTUM CYTOLOGY

The examination of expectorated sputum after staining by modified Papanicolaou techniques is an effective means of establishing the presence of lung cancer. Depending on the amount of sputum produced, the quality of the technical procedures during the preparation of the specimen and the number and character of the cells seen under the microscope, it is possible in many patients to determine the presence of malignancy as well as the cell type. In a series reported by Umiker,[18] sputum cytology diagnosed malignancy in 65.2% of the patients with lung cancer. Spontaneous cough sputum is the most valuable specimen for routine examination. The unfixed sputum should be transported to the laboratory promptly, though it may be kept at room temperature for a few hours without damage to the cells. Pulmonary obstruction due to blockage of the airways may result in a negative cytologic specimen even in the presence of large lung cancers. Additional closure caused by inflammation or mucosal edema or inspissated mucus in the peripheral airways may prohibit malignant cells from being expectorated. In these patients, a course of antibiotics, bronchodilators, and expectorants may reduce obstruction and increase pulmonary flow.

For those patients who cannot produce satisfactory sputum samples or expectorate pulmonary secretions, inducing sputum with water, saline, or mucolitic agents may enable them to bring up secretions that adhere to the air passages. Ultrasonic nebulizers deliver a volume of mist that contains many droplets $<5\mu$ in diameter, which may cleanse the airway but which may also destroy malignant cells.

Adequate specimens for cytologic examination of sputum can be obtained from nearly all patients in a high-risk group as was shown in the preliminary assessment of the Mayo Lung Project (see page 72). A 3-day collection of spontaneous, deep cough sputum was carried out in 488 patients: 470 specimens were satisfactory initially, and of the 18 unsatisfactory specimens 17 were satisfactory on repeat collection. The remaining patient had induced sputum. Only one patient did not produce induced sputum. In the Mayo Lung Project, a complicated classification of cytologic sputum findings is used, with specimens classified as unsatisfactory, or negative if normal cells are present, or as intermediate if metaplastic squamous cells are present with a slight to moderate degree of atypia. Marked irregularities and the presence of cancer cells are indications for further investigation of the patient's condition.

Erozan and Frost[5] reported a similar study, and found that 97.8% of the specimens from asymptomatic patients who were screened were satisfactory using the ultrasonic physiologic aerosol induction technique. They noted that the quality of this technique is good. Of 25 patients who were examined by bronchoscopy on the basis of abnormal cytology and normal chest x-rays, 9 were cytologically diagnosed as having cancer, and the site was located in all. The material from the remaining 16 patients was interpreted as markedly atypical metaplasia, and cancer was not found at this time. The cytologic diagnosis from sputum specimens achieved an accurate diagnosis of lung cancer of up to 75%. When suspicious, inconclusive, and atypical categories are included, 95% of proven lung cancers may be diagnosed by sputum specimens.

In a study of malignancy-associated changes in oral and bronchial epithelial cells from sputum specimens, Rilke and Pilotti[15] found that changes could be described consistently in normal appearing differentiated cells with mature cytoplasm in which there was a slightly increased nuclear cytoplasmatic ratio, and deeply stained, small chromocenters which demarcated round or oval-shaped clear areas of uniform size. They described these changes as "malignancy associated changes type A," and noted a 97.3% coincidence of such changes with malignant tumors. In 2.7% of the examined patients, in whom no malignancy of the lung was found, these changes have persisted for at least 2 years. It is believed that these changes may appear prior to frank tumor growth, and research in this area is being pursued actively. It is anticipated that the yield of positive cytologic specimens from patients with lung cancer will be higher than the above-mentioned figure of 65% once the results of a prospective study of the type done by the Mayo Lung Project are available.

Although the presence of cancer cells in the sputum of a patient with a clinical or radiographic diagnosis of lung cancer may suffice to prove the presence of malignancy, localization of the tumor may depend on x-rays combined with one of the following procedures.

BRONCHOSCOPY

A bronchoscopic examination using the straight Jackson bronchoscope provides important data even in the presence of preoperative cytologic proof of cancer. Direct inspection of the main stem and the segmental bronchi yields information about the extent of an intrabronchial lesion and its possible multiplicity. At the same time, a biopsy of lesions can be performed for histologic examination, and bronchial washings may be obtained if desired.

In Umiker's[18] series, bronchoscopic biopsy established the diagnosis of lung cancer in 45.7% of patients, and bronchial washings produced a diagnosis of malignancy in 43.8%. This compares with 65.2% for sputum collections, which are usually obtained from more extensive segments of bronchial mucosa than the bronchial washings during bronchoscopy. The combined diagnostic accuracy of bronchoscopic biopsy and bronchial washings produced histologic evidence of lung cancer in 64.7% of the patients studied.

In peripheral lesions, bronchial brushing has been diagnostic in two-thirds of patients with lesions that are not visible through the Jackson bronchoscope (Fig. 1) according to Fennessy et al.[6] It involves catheterization of the bronchi under fluoroscopic control with the same type of topical anesthesia used in bronchoscopy. A nylon Fennessy bronchial brush is applied to the lesion, multiple samples are obtained, and smears are made on glass slides for cytologic study. In connection with bronchial washings, this technique provided an overall accuracy of 77% in the diagnosis of lung cancer. A positive diagnosis was also obtained in 53% of patients with pulmonary metastatic disease from other primary tumor and in 33% of patients with pulmonary lymphoma. Complications were slight, with one pneumothorax occurring in over 300 examinations. The problem of dislodgement of part of the brush in the periphery of the lobe required recognition of this complication immediately, to allow removal of the missing parts with a catheter. A correct diagnosis of malignant and nonmalignant cavitating lesions of the lung was obtained by bronchial brush biopsy in 15 of 25 patients in whom cavitary lung disease could not be diagnosed short of surgical exploration.[8]

The recent introduction of flexible fiberoptic bronchoscopes (see Fig. 2) has added the peripheral bronchi to the area that can be inspected by the bronchoesophagologist. The flexible bronchofibroscope is approximately 5 mm in diameter and can bend up to 180° for insertion into the fine bronchi of the various lobes of the lungs. Inspection and biopsy are possible, and photographs can be taken of the observed area. The fibroscope is especially effective in diagnosing cancer in the upper lobes of the lungs, where it is difficult to inspect the bronchial tree with the straight Jackson bronchoscope.

Marsh et al.[12] have defined the indications for use of the bronchofibroscope as follows: (1) in patients with mechanical problems involving the neck and jaw; (2) in patients with hemoptysis; (3) in the presence of thoracic aortic aneurysm; (4) in peripheral, upper lobe, and small hilar tumors; (5) in x-ray negative sputum-positive tumors where detailed study of the segment is required. They also indicated that the Jackson bronchoscope is best used in patients with evidence of major airway disease, or when differential cytology is required, as in small children and in suspected foreign bodies.

Lukeman[11] examined the correlation of cytologic with

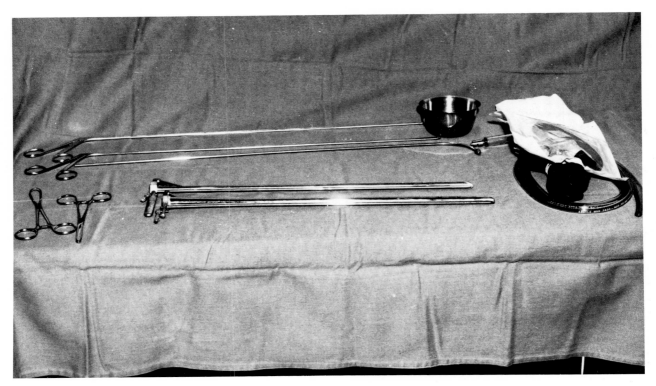

Fig. 1.   Jackson bronchoscope.

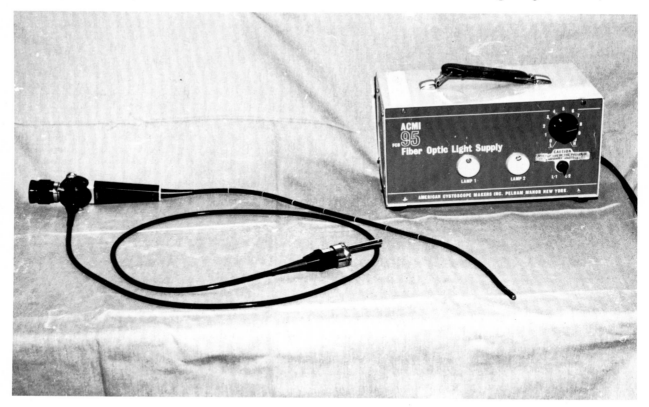

Fig. 2.   Fiberoptic bronchoscope.

histologic diagnosis. Although cytologic studies were positive in 98% of 103 cases of primary lung cancer, a specific histologic diagnosis with regard to cell type was confirmed by cytology in 75% of the cases. Recently, an extension of bronchoscopic examination was described by transbronchoscopic lung biopsy. Of 378 specimens in 450 patients that were considered histologically adequate, 21 specimens from diffuse pulmonary disease showed metastatic cancer, 10 indicated alveolar cell carcinoma, and 4 lymphoma. Although bleeding was always adequately controlled and mediastinal emphysema produced no major problems, 1 patient died.

PERCUTANEOUS PULMONARY AND PLEURAL BIOPSY

In patients with suspicious, undiagnosed peripheral lung lesions on x-ray, who are physically able to lie flat for at least 10 minutes, percutaneous biopsy can be performed under fluoroscopic control. If contraindications such as bleeding, lack of cooperation, bullous emphysema, and severe pulmonary hypertension are avoided, complications can be kept to a minimum. In the series of Zelch et al.,[19] 3% of patients had transient hemoptysis, 3% had a large pneumothorax, 11% had a small pneumothorax, and 1% each had hemithorax or subcutane-

ous emphysema with no serious permanent morbidity. The authors did not encounter any dissemination of the tumor through the needle tract in 208 patients subjected to needle biopsy, of whom 139 had malignant lesions. The needle biopsy was falsely negative in 15 of the 139 patients who were diagnosed on the basis of other pathologic information. Fontana et al.[7] obtained positive biopsies in 78% of 83 cases of lung cancer. Pneumothorax occurred in 57% of the procedures and 17% of all patients required pleural suction to treat pneumothorax. No deaths followed the procedure. Pleural biopsy is useful in patients with recurrent pleural effusions in whom needle biopsy of a peripheral lung lesion is inadvisable. If large pleural effusions are present, a pleural biopsy will frequently yield information about the presence of lung cancer or metastatic malignancy involving the pleural cavity.

SCALENE NODE BIOPSY

If palpable adenopathy is present in cervical, scalene, or supraclavicular lymph nodes, biopsy in a patient with other features of lung cancer will provide a positive histologic diagnosis of bronchogenic carcinoma in about 90% of patients.[13] In the absence of palpable scalene nodes, the results of a biopsy of these nodes usually yield significant information in about 10%. The aggressiveness of the surgeon plays a major role in how many nodes are removed, and scalene node dissections may approach biopsies of the upper mediastinum, with up to 26% positive biopsies obtained from nonpalpable scalene nodes by some investigators.[3]

MEDIASTINOSCOPY

Mediastinoscopy has achieved a dominant place in the histologic diagnosis of cancer of the lung. Furthermore, metastatic malignancy and contraindications to surgery are established at the same time. Usually performed at time of bronchoscopy, a number of recent studies have produced histologic evidence of the presence of cancer in 6.6 to 20% of patients who would otherwise have undergone an exploratory thoracotomy. Mediastinal biopsies were positive in 17 to 35% of patients with epidermoid carcinoma, in 67% of patients with adenocarcinoma, and in 70% of patients with oat cell carcinoma.[4, 9,14,16]

Table 1 indicates the frequency of ipsilateral, contralateral, and bilateral involvement and the importance of obtaining bilateral mediastinal biopsies. The resection rate after negative mediastinal biopsy in patients who are otherwise eligible for surgery has been raised to 96% with judicious use of mediastinal biopsies in prethoracotomy workup. Among several hundred patients,[17] one death was attributed to mediastinoscopy. Complications involving paralysis of the recurrent nerve, cardiac arrest, serious wound infections, severe pneumothorax, and bleeding, all of which required treatment but did not lead to permanent disability, were found in 15 out of 637 patients (2.5%), and 3 patients had implantation of tumor in the incision.

BONE MARROW BIOPSY

Bone marrow biopsy of the posterior iliac crest was performed in 150 consecutive patients by Hansen and Muggia.[10] Of 55 patients with epidermoid carcinoma, 2 (3.4%) had positive bone marrow examination. Of 27

TABLE 1. RESULTS OF MEDIASTINAL BIOPSIES[9]

83 Right-sided lesions	
Ipsilateral positive mediastinal biopsy	23%
Bilateral positive biopsy	30%
Contralateral biopsy, only positive	1.2%
61 Left-sided lesions	
Ipsilateral positive mediastinal biopsy	20%
Bilateral positive mediastinal biopsy	15%
Contralateral biopsy, only positive	11.5%

patients with adenocarcinoma, 5 were positive (18.5%), of 40 patients with large cell carcinoma, 5 were positive (12.5%), and of 28 patients with oat cell carcinoma 13 were positive (46.4%). Thus the overall incidence was 25 of 150 patients for 16.6% involvement. Patients with no demonstrable disease outside one hemithorax were considered to have limited disease, with an incidence of 2% bone marrow involvement for epidermoid carcinoma, 8% for large cell carcinoma, 16% for adenocarcinoma, and 40% for small cell carcinoma. The remainder of positive findings occurred in patients with more extensive disease. Only 16% of patients with positive bone marrow examination had x-ray evidence of bone metastasis, whereas 69% had positive bone scans. Positive bone marrow aspirations indicated a poor prognosis following chemotherapy as a primary means of treatment of these patients, compared to patients who had negative bone marrow biopsies and who were treated by other methods.

PERITONEOSCOPY

Peritoneoscopy with liver biopsy under direct observation was performed in 58 patients, with 4 (7%) positive for metastatic involvement of the liver in small cell carcinoma.[10] Abnormal liver function tests, in many patients on the basis of nonmalignant involvement of the liver, were present in 72%, positive technetium liver scans in 17%, and suspicious technetium liver scans in 21% of the 58 patients.

ABDOMINAL METASTASIS

The results of exploratory laparotomy prior to thoracotomy for lung cancer have been described by Bell.[2] The author reported on a group of patients exposed to exploratory laparotomy prior to thoracotomy for bronchogenic carcinoma; patient selection was based on indications for thoracotomy with exclusion of all patients with known metastasis outside the hemithorax. Recurrent and phrenic nerve paralysis were considered contraindications to thoracotomy, as was hilar node enlargement. The laparotomy immediately preceded an anticipated thoracotomy, and involved inspection and palpation of the liver, omentum, superior mesenteric, celiac, and portal lymph nodes, adrenal glands, and kidneys. Abnormal lymph nodes and all suspected metastases were biopsied. There were 72 patients in this series with proven bronchogenic carcinoma, of whom 34 were found to have epidermoid carcinoma. Of these 22.5% had evidence of abdominal metastasis. Of 15 patients with oat cell carcinoma, abdominal metastasis was present in 33%, and of 9 patients with adenocarcinoma of the lung, 1 revealed evidence of abdominal metastasis. The remainder had bronchioloalveolar or metastatic lung cancer, and revealed no evidence of abdominal involvement. The incidence of abdominal metastasis amounted to 18.8% in all patients with cancer. The liver was the involved organ in 82% of the patients with involvement below the diaphragm, and there were 5 patients (31% of those with abdominal metastasis) with metastatic upper abdominal lymph nodes. Nonpalpable microscopic metastases were found in 2 patients in the kidneys and adrenal glands.

EXPLORATORY THORACOTOMY

The advent of mediastinoscopy has led to a significant decrease in diagnostic or exploratory thoracotomies. There are few, if any, patients in whom a diagnosis is not arrived at following biopsy procedures, and who are candidates for curative surgery on the basis of their general medical condition, pulmonary functions, and the absence of distant metastatic spread. The risk of mortality from diagnostic thoracotomy without major resection is approximately 1 to 3%, and clinical judgment, therefore, indicates that this risk is unwarranted in a patient in whom a significant cure rate cannot be expected. Careful follow-up with chest x-ray, sputum and clinical examinations, especially all the scalene nodes, and indirect laryngoscopy will usually reveal continued growth of an apparently stationary lesion within a reasonable period of time, particularly in the disabled elderly patient who is a poor surgical risk.

When positive sputum cytology or positive histologic diagnosis by limited biopsy procedures cannot be obtained, radiotherapy without histologic proof of the presence of tumor may be administered. If strict criteria are applied, the diagnosis will rarely be incorrect. Exploratory thoracotomy should be resorted to in all patients in whom long-term survival can be expected from a curative surgical procedure, if proof of the diagnosis is not achieved by more limited procedures.

In summary, bronchogenic carcinoma can be diagnosed by sputum examination in 67 to 85% of epidermoid carcinomas, in 65 to 70% of small cell carcinomas, and in approximately 55% of adenocarcinomas. When other techniques have failed, washings and transthoracic needle aspiration techniques under fluoroscopic control will usually provide the diagnosis on peripheral neoplasm with pulmonary densities visible on x-ray. There is increasing evidence that fiberoptic bronchoscopy can localize pulmonary malignancy in the majority of patients who have a positive sputum cytology with negative chest x-rays.

REFERENCES

1. Anderson, H. A., and Fontana, R. S.: Transbronchoscopic lung biopsy for diffuse pulmonary diseases: technique and results in 450 cases. *Chest* **62**:125–128, 1972.

2. Bell, J. W.: Open abdominal biopsy before thoracotomy for lung cancer. *Geriatrics* **20**:715–727, 1965.

3. Brantigan, O. C., and Moszkowski, E.: Bilateral biopsy of nonpalpable cervical lymph nodes. *Dis. Chest* **50**:464–469, 1966.

4. Delarue, N. C., Sanders, D. E., and Silverg, S. A.: Complimentary value of pulmonary angiography and mediastinoscopy in individualizing treatment for patients with lung cancer. *Cancer* **26**:1370–1378, 1970.

5. Erozan, Y. S., and Frost, J. K.: Cytopathological diagnosis of lung cancer. *Semin. Oncol.*: 191–198, 1974.

6. Fennessy, J. J., Fry, W. A., Manalo-Estrella, P., and Hidvegi, D. V. S. F.: The bronchial brushing technique for obtaining cytologic specimens from peripheral lung lesions. *Acta Cytol.* **14**:25–30, 1970.

7. Fontana, R., Miller, W., Beabout, J., Payne, W., and Harrison, E.: Transthoracic needle aspiration of discrete pulmonary lesions: experience in 100 cases. *Med. Clin. North Am.* **54**:961–971. 1970.

8. Forrest, J. V.: Bronchial brush biopsy in lung cavities. *Radiology* **106**:69–72, 1973.

9. Goldberg, E. A., Glicksman, A., Khan, F., and Nickson, J.: Mediastinoscopy for assessing mediastinal spread in clinical staging of carcinoma of the lung. *Cancer* **25**:347–353, 1970.

10. Hansen, H., and Muggia, F.: Staging of inoperable patient with bronchogenic carcinoma with special reference to bone marrow examination and peritoneoscopy. *Cancer* **30**:1395–1401, 1972.

11. Lukeman, J. M.: Reliability of cytologic diagnosis in cancer of the lung. *Cancer Chemother. Rep. (P. 3)* **4**:79–93, 1973.

12. Marsh, B. R., Frost, J. K., Erozan, Y. S., and Carter, D.: Role of fiberoptic bronchoscopy in lung cancer. *Semin. Oncol.* **1**:199–203, 1974.

13. Palumbo, L. T., and Sharpe, W. S.: Scalene node biopsy, correlation with other diagnostic procedures in 550 cases. *Arch. Surg.* **98**:90–93, 1969.

14. Pearson, F. G.: Evaluation of mediastinoscopy in management of presumably operable bronchial carcinoma. *J. Thorac. Cardiovasc. Surg.* **55**:617–625, 1968.

15. Rilke, F., and Pilotti, F.: Data on malignancy associated changes in oral and bronchial epithelial cells in sputum specimens: their possible utilization for identification and follow-up of high risk groups. *Cancer Chemother. Rep. (P. 3)* **4**:73–78, 1973.

16. Sarin, C. L., and Hohl-Oser, H. C.: Mediastinoscopy: a clinical evaluation of 400 consecutive cases. *Thorax* **24**:585–588, 1969.

17. Trinkle, J. K., Bryant, L. R., Hiller, A. J., and Playforth, R. H.: Mediastinoscopy: experience with 300 consecutive cases. *J. Thorac. Cardiovasc. Surg.* **60**:297–300, 1970.

18. Umiker, W. O.: Relative accuracy of various procedures in the diagnosis of bronchogenic carcinoma. *J. A. M. A.* **195**:6–7, 1966.

19. Zelch, J. V., Lalli, A. F., McCormack, L. J., and Belovich, D. M.: Aspiration biopsy in diagnosis of pulmonary nodule. *Chest* **63**:149–152, 1973.

Chapter Twelve

The Diagnosis of Metastatic Spread of Cancer of the Lung

PULMONARY METASTASIS FROM CARCINOMA OF THE LUNG

The chest x-ray, including body section radiography of specific areas or of the entire lung, can detect metastatic lesions of the lung of approximately 1 to 2 cm in diameter. The diagnosis of lymphangitic spread of cancer of the lung is considerably more difficult, since various changes in cardiac and pulmonary perfusion status may provide misinformation. Pulmonary congestion, right heart failure on the basis of obstruction of the pulmonary artery due to lung cancer or its metastasis, and other causes of impairment of the circulatory system may lead to misdiagnosis on the basis of a chest x-ray.

Lung scanning provides information about pulmonary perfusion of the lungs, and it may indicate obstruction of the pulmonary artery due to metastatic disease in the presence of a normal or minimal chest x-ray finding.

LYMPH NODE INVOLVEMENT IN CANCER OF THE LUNG

No significant information is expected from lower extremity lymphangiography, and lymph node scanning has not been applied widely in lung cancer. Information regarding lymph node involvement is usually derived from regular chest x-rays, tomograms of the mediastinum, esophagrams, and biopsies of the mediastinal or supraclavicular lymph nodes. Mediastinal biopsy has been described on page 123.

LIVER METASTASIS

The liver is the most frequent site of metastasis in 42% of untreated patients, and is among the most difficult to diagnose. Liver scanning, one of the main methods of diagnosing liver metastasis, may be typical of metastasis and has been shown to indicate unsuspected liver metastasis in 5% of the patients reported upon by Hayes et al.[5] An additional 8% of the scans were equivocal. The use of enzyme studies, for example, SGOT, SGPT, LDH, and alkaline phosphatase is of value in diagnosis of liver metastasis if underlying preexisting liver damage can be excluded. Therefore, the use of these biochemical methods of diagnosing liver abnormality in patients with lung cancer may indicate metastasis if previous normal studies are available and an abnormal pattern is detected. The use of multiple enzyme studies, including ubiquitous enzymes which are not usually employed in routine biochemical studies of patients, may indicate the presence of liver metastasis in over 50% of patients. Again, underlying liver disease such as cirrhosis may be difficult to exclude, and a liver biopsy by the percutaneous needle method should be performed in all patients in whom liver metastasis is suspected, either on clinical grounds because of palpable or nodular liver enlargement or on the basis of abnormal scan findings or biochemical testing. Hansen and Muggia[4] reported that of 58 patients 72% had abnormal liver function tests. Many of these were shown to be on the basis of nonmalignant liver disease, since only 7% of the patients had positive liver biopsies, with 17% of the 99 m technetium sulphur colloid scans positive for metastasis and 21% suspicious. Liver biopsies obtained on peritoneoscopy have been described on page 123.

BRAIN METASTASIS

The brain is one of the most frequent sites of metastasis in patients in whom the primary tumor has been successfully treated either by surgery or by other methods. In asymptomatic patients, Hayes et al.[5] obtained positive scans with metastatic disease in only 4% of the patients. A prospective study by Pedersen et al.[11] involving neurologic examination, electroencephalography, 99 m technetium pertechnetate brain scanning, and lumbar puncture before thoracotomy in 63 consecutive patients with 39 epidermoid carcinomas, 15 oat cell carcinomas, 5 adenocarcinomas, and 4 unclassified tumors failed to discover intracranial metastasis in 5 patients. In 10 patients, although metastasis was suspected on the basis of the aforementioned examinations, it was later negated either by autopsy or follow-up examination.

There were 18 patients with central nervous system (CNS) signs, and 45 patients who lacked these symptoms. In 4 patients neurologic examination revealed a unilateral hemispheric lesion, and in 5 patients cerebellopontile lesions. Six patients (10%) had symptoms of dizziness and headaches. Diplopia, focal sensory epileptic seizures, or dysgraphic symptoms were noted by 1 patient.

The electroencephalogram showed focal signs in 8 cases, unilateral slow activity in 4 and bilateral slow activity with localized preponderance in the other 4. In 4 cases the EEG abnormality was the only focal sign.

Brain scanning disclosed focal accumulation in 6 patients (10%). In 4 of these 6 patients the brain scan was the only focal sign.

A lumbar puncture was performed in 45 patients. The spinal fluid cytology was negative in all. Less than 10 white cells/ml were found in all but 2 patients, including 7 who had verified or probable intracranial metastasis. Protein values were more than 50 mg/100 ml in 2 cases, 1 with probable intracranial metastasis.

Follow-up was by clinical examination in 76% of the 41 living patients, and by autopsy in 36% of 22 symptomatic patients, in whom the primary tumor could not be treated surgically.

Thus, 41 of 63 patients had adequate follow-up information, and in 8% of these intracranial metastases were found later despite negative findings on initial examination. Among patients with false positive signs and symptoms, clinical signs and EEG findings were more frequently associated with lack of proof of metastatic malignancy in the CNS than was the brain scan, since only 1 patient had a false positive scan. The differentiation of carcinomatous encephalopathy, the CNS equivalent of carcinomatous neuromyopathy, makes evaluation of the follow-up of the 10 patients with false positive signs and symptoms difficult.

The significance of this study is that positive findings do not necessarily indicate the presence of metastatic malignancy, as based on the patients' later clinical course. In general, brain scans are positive for metastatic disease in about 90% of patients. Cerebral angiography and computerized transaxial tomography (EMi scans) allow the diagnosis in the remaining 10% of patients.

BONE METASTASIS

Bone metastasis constitutes 35–40% of cases, with involvement in distant sites in both treated and untreated patients. Bone metastasis is predominantly osteolytic in epidermoid carcinoma, whereas osteoblastic metastasis is known to occur occasionally in patients with small cell or adenocarcinoma. In a series published by Napoli et al.,[9] 38 of 110 patients (35%) revealed evidence of bone involvement on initial x-ray examination. In 10 patients (9%) bone involvement was shown by local destruction of ribs or spine in the thoracic area on the x-rays. In 28 patients (26%) distant metastases outside the thorax were demonstrated. Of the 38 patients with bone metastasis, 50% presented initially with radiographic evidence of bone involvement; the remainder developed radiographic changes during their observation period. Nine patients (9%) with oat cell carcinoma and with adenocarcinoma had osteoblastic metastasis, and all had evidence of bone marrow involvement on bone marrow biopsy (see page 123). Seven of the 9 patients had strontium 85 bone scans which were positive for metastatic disease.

Studies in 82 patients with lung cancer have been reported by Muggia and Schervu.[8] Radionuclide scans revealed bone involvement in 69.2% which was proven on bone marrow biopsy. An additional 15.8% of the scans were positive in the absence of tumor identification on bone marrow biopsies. Bender and Hansen[1] reported no hypercalcemia in 35 patients with small cell carcinoma metastatic to bone, and that it occurred in only

1 of 40 patients with bone metastasis from adenocarcinoma. Six of 47 patients with large cell undifferentiated carcinoma and 18 of 78 patients with epidermoid carcinoma had hypercalcemia; however, osseous metastases were documented in only 6 of the latter group and in 4 patients with large cell carcinoma. Presumably these tumors may produce hypercalcemic humoral substances. The relationship between these substances and the occurrence of destructive bone lesions in epidermoid carcinoma because of increased local bone absorption is not yet established.

Although x-ray examination of painful areas frequently produced evidence of metastatic disease once lung cancer had been diagnosed, the routine use of bone surveys disclosed metastatic disease in approximately 15% of the patients studied. Bone scanning with 99 m technetium diphosphonate has added to the accuracy of diagnosis of bone metastasis in an additional 19 to 32% of 259 patients studied by Osmond et al.[10] Seventeen percent of the patients had metastasis on x-ray bone survey. Six patients (2%) had negative scans and positive x-rays, but only 2 of these patients had metastasis. Often the x-rays were necessary to interpret the bone scans accurately.

The differential diagnosis of positive scans includes many benign changes and Paget's disease in the population under observation. In a series reported by Charkes and Sklaroff,[2] 80% of the patients with positive scans in whom x-rays revealed evidence of metastatic lesions from a known primary tumor showed metastatic malignancy on biopsy examination of the suspected areas.

CIRCULATING TUMOR CELLS

The prognostic significance of circulating tumor cells has been evaluated in a long-term follow-up study by Drye et al.[3] The majority of patients had cancer of the breast or gastrointestinal tract, but there was one patient with cancer of the lung in whom circulating cancer cells were identified in the peripheral blood 3½ months before clinical evidence of recurrence was observed following initial surgery. Tumor cells were obtained from the thoracic duct lymph by Watne et al.[12] The authors studied 6 patients with lung cancer and found tumor cells in 2. An additional 14 patients with lung cancer were studied at autopsy, and in 3 of these tumor cells were present in the thoracic duct lymph. All patients had advanced disease and were seen prior to initiating palliative chemotherapy.

Studies regarding the presence of tumor cells in the peripheral blood of patients with lung cancer remain scarce, partly because of difficulties in histologic identification of tumor cells. The technique lacks clinical significance at this time.

ADRENAL METASTASIS

The high incidence of adrenal metastasis in apparently localized carcinoma of the lung of all histologic types (see page 58) has led to the development of investigative techniques for their early diagnosis. Although radiographic studies of adrenal venography and arteriography are not suitable for screening purposes because of technical difficulties and associated morbidity, the introduction of the radionuclide ^{131}I-19-iodo-chlorestrol with uptake and retention in the adrenal gland and cortical tumors may have prospects for screening.[7] Optimum scanning is obtained approximately 5 to 14 days after the administration of the isotope. At present, data are lack-

ing about the use of this isotope for the diagnosis of metastatic disease in the adrenal gland.

In summary, a breakthrough in the early diagnosis of metastatic lung cancer will depend upon a better understanding of the mode of dissemination. Radionuclide studies such as radioactive gallium citrate and radioactive labelled anti-CEA (carcinoembryonic antigen) antibodies, which have shown promising results in pilot studies, may provide a new path to early diagnosis of distant metastatic spread in bronchial carcinoma. On the basis of our present system of diagnostic workup, patients with histologically established lung cancer which is limited to the thorax must be carefully examined for metastasis in the adrenal glands, lung, brain, bone, and liver. In patients with undifferentiated carcinomas, bone marrow involvement must also be excluded.

The diagnosis of metastases to pleura, scalene nodes, mediastinum, bone marrow and abdomen is described on pp. 122ff.

REFERENCES

1. Bender, R. A., and Hensen, H. H.: Hypercalcemia and bronchogenic carcinoma—a prospective study of 200 patients. *Ann. Intern. Med.* 80:205–208, 1974.

2. Charkes, N. D., and Sklaroff, D. M.: The osseous system. In *Clinical Scintillation Scanning*, Harper and Row, New York, 1969.

3. Drye, J. C., Rumage, W. T., and Anderson, D.: Prognostic import of circulating cancer cells after curative surgery: a long time follow-up study. *Ann. Surg.* 155:733–740, 1962.

4. Hansen, H., and Muggia, F.: Staging of inoperable patients with bronchogenic carcinoma with special reference to bone marrow examination and peritoneoscopy. *Cancer* 30:1395–1401, 1972.

5. Hayes, T. P., Davis, L. W., and Raventos, A.: Brain and liver scans in the evaluation of lung cancer patients. *Cancer* 27:362–363, 1971.

6. Jereb, M., Jereb, D., and Unge, G.: Radionuclear selenite for scintigraphic demonstration of lung cancer and metastasis in the mediastinum: a preliminary report. *Scand. J. Respir. Dis.* 53:331–337, 1972.

7. Kirschner, A. S., Ice, R. D., and Beierwalters, W. H.: Radiation dosimetry of ^{131}I-19-iodo-chlorestrol. *J. Nucl. Med.* 14:713–717, 1973.

8. Muggia, F. M., and Schervu, L. R.: Lung cancer: diagnosis in metastatic sites. *Semin. Oncol.* 1:217–228, 1974.

9. Napoli, L. D., Hansen, H. H., Muggia, F. M., and Twigg, H. L.: The incidence of osseous involvement in lung cancer, with special reference to the development of osteoblastic changes. *Radiology* 108:17–21, 1973.

10. Osmond, J. D., Pendergrass, H. P., and Potsaid, M. S.: Technetium-99m diphosphonate (HEDSPA)—a new bone seeking radiopharmaceutical: clinical experience with 140 cases of metastatic carcinoma of prostate, breast and lung. *Am. J. Roentgenol. Radium Ther. Nucl. Med.* In preparation.

11. Pedersen, H. E., Kjelms, E., Struve-Christensen, E., and Dyrbye, M.: Intracranial metastasis from cancer of the lung. A prospective study of the diagnostic validity of positive and negative findings in neurological examination, electroencephalography, 99m Tc brain scanning, and lumbar puncture before thoracotomy. *J. Thorac. Cardiovasc. Surg.* 65:159–164, 1973.

12. Watne, A. L., Imeran, H., and Moore, G. E.: Clinical and autopsy study of tumor cells in thoracic duct lymph. *Surg. Gynecol. Obstet.* 110:339–345, 1960.

The Surgical Treatment of Cancer of the Lung

The evolution of thoracic surgery has been greatly influenced by the decrease in operative mortality and morbidity which followed the introduction of safe anesthetic techniques, the use of antibiotics and improvement in techniques of blood and fluid replacement, and the development of effective treatment of nonmalignant pulmonary disease. Operative mortality has gradually fallen to acceptable levels and has allowed the thoracic surgeon to concentrate more on the tumor and its manifestations. Thoracic surgery has grown from a technical specialty concerned with details of surgical procedures to an intellectual specialty in which surgical procedures are part of an overall treatment program for patients with bronchogenic carcinoma. Paraphrasing the words of Alfred North Whitehead: thoracic surgery, as some other features of life in our day, has matured to the stage of generalization where freedom reigns and expertise fuses with intellect.

Staging procedures described in previous chapters have defined the indications for curative and palliative thoracic surgical procedures. Treatment that may be used in combination with surgery, such as radiation therapy, chemotherapy, and immunotherapy will be dealt with in later chapters.

CURATIVE SURGERY

In curative operations initial evaluation of the patient and the tumor indicates that the aim of surgery is to provide the maximum likelihood of cure, by operation alone or by a surgical procedure with adjunct treatment by radiation therapy or chemotherapy.

The following absolute contraindications to curative surgery according to Nealon[24] are generally accepted in the surgical community: (1) Spread of the tumor beyond the hemithorax; (2) central nervous system or spinal cord involvement; (3) spread of the tumor to supraclavicular or axillary lymph nodes; (4) liver metastasis; (5) demonstration of neoplastic cells in pleural fluid; (6) paralysis of the recurrent laryngeal nerve; (7) inability of the patient to tolerate the operation; (8) refusal of the patient to submit to the operation. Most surgeons would also add mediastinal lymph node involvement to this list, including phrenic nerve paralysis. Oat cell carcinomas are usually not considered eligible for curative surgery.

The curative procedures consist of segmental resection, lobectomy, and pneumonectomy. If the diagnosis of lung cancer has been established histologically prior to taking the patient to the operating room for a resection, the decision about the type of surgery to be performed depends solely on the extent of the disease upon opening the thorax. If the histopathological diagnosis has not been obtained preoperatively, the surgeon should be prepared to perform a frozen section, as it is generally accepted that a curative resection should not be performed for oat cell carcinoma because of the frequency of subclinical metastasis. If the tumor is unresectable upon entering the thorax, the surgeon should still perform a biopsy except when there is a life-threatening emergency. It is very important for the radiation therapist and the chemotherapist to have a histologic diagnosis to guide subsequent treatment. Simple excisions may be performed if a benign tumor or a nonspecific lesion such as lipoid pneumonia is encountered on exploratory thoracotomy. Needle biopsy of the pleura or aspiration biopsy of the lung lesion do not argue against curative surgery if the patient is otherwise eligible for such a procedure.[7] General principles of cancer surgery should apply in all operations including as little manipulation of the tumor as possible, early clamping of the venous return, and resection of lymph nodes en bloc with the primary tumor if indicated.

Preoperative workup must determine whether a patient can be expected to survive the planned procedure. In this regard physiologic age is much more important than chronologic age, and serious reduction of pulmonary reserve as well as cardiovascular, renal, or hepatic disease are major contraindications to resectional pulmonary procedures. Usually, however, criteria are taken liberally and cannot be definitely fixed in view of the seriousness of the prognosis in cancer of the lung. Among criteria which can be used in assessing the risk over and above that deriving from anesthesia; uncorrected poor nutritional status, anemia or dehydration, and myocardial infarction within 6 months of diagnosis are usually regarded as contraindications to thoracic surgery. In a group of patients who underwent general anesthesia within 3 months following myocardial infarction, 37% had a recurrent myocardial infarction within the first postoperative week; the mortality was 54%. Pulmonary hypertension, uncontrolled emphysema, and serious coronary insufficiency should be corrected before entering the thorax for resection.[23]

It is usually considered that a forced expiratory volume (FEV$_1$) of 2.5 liters or more indicates that the patient can tolerate pneumonectomy. With FEV$_1$ of less than 1 liter, the patient cannot tolerate any loss of functional lung tissue. In patients with intermediate FEV$_1$, studies such as ^{133}Xe lung scans may provide the necessary preoperative information. Also, if the percentage of ventilation to the non-tumor-bearing lung multiplied by the FEV$_1$ equals 1 liter or more of flow, pneumonectomy is functionally tolerated. Miller[21] examined a group of dyspneic surgical candidates preoperatively, and noted that 90% of them survived if their maximum breathing capacity was greater than 40% of normal. All of the patients in whom maximum breathing capacity was less than 40% prior to pulmonary surgery suffered fatal postoperative pulmonary complications.

Segmental resection is the most conservative procedure that can sometimes be employed in the treatment of cancer, especially in patients who have borderline impaired respiratory reserve and in whom a peripheral solitary lesion is found. In general, however, segmental resection is performed when the lesion is thought to be benign, after a frozen section in the operating room, whereas the procedures of choice for malignancy are more extensive. A limited series of 17 patients with bronchogenic carcinoma reported by Le Roux[20] was managed by segmental resection, and 5 patients remained free of tumor for 5 years. If there is a suspicion of cancer, a biopsy of mediastinal lymph nodes should be performed. Occasionally, when the lesion is very superficial and small, a wedge resection may remove the primary tumor completely. The Beattie and Martini[2] series produced a 5-year survival in 4 out of 17 selected patients with lung cancer after wedge resection. Other reports such as that by Overholt et al.,[26] with a 5-year survival of 10%, are not as encouraging with reference to wedge resection and segmental resection, therefore, these operations do not as a rule form part of the standard procedures in the curative treatment of lung cancer.

Lobectomy as a preferred mode of treatment has been advanced by some of our outstanding thoracic surgeons, such as Paulson.[27] The advantage of lobectomy over pneumonectomy lies in the safety of the operation and the retention of better pulmonary function. These advantages have been demonstrated by the postoperative mortality rate which was 10% for patients after pneumonectomy in the series of Overholt et al.[26] but only 1% for patients undergoing lobectomy. They felt that lobectomy is indicated if a lesion is limited to one lobe without lymphatic extension or involvement of lymph nodes, especially when the pulmonary function will not permit pneumonectomy. Occasionally this procedure is performed in patients with pulmonary hypertension and peripheral lung cancer. When there is extension of the tumor to the chest wall, mediastinum, or diaphragm, the probability of recurrence in this area of extension indicates the need for additional resection of adjacent structures in such patients, or other change in treatment planning.

Anatomically the right upper lobe of the lung is best suited for an adequate lobectomy for cancer. The lower and middle lobes contain lymphatics which pass through the upper lobe and make an adequate though limited cancer operation more difficult. A problem which is even more debatable than the question of whether a pneumonectomy or lobectomy should be performed is that of lymph node dissection with lobectomy. The so-called "radical lobectomy" includes an en bloc resection of adjacent mediastinal lymph nodes. Although the procedure itself is often difficult to carry out within anatomic landmarks or boundaries, it has been suggested by Cahan and Beattie[6] that the term "radical" as distinguished from "simple" be used for surgical procedures that include a resection of local lymph nodes. In their series, 64 patients were submitted to simple lobectomy, 4 of whom were classified as operative deaths, and 48 patients underwent radical lobectomy, 5 of whom died in the immediate postoperative period. Sixteen patients (27%) survived 5 years after simple lobectomy, and 19 patients (44%) survived 5 years following radical lobectomy. There was an increase in survival among the patients with metastatic lymph nodes proven on the surgical specimen: 8% survived after simple lobectomy and 19% survived after radical lobectomy with excision of the adjacent mediastinal lymph nodes. Even among those patients in whom only negative lymph nodes could be identified in a surgical specimen, only 30% survived after simple lobectomy compared to 60% after radical lobectomy. Similar results are reported by Overholt et al.[26] who showed a 5-year survival of 49% among patients after lobectomy with nodes free of metastatic cancer, whereas there were only 30% surviving 5 years among the patients in whom lymph nodes were shown to be involved by metastasis on histologic section.

Although data regarding the histologic subgroups in these series are not available, few if any patients with oat cell carcinoma are included, and the results of surgery for oat cell cancer[16,19] have been uniformly worse by far than for epidermoid carcinoma and adenocarcinoma.

Other authors, Nealon[24] and Paulson[27] among them, question the validity of increased survival in patients who have lymph node dissection in association with lobectomy and feel that the value of lymph node dissection is mostly in prognostication because in their studies the majority of these patients did poorly.

In the past, pneumonectomies were the procedure preferred by most thoracic surgeons. The recent advent of mediastinoscopy and the exclusion of many previously unresected patients has led to an increase in resectability rate to 97% of those submitted to thoracotomy.[9] Lobectomy has become a more favored procedure, probably because mediastinoscopies exclude many of the patients who were previously diagnosed as having mediastinal involvement on pneumonectomy and mediastinal dissection. In order to resect mediastinal lymph nodes on thoracotomy, more extensive operations are necessary with resultant significant increase in morbidity as compared to resection of hilar and intrapulmonary lymph nodes only. Intrapulmonary and hilar nodes can be partially resected in conjunction with lobectomy without a significant increase in morbidity. A comparison of results in selected patients treated by a variety of surgical procedures is given in Table 1.

Pneumonectomy is usually indicated for two reasons: one group of thoracic surgeons believes that pneumonectomy is the preferred procedure and that it should be performed whenever possible, that is whenever the patient is able to withstand the immediate and late effects of the operation, with regard to both postoperative complications and the long-lasting respiratory deficit arising from a pneumonectomy. A second group of surgeons feels that pneumonectomy is indicated in tumors extending beyond one lobe, and in patients in whom the tumor extends toward or into a hilum where lobectomy is not sufficient to adequately remove the disease. Because of the anatomic relationship of lymph nodes to lung, more pneumonectomies are performed for lower and middle lobe tumors than for upper lobe lesions.

The distinction between simple pneumonectomy in which only an occasional lymph node is biopsied and radical pneumonectomy in which an en bloc resection including the mediastinal nodes is attempted is similar to that discussed under lobectomy. The location of the lesion becomes significant in this regard, since the radical pneumonectomy is more difficult to perform on the left side where the large vessels interfere with an adequate resection of the mediastinal lymph nodes.

In our experience, the complete removal of tumor is necessary because patients with transsected tumor do poorly, and rapidly develop local and distant metastases. If staging is carried out, patients with $T_1N_0M_0$ tumors, excluding oat cell carcinoma, should be submitted to curative surgery if medically eligible. Any higher primary tumor stage as well as nodal or other metastatic spread indicates the need for a different form of treatment. As discussed earlier, there is no general agreement among thoracic surgeons, however, because limited lymph node involvement is at times not felt to be a contraindication to curative surgery, and in the series reported in Table 1 resections under such circumstances may produce respectable results in selected patients.

PALLIATIVE SURGERY

Although rarely practiced by most thoracic surgeons, palliative resections are occasionally indicated. Long-term results are generally poor. Dillon and Postlethwait[10] indicated that in 22 patients palliative pneumonectomy was performed for symptomatic invasion of the pleura and massive lymph adenopathy. All 22 patients died within a year and the operative mortality was 21%. There were 14 lobectomies for palliation because of persistent infection or intractable hemorrhage; 11 of these patients were dead within 1 year, all 14 died within 2 years. The average survival time for patients with lung cancer who underwent pneumonectomy for palliation was 5.7 months, whereas patients who underwent lobectomy for palliation survived an average of 11 months.

SPECIAL PROCEDURES IN THE SURGICAL TREATMENT OF LUNG CANCER

There is a significant number of modifications of the standard procedures of lobectomy and pneumonectomy. Paulson et al.[28] have described how lobectomy is justifiable selectively, provided that the lymphatic regions of

TABLE 1. FIVE-YEAR SURVIVAL FOLLOWING SURGERY FOR CANCER OF THE LUNG

	Overholt et al[26]	Nealon[24]	Cahan and Beattie[6]	Paulson et al[28]
Lobectomy, lymph nodes free	49%	40%[a]	30–60%[c]	45%[b]
Lobectomy, lymph nodes involved	30%	10%[a]	8–19%[c]	
Pneumonectomy, lymph nodes free	39%		55%	17%[b]
Pneumonectomy, lymph nodes involved	25%		19–29%[c]	
Wedge resection			20%	
Chest wall involvement		10%	10%	
Pericardiectomy as part of resection			30%	
Operative mortality, lobectomy			6–10%[c]	4%
Operative mortality, pneumonectomy			21–30%[c]	9%
Operative mortality, exploration only				5%

[a] Includes pneumonectomy.
[b] Includes lymph nodes involved.
[c] Simple versus radical surgery.

the hilum are removed and bronchoplastic procedures with removal of portions of the main stem bronchi and subsequent closure or anastomosis with peripheral bronchi are performed. In epidermoid carcinoma, 33% of their patients did not have hilar lymphatic involvement but there was tumor infiltration of intrapulmonary nodes. Their series consisted of 54 patients treated by lobectomy with a margin of 1.5 to 2 cm beyond visible carcinoma, mostly right upper lobe lesions. The advantage of preservation of the middle and lower lobes is quoted as the main benefit derived from the procedure. Occasionally, sleeve resections of the pulmonary artery were combined with the bronchoplastic procedure. The patients were selected on the basis of limited tumor shown on body section x-rays, bronchoscopic examination, mediastinal biopsies, and also on the basis of their general medical and pulmonary functions. With the presence of significant hilar node involvement or known mediastinal involvement from mediastinoscopy, a limited bronchoplastic procedure was felt to be contraindicated.

Twenty-two of their 54 patients had lymph node involvement. A 4-year survival of 39% was achieved. It should be emphasized that these patients frequently underwent preoperative radiation therapy of about 3000 to 4000 rads for 3 to 4 weeks. Similar results, however, have been reported with sleeve resection in the absence of preoperative radiation therapy by Rees and Paneth[30] and Jensik et al.[15] in selected patients. The importance of frozen section microscopy to determine margins of resection in the operating room was emphasized by Hansen.[13]

Extended procedures involving the heart and great blood vessels, the thoracic wall, and the pleura have been described in an attempt to develop curative procedures that involve resection of major portions of the thorax. The treatment of tumors involving the thoracic wall by thoracoplasty and bronchoplastic procedures was reported by Geha et al.[11] in 41 patients with en bloc resection with thoracoplasty. Twelve of these patients survived 5 years. The survival rate ranged from 60% for adenocarcinoma to 10% for large cell undifferentiated carcinoma. Successful removal of the intrathoracic trachea, carina, and main stem bronchi with subsequent replacement by a molded silastic prosthesis has been described in one long-term survivor.[25]

The difficulties in extending operability in lung cancer to the heart and great vessels has been discussed by Bailey et al.[1] The use of an extracorporeal bypass of the cardiopulmonary system has been suggested, but only 3 patients have been reported in the literature who survived this procedure indicating that such procedures are not likely to be accepted as routine treatment of cancer of the lung.

In view of the rising incidence of lun the older population, patients with l quently are 70 years of age or older. patients reported upon by Golebiowski that with careful preoperative workup anu uperative anu postoperative management as well as appropriate treatment of complicating conditions, pulmonary resection may be carried out without undue mortality. Plested et al.[29] were able to show that initial excisional biopsy of a solitary pulmonary nodule does not jeopardize the prognosis in patients who later undergo lobectomy or pneumonectomy. In these authors' hands, 131 patients with solitary pulmonary nodules were diagnosed by wedge resection or by subsegmental anatomic resection, if there were nodules 3 cm or less in diameter. The excisional biopsies were followed by lobectomy or pneumonectomy when the pathologic diagnosis was established. The 5-year survival in 76 patients thus treated was 62%, compared to a 5-year survival of 40% among 54 patients who were initially treated by lobectomy and pneumonectomy.

PROGNOSTIC FACTORS IN THE SURGICAL TREATMENT OF CANCER OF THE LUNG

The evidence from information obtained at the Sloan-Kettering Memorial Cancer Center[36] and from the National Institutes of Health[8] indicates that the female sex has a better survival than the male sex following surgical treatment of lung cancer. This is based on the better survival in patients with adenocarcinoma among whom women predominate, whereas the survival rate among the epidermoid carcinoma is approximately equal between female and male patients.[33] The average age of patients surviving lung cancer is younger than that of patients who die of their tumor, especially female patients. In the Memorial Hospital series the median age for female patients surviving 10 years after treatment of lung cancer was 39.5 years, and for males 55.7. The median age of all patients seen at Memorial Hospital was 57.2 years for women, and 59.4 years for men.

The relationship between cell type and prognosis has been evaluated by Rienhoff et al.,[31] who reported on 550 cases of lung cancer treated surgically at Johns Hopkins Hospital between 1933 and 1958. Survival in bronchiolo-alveolar carcinoma was 87% at 5 years, whereas that for adenocarcinoma was 25% and for squamous cell carcinoma 21%. Patients with undifferentiated carcinoma, including large and small cell types, had a 5-year survival of 7%. Similar figures were reported in a review by Lee.[18] In addition to lymph node involvement referred to previously, blood vessel invasion is a significant factor in prognosis. If both lymph nodes and blood vessels were free of tumor involvement, a 5-year survival of 50% was obtained by Rienhoff and co-workers, but a group of patients in whom both of these factors were positive had a 5-year survival of only 13%. The site of origin of the tumor may have some influence on the prognosis, with a 5-year survival rate for tumors originating from the left lung at 36%, higher than for those originating from the right lung with 30%. Although these data from the Memorial Hospital series are not statistically significant, at the American Oncologic Hospital the 5-year survival of patients treated by radiation therapy was 2.5% for right-sided lesions, and 8% for left-sided lesions. The Memorial Hospital series also suggested that upper lobe lesions have a better prognosis than lower lobe lesions, a fact which could not be substantiated from the American Oncologic Hospital data. The stage of the patient's tumor determines the prognosis, as shown by Mountain et al.[22] (see page 118).

Closely related to the staging is the size of the primary lesion. Jackman et al.[14] and Steele and Buell[5,32] analyzed 478 patients whose pathology included squamous cell carcinoma, adenocarcinoma, and undifferentiated carcinoma; there were no patients with oat cell carcinoma. In patients with lesions under 2 cm in diameter the 5-year survival was 68% and 57% respectively, whereas 2 to 4 cm lesions produced a 5-year survival of 43.5% and 42%. For the larger lesions measuring 4 to 6 cm diameter in Steele's report, a 5-year survival of 32% was obtained. This explains the fact that results of lobectomies have revealed superior 5-year survivals (25 to 35%) when compared to those in pneumonectomies (12 to 26%). Since lobectomies are frequently performed for smaller tumors, the more limited operation is done on more favorable patient material. Stoloff[34] reported that of 132 patients whose tumor was located in a main stem bronchus and biopsied by bronchoscopy only 1 survived for 1 year. The 5-year survival in patients without involvement of the main stem bronchus but with involvement of a peripheral bronchi was 13% of 728 patients.

The causes of death for 5- and 10-year survivors were analyzed by Watson.[36] A common cause of death was cardiovascular complication, possibly a combination of factors of the age of the patient with compensatory emphysema, pulmonary fibrosis, cor pulmonale, and pulmonary hypertension. On the other hand, 23% of 61 five-year survivors and 14% of 56 ten-year survivors had a recurrence of lung cancer. Surgery is expected to fail to control the tumor in the hemithorax operated upon in 42% of the patients.[17] This has led to adjunct treatment in the form of postoperative and preoperative radiation therapy as well as chemotherapy which is discussed elsewhere in this book.

Closely related is the presence or absence of symptoms prior to diagnosis and treatment of lung cancer. The smaller the lesion in the lung, the smaller the likelihood of symptoms, thus correlating size and symptomatology in cancer of the lung. This relationship to survival has been emphasized by Berndt[3] who reported 12.5% five-year survivors among 183 patients who were asymptomatic at the time of diagnosis as compared to 6.0% among the 1747 patients who had symptoms.

A significant relationship exists between growth rate and survival after surgical treatment of lung cancer.[37] Among 19 patients, a rapid growth rate with doubling times between 1.8 and 3.9 months yielded an average survival of 26 months, whereas patients with tumors of slow growth rates (6.7 to 10.0 months doubling time) had an average survival of 54 months.

In summary one can quote Boyd[4] who stated: "When resection can be achieved in any bronchogenic carcinoma characterized by a long history, it is justified and operability should be pushed to the ultimate level of safety. For all others, which are unfortunately the majority of cases seen in practice, lobectomy is as effective as extended resection and much safer." Boyd was referring to epidermoid carcinomas without gross involvement of lymph nodes on preoperative evaluation. A judicious set of indications for lobectomy and pneumonectomy, possibly associated with lymph node dissections, will balance and bring out in the patient's favor the contradictory events of decreased life expectancy because of the surgical procedure as compared to the increased life expectancy if the tumor can be effectively treated. The fact that so many different surgical procedures and adjunct measures such as radiotherapy and chemotherapy are being used in the treatment of lung cancer indicates that no one optimal treatment has yet been found. The prognosis for the patient with lung cancer with a small peripheral epidermoid carcinoma is relatively good but deteriorates rapidly as the disease progresses, with successive increase in size of the local lesion, involvement of mediastinal lymph nodes and, finally, dissemination of the tumor to extrathoracic and distant metastatic sites. Although on the whole a limited improvement in survival rates of patients with lung cancer may be expected from the efforts previously described with reference to early detection, it is probable that more drastic measures, such as limitation of smoking and air pollution will be necessary to decrease the impact of this disease on the entire population. Until such time when cancer of the lung becomes a rare disease, in the opinion of those intimately involved in the management of patients with lung cancer a logical progression of staging procedures is necessary to define the extent of the patient's disease prior to initiation of treatment. There also should be a logical system of possible adjunct measures. If hard data are not available, the treatment should be decided on the basis of known data and experience. If other facts are obtained, the treatment may have to be altered to a significant degree.

Although surgical treatment provides the best available therapy for patients with lung cancer at the present time, a significant number of patients can be treated effectively by other means, especially radiation therapy. Such treatment should be directed toward permanent control of the primary tumor, possibly defined as cure,

if it is possible or probable that this can be achieved with an acceptable rate of complications. On the other hand, patients with lung cancer may be expected to live for prolonged periods of time even though the chance of cure is very small. These patients benefit from treatment directed toward their symptoms and the control of significant present or foreseeable effects of the tumor on their health as well as their social and economic circumstances. Radiation therapy is one of the more significant treatment methods used in patients who are ineligible for curative surgical resection.

REFERENCES

1. Bailey, C. P., Schechter, D. C., and Folk, F. S.: Extending operability in lung cancer involving the heart and great vessels. *Ann. Thorac. Surg.* **11**:140–150, 1971.

2. Beattie, E. J., and Martini, N.: Extended radical surgery for lung cancer. *Proc. Sixth Natl. Cancer Conf.*, Lippincott, Philadelphia, 1970.

3. Berndt, H.: Results of treatment of accidentally discovered and symptomless bronchial carcinomas. *Dtsch. Med. Wochenschr.* **94**:1559, 1969.

4. Boyd, D.: Is extending radical resection superior to lobectomy in treating resectable bronchial cancer? *J. A. M. A.* **195**:15, 1966.

5. Buell, P. E.: Importance of tumor size in prognosis for resected bronchogenic carcinoma. *J. Surg. Oncol.* **3**:539–551, 1971.

6. Cahan, W. G., and Beattie, E. J.: Lymph node dissections in lung cancer. *Clin. Bull. Memorial Sloan-Kettering Cancer Cent.* **2**:123–126, 1972.

7. Cliffton, E. E., and Luomanen, R. K. J.: Surgical treatment. In *Lung Cancer*, C. V. Mosby, St. Louis, 1968.

8. Connelly, R. R., Cutler, S. J., and Baylis, P.: End results in cancer of the lung: comparison of male and female patients. *J. Natl. Cancer Inst.* **36**:277–287, 1966.

9. Delarue, N. G., Sanders, D. E., and Silverberg, S. A.: Complementary value of pulmonary angiography and mediastinoscopy in individualizing treatment for patients with lung cancer. *Cancer* **26**:1370–1378, 1970.

10. Dillon, M. L., and Postlethwait, R. W.: Carcinoma of the lung. *Ann. Thorac. Surg.* **11**:193–200, 1971.

11. Geha, A. S., Bernatz, P. E., and Woolner, L. B.: Bronchogenic carcinoma involving the thoracic wall: Surgical treatment and prognostic significance. *J. Thorac. Cardiovasc. Surg.* **54**:394–402, 1967.

12. Golebiowski, A.: Pulmonary resection in patients over 70 years of age. *J. Thorac. Cardiovasc. Surg.* **61**:265–270, 1971.

13. Hansen, J. L.: Frozen section microscopy of the bronchial stump in surgery for cancer in the lung. *Acta Pathol. Microbiol. Scand.* **212**:112–113, 1970.

14. Jackman, R. J., Good, A., Clagett, O. T., and Woolner, L.: Survival rates in peripheral bronchogenic carcinoma four centimeters in diameter presenting as solitary pulmonary nodules. *J. Thorac. Cardiovasc. Surg.* **57**:1–8, 1969.

15. Jensik, R. J., Faber, L., Milloy, F. J., and Amato, J. J.: Sleeve lobectomy for carcinoma: a ten year experience. *J. Thorac. Cardiovasc. Surg.* **64**:400–412, 1972.

16. Kato, Y., Ferguson, T. B., Bennett, D. E., and Burford, T. H.: Oat cell carcinoma of the lung. A review of 138 cases. *Cancer* **23**:517–524, 1969.

17. Kern, W. H., Jones, J. C., and Chapman, N. D.: Pathology of bronchogenic carcinoma in long-term survivors *Cancer* **21**:772–780, 1968.

18. Lee, Yeu-tsu: Prognostic factors in surgical treatment of bronchogenic carcinoma. *Surg. Gynecol. Obstet.* **135**:961–975, 1972.

19. Lennox, S. C., Flavell, G., Pollock, D. J., Thompson, V. C., and Wilkins, J. L.: Results of resection for oat cell carcinoma of the lung. *Lancet* **2**:925–927, 1968.

20. Le Roux, B. Y.: Management of bronchial carcinoma by segmental resection *Thorax* **27**:70–74, 1972.

21. Miller, R. D.: Preoperative Pulmonary Evaluation of the Dyspneic Surgical Candidate. *Surg. Clin. North Am.* **53**:805–812, 1973.

22. Mountain, C. F., Carr, D. T., and Anderson, W. A. D.: A system for the clinical staging of lung cancer. *Am. J. Roentgenol. Radium Ther. Nucl. Med.* **120**:130–138, 1974.

23. Mountain, C. F. L.: Surgical therapy. In *Lung Cancer: Biologic, Physiologic and Technical Determinates*. Semin. Oncol. **1**:253–258, 1974.

24. Nealon, T. F.: Choice of operation and technique for cancer of the lung. *Proc. Sixth Natl. Cancer. Conf.*, Lippincott, Philadelphia, 1970.

25. Neville, W. E., Hamouda, F., Anderson, J., and Dwan, F. M.: Replacement of the intrathoracic trachea and both stem bronchi with a molded silastic prothesis. *J. Thorac. Cardiovasc. Surg.* **63**:569–576, 1972.

26. Overholt, R. H., Oliynyk, P. N., and Cady, B.: The current status of primary carcinoma of the lung. *Prog. Clin. Cancer* **4**:211–222, 1970.

27. Paulson, L.: Philosophy of treatment for bronchogenic carcinoma *Ann. Thorac. Surg.* **5**:289–299, 1968.

28. Paulson, D. L., Urschel, H. C., McNamara, J. J., and Shaw, R. R.: Bronchoplastic procedures for bronchogenic carcinoma. *J. Thorac. Cardiovasc. Surg.* **59**:38–48, 1970.

29. Plested, W. G., Miller, T. A., Steele, J. D., and Buell, P.: Influence on survival of excisional biopsy preceding lobectomy or pneumonectomy for primary bronchogenic carcinomas presenting as solitary nodules. *Ann. Thorac. Surg.* **7**:486–490, 1969.

30. Rees, G. M., and Paneth, M.: Lobectomy with sleeve resection in the treatment of bronchial tumours. *Thorax* **25**:160–164, 1970.

31. Rienhoff, W. F., Taalbert, G. A., and Wood, S.: Bronchogenic

carcinoma: a study of cases treated at Johns Hopkins Hospital from 1933 to 1958. *Ann. Surg.* **161**:674–687, 1965,

32. Steele, J. D., and Buell, P.: A symptomatic solitary pulmonary nodule. Host survival, tumor size, and growth rate. *J. Thorac. Cardiovasc. Surg.* **65**:140–151, 1973.

33. Steensberg, J.: Survival in males with surgically treated localized cancer of the lung. *Cancer* **22**:1–7, 1968.

34. Stoloff, I. L.: The prognostic value of bronchoscopy in primary lung cancer. *J. A. M. A.* **227**:299–301, 1974.

35. Tarhan, S., and Moffitt, E. A.: Principles of thoracic anesthesia. *Surg. Clin. North Am.* **53**:813–817, 1973.

36. Watson, W. L.: *Lung Cancer,* C. V. Mosby, St. Louis, 1968.

37. Weiss, W., Boucot, K. R., and Cooper, D. A.: Survival of men with peripheral lung cancer in relation to histologic characteristics and growth rate. *Am. Rev. Respir. Dis.* **98**:75–86, 1968.

Chapter Fourteen

"Curative"
Radiation Therapy

External beam radiation therapy for inoperable cancer to cure a patient of his tumor has depended largely on the design machines that produce beams of ionizing radiation which make it possible to deliver a high amount of radiation in the thoracic cavity. Thus it is not surprising that one of the first large series of roentgen therapy for cancer of the lung was published as recently as 1940.[18] In the discussion of this paper, Dr. Maurice Lenz of New York stated that in the past vigorous irradiation was considered impractical in cases of inoperable lung cancer because of the concomitant injury to large volumes of normal lung tissue which had to be included in the treatment portals. Added to this was the danger of empyema if an abscess cavity was associated with the cancer, especially if it was situated in an atelectatic lobe. The dosage administered in bronchogenic carcinoma had been much less than that proven adequate for similar carcinomas in more accessible locations, and Dr. Lenz felt that the entire dose should be administered in a single course of treatment, since the so-called "retrogressive changes in the normal tissues" following irradiation made administration of adequate x-ray dosages impossible at a later time.

The authors classified their treatment technique as moderate if treatment was administered with anterior and posterior mediastinal fields using x-ray equipment as 135 kV with 560 R delivered in 20 minutes, while "massive technique" was delivered using cross-firing pairs of anterior and posterior thoracic fields, at 200 kV with 560 R delivered in 20 minutes. "Fractional treatment" was given with the factors for massive treatment, but with fewer minutes per treatment, up to the same total dose. A fourth method of protracted fractionation was given using 4 to 6 fields at 200 kV at 50 cm TSD with a Thoraeus filter giving 150 to 200 R per field for a total dose of 2000 to 3000 R.

The authors divided a group of 250 patients with inoperable bronchogenic carcinoma into equal numbers; half were treated by x-ray therapy and the other half by conservative measures only. The groups were equally divided by grade of epidermoid carcinoma or adenocarcinoma, extent of the disease, and location of the primary tumor in the lung. Approximately 50% of the patients under radiotherapy received treatment with a single course, massive dose. The remainder received two or more courses of fractional technique, but only 4 patients were treated by the so-called protracted fractional method.

Of the treated group of patients, 25 (20%) survived 1 year, whereas only 3 patients lived a year or more without specific treatment after histologic proof of diagnosis. Of the patients who underwent some form of x-ray therapy, 30% died within 4 months of relentlessly progressive cancer. On the other hand, there were 6 patients who survived 4 years or more, and 5 who survived 5 years or more. The longest survivor lived for 146 months after treatment. It is of interest that all the survivors had adenocarcinomas of various grades, which were located in the right lung. They were equally divided among male and female patients. Most received a single course of treatment, but 1 patient received seven courses. The conclusions from this early work were summarized by Dr. Lenz, who stated: "that such carefully substantiated study as set forth by Drs. Leddy and Moersch will hopefully convince the clinician of the importance of sending earlier cases of carcinoma of the lung for roentgen therapy, and this offers the only hope for improvement in therapeutic results."

The rapid advances in radiotherapeutic technology following World War II have led to an elaborate bibliography dealing with curative radiation therapy of lung cancer. Unfortunately, even in recent large series of patients with radical radiotherapy for inoperable lung cancer, only a slight improvement in survival has been achieved since Leddy and Moersch first published their 10% 5-year survival study.

A philosophy of curative x-ray treatment for bronchogenic carcinoma may be based on some of the experience gained during trials of preoperative radiation therapy followed by surgery. In an early trial using orthovoltage x-ray therapy preoperatively for 4700 rads average dose, Bromley and Szur[6] demonstrated that 40% of the primary tumors were controlled by this type of radiotherapy. Bloedorn[3] and Mallams et al.[20] also showed that approximately 35% of the primary tumors treated by supervoltage x-ray for 3000 to 6000 rads could be controlled locally. In an autopsy series of patients treated by radiotherapy,[28] no residual tumor was found in 18 of 60 patients (30%) with all histologic groups of lung cancer. Microscopic foci of cancer occurred in 23%, and viable gross tumor in 47% after 4800 to 6250 rads tumor dose. All patients had assessment of their tumor size before treatment.

We have used the following indications for curative supervoltage radiation therapy of lung cancer:

1. Technically operable disease, usually localized tumor, in patients with medical contraindications to surgery such as recent coronary infarctions, and other reasons for increased surgical risk.

2. Locally advanced bronchogenic carcinoma involving one lung, either because of large size, extension of the tumor to the mediastinum, or involvement of mediastinal lymph nodes or hilar adenopathy.

3. Oat cell carcinoma, if limited to one lung and the homolateral mediastinal lymph nodes.

4. Patients with unilateral lesions with vocal cord or phrenic nerve paralysis.

5. Patients with supraclavicular metastasis with limited tumor in the lung, when a nonpalpable supraclavicular node is proven by biopsy and involved with malignancy.

6. Patients with limited tumor localized in one lung, and Horner's syndrome.

7. Patients with unilateral tumor growing to within 1 cm or less of the carina.

Contraindications to curative radiation therapy are the following:

1. Distant extrathoracic metastasis, such as bone involvement, excluding limited bone involvement in contiguity with superior sulcus tumors.
2. Pleural effusion positive for malignant cells.
3. Bilateral pulmonary or mediastinal involvement.
4. Multiple unilateral pulmonary lesions.
5. Bronchoesophageal fistula or sinus tract.
6. Coexisting life-threatening second malignancy.
7. Severe respiratory disability.

The workup must include studies which confirm that the tumor is limited to the lung and mediastinum. Aside from chest x-ray and tomogram of the lesion, the following may be necessary: tomograms of both lungs, liver function studies and liver scan, brain scan, bone survey and/or bone scan. X-rays should be obtained of all symptomatic areas that suggest the presence of bone metastasis, even if they are associated with a fairly long history of pain. A biopsy of palpable and clinically significant lymph nodes should be performed, especially if they are located in the axilla, neck, or supraclavicular region. It is best to proceed on the assumption that any symptoms may be related to bronchogenic carcinoma, and must be proven to be due to an associated nonmalignant disease.

Since patient selection is as important in curative radiation therapy as it is in surgical curative resection in lung cancer, treatment should not be undertaken before pertinent studies for staging of the patient's disease are completed. It is then necessary to define the target volume to be treated, the dose to be delivered to known areas of involvement and also to suspected lymph nodes or likely areas of extension, and to design a treatment plan in which normal tissue tolerance limits will not be exceeded. Since pulmonary function is always interfered with if an adequate dose of radiation therapy is given, pulmonary function tests should precede the decision regarding treatment whenever any type of pulmonary respiratory disease is present or suspected. From the radiation therapist's point of view, bronchogenic carcinoma should

be divided into three anatomic groups, all of which require a different therapeutic approach.

1. Peripheral lesions. These lesions occasionally appear as "coin" lesions and are usually solitary masses of variable size entirely surrounded by lung tissue. Occasionally, they abut the parietal pleura. For epidermoid carcinoma, the incidence of mediastinal lymph node metastasis increases from about 25 to 50% as the tumor size increases from about 2 to about 10 cm. In anaplastic carcinoma these lesions are very rare, since most of them present as relatively large lesions or with mediastinal adenopathy, which occurs in 90% or more of these tumors. Adenocarcinoma shows lymph node involvement in approximately the same percentage as epidermoid carcinoma. Bronchioloalveolar carcinoma may present in this fashion, occasionally with multiple lesions, and lymph node involvement with this histology is quite rare occuring in approximately 10 to 15% of cases.

2. Hilar and parahilar lesions. This is one of the commonest manifestations of bronchogenic carcinoma, reported in up to 75% of some series.[4] The lesions usually originate from main stem bronchi, frequently obstruct the bronchus, and grow around the hilum into the mediastinum. Lymph node metastasis are present in 60 to 70% of patients with epidermoid carcinoma and adenocarcinoma; they are always involved in patients with oat cell carcinoma. The mass is frequently difficult to separate radiographically from the mediastinum, and the primary tumor and the mediastinal adenopathy may form a single tumor mass which is attached to normal mediastinal structures. Atelectasis, partial or complete, may be present.

3. Apical location. Apical lung tumors form a separate group because of their anatomic location and because of certain clinical features. They are generally epidermoid carcinomas of a low grade of differentiation with a relatively slow growth rate and relatively low incidence of metastasis.[24] The tumors are often described as superior sulcus tumors because they arise in a vestigial fissure formed during the embryologic development of the right upper lobe of the lung because of migration of the azygos vein. The clinical syndrome which was first described by Pancoast[23] and carries his name consists of severe pain in the shoulder along the ulnar nerve distribution because of involvement of the nerve roots of segments C8 and D1, together with x-ray evidence of a tumor in the apex of the lung with or without bone destruction, and Horner's syndrome. This syndrome is characterized by: drooping of the upper eyelid, exophthalmus, myosis, and loss of perspiration of the affected side because of tumor involvement of the cervical sympathetic chain. Epidermoid carcinoma predominates

among the histologic diagnosis, and involvement of mediastinal lymph nodes occurs in approximately 30% of cases.

The technique of radiation therapy varies with this anatomic classification. Treatment should not be initiated until at least one week has elapsed since surgery and healing of any surgical incisions is progressing well, preferably with removal of sutures. Associated infections, such as abscess and/or tuberculosis should be treated aggressively by appropriate antibiotic therapy, and the patient should have near normal temperature.

Adequate treatment planning is necessary to achieve maximum benefit from treatment, and portal localizing films are indispensable. They are obtained on a radiographic unit which permits exact duplication of the treatment setup. The exact source or target skin distance and positioning of the radiographic tube around the patient to duplicate treatment procedures are necessary. The collimator of the diagnostic x-ray unit should be of good quality and define the field size accurately. A field-size scale for the treatment distance is necessary.

If a supervoltage unit is used for localizing purposes, special cassettes are required to supply optimum detail especially if sources of large diameters are used in cobalt irradiators. We have found that cardboard cassettes lined with 1/8 inch of lead and using Kodak M industrial film will produce acceptable localizing x-rays with reference to differences in density between air and soft tissue and bone, although they are inferior in quality to those obtained with a diagnostic x-ray unit. Linear accelerators produce an x-ray beam of high megavoltage, and the smaller target may produce radiographs for localizing purposes that are almost equal to those obtained with a radiographic tube. (For examples of localizing films, see Figs. 1,2,3.)

It is necessary to have a good system of treatment that will make it possible to duplicate portal setups from day to day on the treatment table. This involves both clear identification of the portal markings on the patient's skin, using a marking ink such as Castellani's tincture applied with a thin marking aid such as the wooden part of a Q-tip. Portal setups should be made so that the entire marking is seen in the light beam localizer of the therapy machine. This allows for closed-circuit television monitoring of the setup with appropriate sensitive lenses from outside the room, using only the localizing light for illumination.

Immobilization is extremely important. It has been our custom to treat all patients supine, since the mobility of the skin of the posterior thorax makes exact opposition of anteroposterior and posteroanterior portal markings very difficult. Treatment with the patient supine

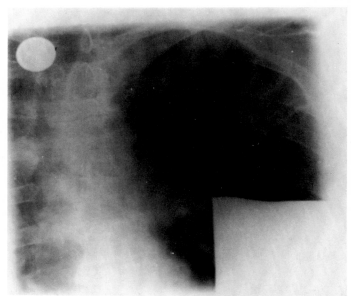

Fig. 1.   Patient W. W. (See Figure 19). Localizing film for parallel opposing cobalt teletherapy portal for a peripheral epidermoid carcinoma. This was treated to 4500 rads in 4½ weeks.

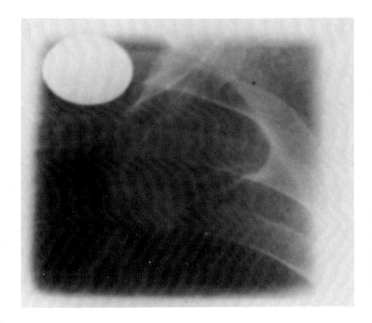

Fig. 2.   Small field to the peripheral lung tumor only which was treated to 6000 rads total tumor dose by parallel opposing portals.

requires an opening in the tabletop of the therapy machine, to allow maximum utilization of the skin-sparing effect of the supervoltage equipment that should be used in all patients eligible for curative radiation therapy. Most manufacturers now provide a tabletop which contains an opening large enough to accept most portals

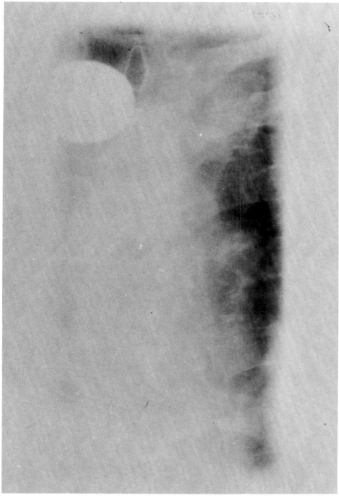

Fig. 3. Small field for the mediastinum, treated by lateral arc rotation to 6000 rads total tumor dose at the mediastinum.

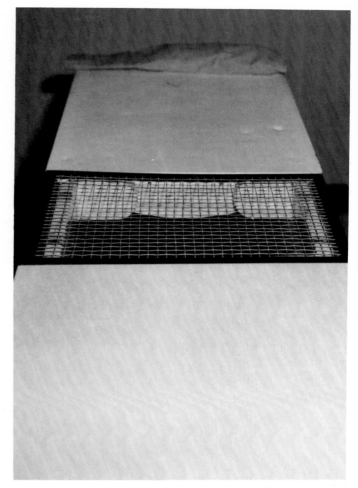

Fig. 4. Table top with tennis racket type opening for treatment of posterior portals with the patient in the supine position.

used in treatment of lung cancer, and is usually covered with an aluminum grid or tennis racket type of support (Fig. 4). Patients may be treated through the table, however, skin reaction will be significant especially if high doses are necessary in the maximum area of each beam and modification of treatment techniques may be necessary to avoid moist desquamation. Immobilization should be arranged by having the patient comfortable and flat, using sandbags if necessary, especially if kyphosis or other skeletal abnormalities make it difficult for the patient to stay in the supine position for prolonged periods. The position of the arms and hands should be well defined, and in our department the usual position of the hands is on the iliac crest anteriorly, so that a standard treatment position is used in all patients. Although it is not necessary in all patients treated for bronchogenic carcinoma, immobilization of the head by head clamps or other devices is often useful. The central axis beam and the outline of the portal should be indicated, as this will lead to a more rapid setup and establishment of the source skin distance.

When cobalt irradiators are employed, secondary blocking should always be used to minimize the penumbra. In most collimators of the John's type, penumbra trimmers can be extended for rectangular fields.

Techniques should be directed toward optimal protection of vital normal tissues. In the treatment of bronchogenic carcinoma these include lung, spinal cord and, probably, pericardium and heart. If a cobalt irradiator is used for treatment, it should have a source skin distance of 70 cm or more. Field-shaping can be achieved using lead blocks obtained commercially or homemade, which should be at least 5 cm in thickness for less than 3% transmission. A suitable arrangement for a widely used cobalt teletherapy machine is shown in Figure 5.

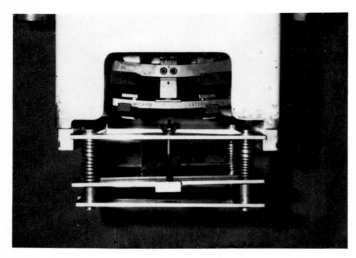

Fig. 5. Secondary blocking in place on a cobalt teletherapy machine. Secondary blocking may also be achieved by the trimmer bars incorporated into the collimator.

For treatment under the table it is necessary to reverse the orientation of the blocks, and a device has been manufactured which will make such treatment possible

(Fig. 6). Penumbra trimmer bars are part of the collimator assembly in most modern teletherapy machines.

Localization carefully duplicates the geometric relationship for the treatment setup. For small changes in field size in relation to the lesion on the x-ray we have found a lead-marked plate on the skin surface useful because it gives a magnification factor at the skin level for changes in the portal arrangement.

For rotation therapy, films must be obtained in orthogonal projections at right angles, and most teletherapy machines lend themselves to use of the table height for day-to-day treatment. The table height is the distance between the tabletop and the center of rotation. In order to obtain the table height from lateral localizing films, a bridge has been designed that allows intrapolation even if the table height is not set exactly at the desired elevation above the tabletop in the first localizing film (Figs. 7,8).

Dose calculations can be made from central axis beam tables; however, they are more accurate if isodoses are obtained especially if any significant degree of field-shaping is entered into. At present it is very difficult to deal with the lack of absorption in lung tissue. This effect is significantly higher for peripheral lesions sur-

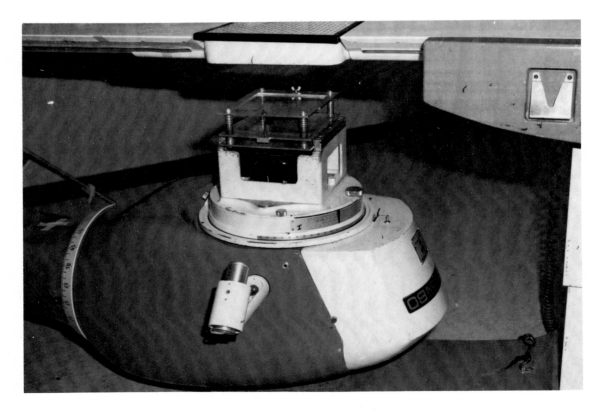

Fig. 6. Device which allows posterior treatment of the patient in the supine position from skin markings on the anterior chest wall. The blocks are set up according to skin markings with the field shaping device anterior to the patient.

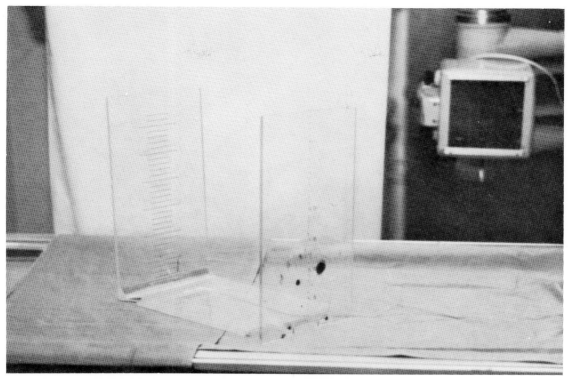

Fig. 7. Table height indicator for localization of lateral or rotation portals. This accurately describes the table height. A marking on the patient's skin, the collimator setting on the machine, and the table height on the treatment couch define the treatment parameters.

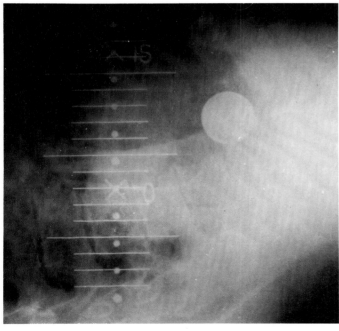

Fig. 8. Lateral table height indicated in a localizing film for rotational treatment of the mediastinum for bronchogenic carcinoma (Table height equals $(10+8)/2=9$ cm).

rounded entirely by normal lung and less so for massive tumors involving the mediastinum, where little lung is transversed by the treatment beam in the central axis position. Computer programs that would account for tissue inhomogeneity require a transverse tomographic unity with transfer of the areas of solid tissue and lung for isodose construction. Even with this aid, it is necessary to perform isodoses in multiple planes to account for the three-dimensional distribution of solid tissue versus lung. Because of all these difficulties, we have disregarded the difference in dose as not being significant so long as appropriate caution is used in evaluating the patient's pulmonary function prior to treatment.

Weekly verification films are necessary to be certain that treatment from day to day and week to week is carried out exactly as planned. The use of Dupont imaging film, or of a similar film of low sensitivity, makes it possible to expose the film in the treatment position during the actual radiation therapy with adequate detail to ascertain that treatment conditions are as planned. Occasionally patients may lose or gain weight, and it may be necessary to recalculate the dose because of changes in physical measurements.

Clinical examination should be carried out weekly

during the course of treatment, especially with reference to changes in the motility of the vocal cords, appearance of palpable adenopathy in the supraclavicular or axillary areas or in the mediastinum, and bone pain or hepatomegaly. Temperature should be obtained routinely, and appropriate antibiotic management must be instituted following culture of the sputum if infection is a problem. It is well to remember that a major cause of death in patients with bronchogenic carcinoma is overwhelming infection.

Chest x-rays should be repeated at least once during the course of the patient's radiation therapy, unless the patient has specific symptoms or x-ray findings that require more frequent studies. As a rule, we obtain chest x-rays in patients treated for cure when 4000 rads have been delivered. This occurs approximately one month following initiation of treatment, and will indicate any significant changes in the radiographic appearance of the tumor; it also permits evaluation of treatment effect at this dose level in a consistent form. If patients have evidence of atelectasis, an x-ray is also obtained at 2000 rads, with the aim of modifying the treatment technique by reducing field size.

Follow-up examinations should be frequent during the first year after treatment, including chest x-rays at least every 3 months initially, and every 6 months thereafter. Other studies are usually obtained on the basis of clinical symptoms or changes in findings on clinical examination, such as hepatomegaly or neurologic symptoms indicating the likelihood of brain metastasis. Bone pain

is also a frequent symptom that indicates the need for additional radiographic or nuclear imaging studies.

Follow-up examinations should include a physical examination that includes indirect laryngoscopy, palpation of the lymph nodes, and abdominal palpation for hepatomegaly. It is especially important to follow the larynx carefully because of an increased incidence of cancer of the vocal cords and other parts of the larynx in patients whose bronchogenic cancer has been arrested for a long time. Pulmonary function studies should be performed as indicated especially in patients with decreased pulmonary function, to avoid acute problems of respiratory decompensation or cardiovascular complications due to decreased pulmonary reserve. If the patient has no significant symptoms, no specific medication is indicated. We have not practiced prophylactic use of corticosteroid medication to delay the onset of pulmonary fibrosis secondary to radiation therapy.

TECHNIQUE OF RADICAL RADIATION THERAPY AT THE AMERICAN ONCOLOGIC HOSPITAL

Peripheral Tumors, Epidermoid and Adenocarcinoma

This group of tumors includes all tumors in the periphery of the lung, surrounded by at least 2 cm of lung tissue and separated from mediastinal and chest wall structures. Treatment is administered to the primary tumor and the mediastinum at least 5 cm below the carina if the lesion is located in the upper lobes, and at least 8 cm below the carina or to a level 2 cm below the lowermost extension of the tumor in the periphery of the lung, if the tumor is located in the middle or lower lobes of the lung. Parallel opposing portals are used, with field-shaping to treat the mediastinum with at least 8 cm in width and with a minimum 2 cm margin around the radiographically visible primary tumor in the periphery of the lung. 4500 rads are delivered in a period of 5 weeks, usually treating both portals daily 5 times a week.

On the basis of the chest x-ray obtained at 4000 rads, a field-size reduction is designed to treat the residual tumor with a 1 cm margin and known mediastinal adenopathy with an additional 1500 rads in 10 treatments. Generally, it is possible to design a suitable treatment plan using lateral arc rotation, which allows one to spare the opposite lung as well as the spinal cord and to include known metastatic disease in the mediastinum and the primary tumor in the same portal. If there is no known metastatic disease in the mediastinum, only the primary tumor will be treated. If a rotation arrangement is impossible or cannot be used because of the location of the tumor, parallel opposing portals

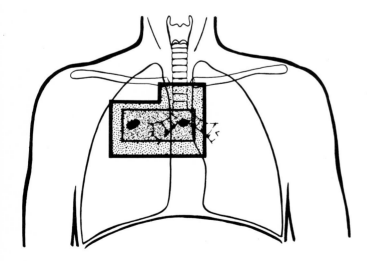

Fig. 9. Schematic of radiotherapy treatment planning for peripheral lung lesions. The mediastinum and primary tumor are treated en bloc to 4500 rads with a large field using parallel opposing technique. A small field is then given to known areas of disease carrying the tumor dose to 6000 rads with a technique which will avoid excessive irradiation of the spinal cord. (Courtesy Lea and Febiger.)

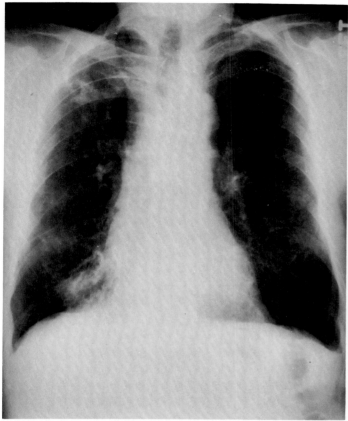

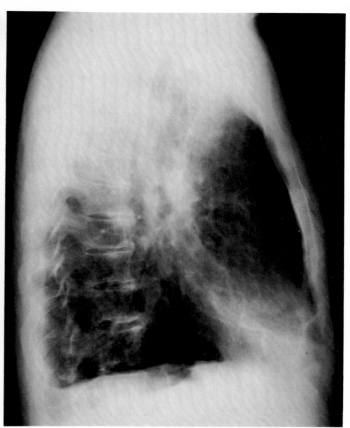

Fig. 10. Patient J. G. Chest x-rays revealing evidence of epidermoid carcinoma of the right upper lobe with mediastinal mass. The patient also has chronic pulmonary disease.

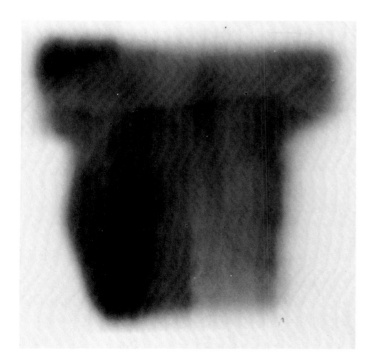

Fig. 11. Localizing film for this patient's treatment plan encompassing the primary tumor, hilar mass and mediastinum.

angled away from the spinal cord will be used. The dose is calculated as a minimum dose to the known areas of involvement. The treatment of the primary tumor and the mediastinum is supplemented by supraclavicular irradiation, if mediastinal lymph nodes have been proven on biopsy or if the supraclavicular nodes are involved. An anterior portal for the supraclavicular area is used, extending from the midclavicle to the lower margin of the thyroid cartilage, with shielding of 2.5 cm width to within 3 cm of the sternal notch. This portal is separated from the mediastinal portal by 0.5 cm for a cobalt irradiator. Treatment is given at the same time as that for the primary tumor and the mediastinum to a dose of 5000 rads delivered in 4 weeks. An additional 1000 to 2000 rads are given with a small field to the known areas of involvement or the area of excision. If neither of these circumstances prevails, no small field or additional treatment is administered.

Hilar and Perihilar Tumors, Epidermoid and Adenocarcinoma

The approach to the treatment of the mediastinum and primary tumor in the immediately adjacent region is

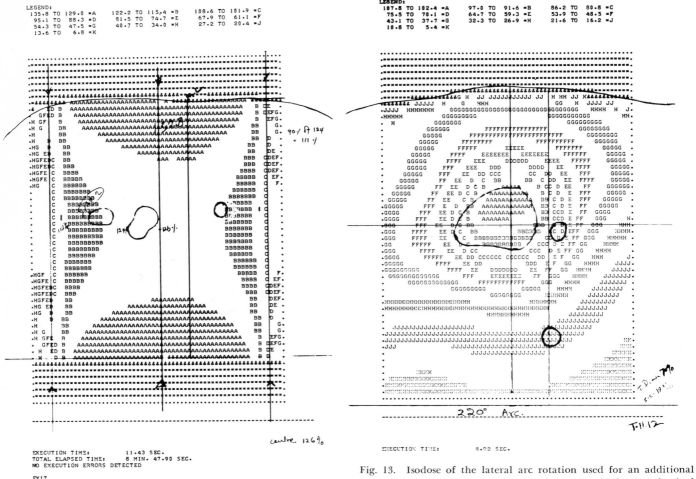

Fig. 12. Computer isodose of the dose distribution using cobalt tele-therapy for a tumor dose of 4500 rads in 5 weeks. Tumor and mediastinum are indicated.

Fig. 13. Isodose of the lateral arc rotation used for an additional 1500 rads with reduced field size. Tumor (near midplane) and spinal cord (posteriorly) are indicated.

similar to that of the peripheral tumors. A treatment portal is set up to extend from the sternal notch to 8 cm below the carina, 4 cm to the opposite of the midline from the site of involvement, and a margin of at least 2 cm around the radiographically visible lesions. 4500 rads are delivered using parallel opposing beams, and are supplemented by an additional dose of 1500 rads using a rotational small field to cover the known areas of involvement. A 360° rotation or a lateral arc usually provides a suitable dose distribution and spares normal tissues insofar as possible, particularly to avoid over-treatment of the spinal cord. Areas of atelectasis should be covered liberally, and repeated chest x-ray will frequently allow delineation of the tumor mass and reduc-

tion of the field size following reexpansion of the atelectatic lung. Supraclavicular portals are treated as mentioned previously.

Apical Tumors

The location of apical tumors with and without Pancoast syndrome and their biologic behavior pose special technique problems. The frequency of involvement of the parietal pleura, chest wall, and supraclavicular nodes makes it desirable to treat all areas to the mediastinum 5 cm below the carina in a single portal. Again, the mediastinal portions should be 8 cm wide, and the treatment portal should extend to 2 cm around the radiographically visible lesion, including partially collapsed lung. This treatment delivers 4500 rads in 5 weeks to the lower mediastinum (Fig. 15). By performing a separate dose calculation in the form of isodoses or with

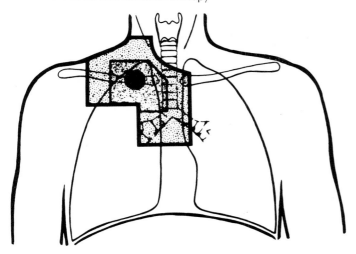

Fig. 14. Schematic of the portal arrangement for treatment of a superior sulcus tumor. (Courtesy Lea and Febiger.)

separate measurements at various levels of the thorax, one can arrive at a dose at the mediastinum, in the area of the sternal notch and also in the supraclavicular region. The larynx should be shielded by appropriate blocking, which should not however cover the sternocleidomastoid muscle. Depending on the involvement of the mediastinal nodes with tumor, small-field therapy should supplement large-field radiotherapy to deliver a total dose of 6000 rads to the primary tumor and known area of mediastinal disease. This can usually be achieved by adding an additional pair of parallel opposing portals. Usually, by the time the lower mediastinum has received 4500 rads, the apical tumor will have received

between 5000 and 5300 rads, therefore the small field will not be required to deliver a dose as high as that in the other anatomic locations. If mediastinoscopy has been positive, the portal should be extended to the opposite supraclavicular area, and dose calculation can then be made to deliver 5000 rads given dose by cobalt teletherapy from an anterior T-shaped portal. A posterior portal supplements the dose to 4500 rads at the midplane of the mediastinum (Figs. 10,11,12,13). Small-field therapy may be required to include an area of supraclavicular adenopathy, if this has been diagnosed as involved on biopsy or by palpation (Fig. 14).

The patient with apical tumor who has evidence of axillary adenopathy shown to be metastatic on biopsy is a special case. In these patients it is necessary to evaluate them carefully for evidence of distant metastasis, especially to the liver. In some patients, the early involvement of the pleura by direct extension will lead to involvement of the right axillary node, and the treatment portal may be extended to include the entire axilla by appropriate arrangement including sites of biopsy as well as the entire axilla. In these patients, the axilla should receive an additional 1500 rad dose using a direct axillary portal.

Patients with brachial plexus involvement secondary to apical tumors have pain extending into the arm. Neither this pain nor bone involvement should contraindicate radiotherapy with curative intent in apical tumors; although the brachial plexus is included in the above-mentioned portal outline, however, it is necessary to be sure to cover all destroyed bone in the portal with an adequate margin. Relief of pain from brachial plexus pressure occurs after the third week of treatment at the earliest, although occasionally it will persist despite radiation therapy.

Oat Cell Carcinoma, Small Cell Carcinoma, and Anaplastic Carcinoma

The treatment is designed to follow the portal outlines previously described for epidermoid and adenocarcinoma. In all of these patients, however, the supraclavicular areas should be treated electively even if no palpable disease is present. Because of the rapid response of these patients to radiation therapy, a chest x-ray should be obtained at 4000 rads, and large-field therapy should be discontinued if adequate regression of the tumor has taken place. Small-field therapy should be started for a tumor dose of 4500 to 5500 rads. Combination of radiotherapy and chemotherapy is the treatment of choice (see Chapter 17). Prophylactic irradiation of the brain to a lower dose may be of value.

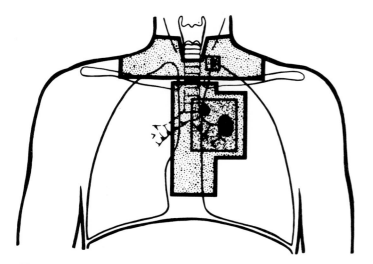

Fig. 15. Schematic for the large and small field in treatment planning in a patient with perihilar anaplastic or oat cell carcinoma of the lung. (Courtesy Lea and Febiger.)

In the dose calculations during treatment planning, a careful definition of the tumor volume (the volume shown by clinical or x-ray findings to be involved with tumor), the target volume (the volume of tissue for which dose calculations are made, including subclinical tumor), and the critical tissues, such as spinal cord, have to be clearly defined in multiple planes. Generally, central axis dose calculations are insufficient and isodoses in multiple planes are necessary. Frequently, compensators or wedges are necessary to obtain homogeneous irradiation.

Among general medical measures before and during x-ray therapy for bronchogenic carcinoma, it is important to correct hematologic abnormalities, such as anemia, after diagnosis of their cause. The subjective and objective symptoms should be on the way toward improvement before initiating radiation therapy. The nutritional status of the patient is important, and dietary supplements should be prescribed if necessary.

Although a histologic or cytologic diagnosis may usually be reached, there is a group of patients illustrated by the following history. Patient H. S. was first seen in April, 1969, with a history of hoarseness of 3 months' duration. Following symptomatic treatment by his family physician, he was referred to an ear, nose, and throat surgeon and, upon laryngoscopy, squamous cell carcinoma involving the right vocal cord was diagnosed. The patient underwent radiation therapy and received 6500 rads from a cobalt irradiator for a period of 6½ weeks. Regular follow-up appointments were undertaken and there was no evidence of current disease in the larynx, nor of cervical adenopathy. Chest x-ray has been persistently within normal limits. About 1 year after treatment of the larynx, however, the patient developed pneumonia and chest x-rays showed an abnormality in the right lung which, upon tomographic examination, proved to be a mass in form of a 1 cm pulmonary coin lesion. No other lesions were identified, nor was there evidence of hepatomegaly, adenopathy, or recurrence of the tumor in the larynx. The patient was hospitalized, sputum studies were obtained, and a bronchoscopy and mediastinoscopy were performed. No histologic diagnosis could be obtained. The remaining workup of the patient was normal except for an electrocardiogram which showed evidence of a recent coronary infarction. The patient was then discharged with a suspected but unproven bronchogenic carcinoma, and chest x-rays were obtained at 6-week intervals. Gradual increase of the lesion on the chest x-ray became evident. Repeat workup including bronchoscopy, bronchial washings, sputum examinations, and radiographic studies failed to reveal the histologic nature of the coin lesion of the right lower lobe of the lung. The patient was not a candidate for thoracotomy because of recent coronary infarction and cardiac decompensation. The tumor nodule had almost doubled in diameter over a period of about 8 months, an increase indicating a volume doubling time of approximately 40 days. The patient was still symptom-free, and there was no evidence of metastatic adenopathy on clinical examination and x-ray studies of the mediastinum.

At this time, two courses of management were available: (1) a further follow-up, in the hope of stabilizing this patient's cardiac condition to allow a thoracotomy for diagnostic purposes because a lung biopsy was considered impossible due to the proximity of the lesion to the mediastinum, the deep location of the coin lesion, and its relatively small size; (2) radiotherapy on the basis of a clinical diagnosis for the presumed squamous cell carcinoma of the lung. The patient underwent such treatment, and subsequent x-rays showed excellent regression of the lesion. He has been free of tumor or metastatic disease for 12 months following the end of his radiotherapy.

It should be emphasized that this patient was an exceptional case. The risk of diagnostic procedures for a lung lesion should exceed the risk of the treatment, and there should be a good probability of correct diagnosis. An additional study to be considered is a bone marrow biopsy to eliminate the possibility of metastatic oat cell carcinoma.

Special considerations are necessary in patients with impaired pulmonary function, considered critical below 60% of the normal vital capacity. In order to minimize pulmonary complication in these patients, the volume of radiation should be restricted insofar as possible, while the other indications and contraindications for radical radiation therapy remain in effect. In these patients, treatment may be administered to a dose of 6000 rads if it is directed only to involved tumor-bearing areas. If there is no known involvement of the immediately adjacent lymph nodes, their treatment portal may be discontinued after 4500 rads. When mediastinal nodes are known to be involved from other studies such as mediastinoscopy, there is no easy solution to the quandary of deciding between treatment of known areas of involvement and the possible side effects. It is recommended that the dose be cut to 5000 or 5500 rads if sufficient response is seen on x-ray. If not, a higher risk of pulmonary complications with possible respiratory decompensation and right heart failure must be accepted.

Stump Recurrences

Recurrences at the bronchial stump after presumably curative surgery without any further treatment should be staged as primary tumors, and are usually diagnosed on bronchoscopy. Treatment is modified because one lung has been partially or completely removed surgically, therefore the other lung must be protected from radiation as much as possible. In such patients, problems arising from pulmonary fibrosis are more severe than in patients who have not undergone surgery. The classification should follow that indicated earlier for curative treatment for the appropriate stage of the recurrent tumor and metastasis, except that radiation therapy should be planned to avoid irradiation of the opposite lung. This usually indicates that radiation should be limited to the homolateral mediastinum, and that great care must be taken in localizing the patient because of extensive postoperative changes which may be expected on chest x-ray.

RESULTS OF "CURATIVE" RADIOTHERAPY AND COMPARISON WITH SURGERY

Traditionally, and with good reason, surgery has been the preferred treatment for patients with operable lung cancer. Smart[33] reported a series of patients identified as operable with 5-year survival rate of 22% in 40 patients with early bronchogenic carcinoma, who were treated with 5000 to 5500 rads for 7 to 8 weeks for epidermoid carcinoma and with 4900 to 5500 rads for oat cell carcinoma. These results were comparable to those in a number of surgical series. There were 27 patients with epidermoid carcinoma, 8 patients with oat cell carcinoma, and 5 patients diagnosed by cytology alone.

A randomized series of 58 patients with bronchogenic carcinoma confined to the thoracic area, without gross evidence of distant metastasis, were reported by Morrison et al.[21] Surgery was compared to radiotherapeutic treatment with a tumor dose of 4500 rads in 4 weeks at five fractions per week. In 37 patients with epidermoid carcinoma, surgery produced a 4-year survival rate of 30% compared to 6% in patients treated by radiation therapy alone, whereas of 19 oat cell carcinomas 10 and 11% respectively survived 1 year after surgery and radiation therapy; however, only 1 patient survived in each group. Another report resulted from a cooperative study by the National Cancer Institute that involved the randomization of preoperative radiation therapy.[27] During the process of randomization, however, 278 operable patients were randomized for surgery only and 74 potentially operable patients received radiation therapy alone. The 3-year survival among these patients amount to 20.1% among the patients treated by surgery alone, and to 9% among the patients treated by radiation therapy only. The majority of these patients had epidermoid carcinoma or adenocarcinoma. The postoperative mortality was 12%. Fox and Scadding[14] treated a group of 144 patients with oat cell carcinoma of the lung randomly by surgery (71 patients) and by radical radiation therapy to at least 5000 rads tumor dose (73 patients). Of the surgical patients, 34 underwent pneumonectomy and 62 of 73 patients received a complete course of radiation therapy. Of the 71 patients treated by radiation therapy 3 (4%) survived 10 years as opposed to only 1 patient in the surgical group who died 6 years after treatment. This patient had been randomized for surgery, but refused operation and received radiation therapy. He was the sole survivor of the surgical group. The mean survival among the surgery patients was 199 days, among the patients assigned to radical radiotherapy 300 days. Among the 62 patients who actually underwent radical radiotherapy, the mean survival was 331 days. The results of these comparative studies are listed in Table 1.

Among the patients with inoperable lung cancer, one group may be found to be unresectable at thoracotomy. A series of 103 such patients was reported by Guttman.[15] These patients were subsequently treated with 2 MeV

TABLE 1. SURGERY VERSUS RADIATION THERAPY IN OPERABLE CANCER OF THE LUNG

Study	Surgery	Radiotherapy
Morrison et al. (4-year survival)[21]		
37 Squamous cell carcinoma	30%	6%
19 Anaplastic carcinoma	10%[a]	11%
Smart (5-year survival)[33]		
40 Operable patients		22.5%
Fox and Scadding (5-year survival)[14]		
144 Oat cell carcinoma	1.4%[a]	4.1%
35 Patients, resected	0%	
62 Patients, radical radiotherapy		4.8%
Cooperative study (3-year survival)[27]		
278 Operable patients	20.1%	
74 Potentially operable patients, radiotherapy only		9.0%

[a] Only 1 patient survived.

x-rays to deliver a tumor dose of 5000 rads over a period of 5 weeks to the entire involved lung and adjacent mediastinum. The 1-year survival was 57%, and 5-year survival was 8.7%. The average survival time for these patients amounted to 27 months, and can be compared with the average survival of about 6 months of untreated patients with advanced lung cancer. A second group of patients who were explored had incomplete resection of the tumor performed at thoracotomy. Guttman[15] reported on 15 such patients and found no 5-year survival and a 9-month survival of 25%, indicating the poor prognosis in patients in whom the tumor had been transsected during surgery. A third group are those who were inoperable and not explored, but in whom the tumor appeared amenable to radiation therapy according to commonly accepted criteria. Columbia University[15] reported 150 such patients with a 5-year survival of 2.5% and a 1-year survival of 40%. Again, treatment consisted of approximately 5000 rads in about 5 weeks. Similar series have been reported from the University of Maryland,[10] with a 5-year survival of 2.7% in 110 patients, from Stanford University,[8] with a 1-year survival of 30% and a 5-year survival of 6%, and by Deeley,[11] who reported on 513 patients with a 1-year survival of 36% and a 5-year survival of 6%. A randomized study with the results in 308 inoperable patients treated by x-ray with doses of 4000 to 5000 rads was reported by Roswit et al.,[29] who achieved a one-year survival of 22.2% as compared to 246 patients who were given an inert placebo and in whom a 1-year survival of 16% was found. Bignall et al.[2] reported a 1-year survival of 19% and a 5-year survival of 1.5% among 2008 inoperable patients treated by radiotherapy. For comparison, 1721 untreated patients had a 5-year survival of 0.3%.

Patients whose disease is diagnosed by mediastinoscopy only are selected because they usually have peripheral lesions and no evidence of extrathoracic metastasis. The American Oncologic Hospital treated 16 such patients at least 2 years prior to a survival analysis. Ten of the 16 died of tumor metastasis within 1 year after radiation therapy, for a 1-year survival of 37.5%. Four additional patients died between the first and second year of survival, for a 2-year survival of 12.5%. One additional patient is alive at present, without evidence of disease under follow-up, and another patient died of metastatic disease 3 years after treatment. We interpret this to mean that although a favorable group of patients has been selected, a larger series of patients is required to show that a better long-term survival of this group of patients may be achieved.

The histology of the tumor treated was examined by investigators at the University of Turku,[22] in whose series 178 patients treated by radiation therapy for inoperable lung cancer had a 1-year survival rate of 31% and

a 3-year survival rate of 10%. A breakdown into epidermoid carcinoma, adenocarcinoma, and oat cell carcinoma revealed that the 1-year survival was 33%, 25%, and 36% respectively. Patients treated with 4000 rads tumor dose or less had a 1-year survival of 11%, whereas 37% of the patients treated with 5000 or 5900 rads survived 1 year. A similar analysis by Caldwell and Bagshaw[8] revealed a 2-year survival of 13% and 48% respectively. Sicher[32] reported a 1-year survival of 3% for patients treated with 2000 to 2999 rads, 7% for 3000 to 3999 rads, 18% for 4000 to 4999 rads, and 21% for 5000 rads or more. A detailed analysis of 688 patients treated by Pierquin et al.[26] shows the relationship between dose of radiation and survival (Figure 16). An optimum dose of about 5500 rads is suggested.

Another significant parameter for evaluating the effectiveness of radiation therapy is the percent of patients who show some objective sign of response of the tumor to treatment. This is a valid approach when comparing data with the results of chemotherapy because of the frequent use of this parameter in patients with advanced disease. On the other hand, the evaluation of pulmonary parenchymal densities, following both radiotherapy and chemotherapy, is inaccurate because nonmalignant changes, such as associated pneumonitis and atelectasis, are difficult to distinguish from primary tumor mass. Also, since endobronchial lesions are not visualized on x-ray, they are not assessed in a review of serial x-rays. Response to treatment is identified as a measurable decrease in tumor size; however, no generally accepted

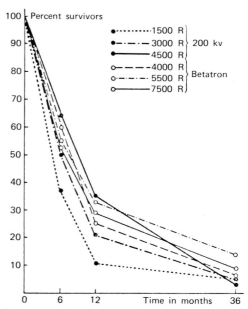

Fig. 16. Relationship between radiation dose and survival in patients with lung cancer. (Courtesy of J. d'electrologie et de radiologie.)

values have been used and each investigator has set his own standards. Usually, partial response is defined as a change in the measurable diameter of radiographically visual tumor by at least 25%, and complete response as the disappearance of radiographically visible lesions. Tumor response has ranged from 54% at 4000 rads to 87% at 6500 rads for histologically proven cancers of the lung, according to Rubin.[31] Reports for tumor response at 5000 rads have varied from 30% to 86%. The dose response is not linear with dose as has been suggested by Pereslegin,[25] whose report includes a bell-shaped dose response curve with a 10% response at 4000 rads, rising to 92% at 6500 rads, then decreasing to 40% at 8500 rads. Neither the exact basis of the tumor response, nor the histologic types were recorded in this study.

The significance of bronchoscopic assessment of tumor response was pointed out by Brouet and co-workers,[7] who noted a 58% objective response to 6000 rads in 6 weeks among 48 patients in whom a 1-year survival of 31% was achieved. This was significantly higher than the assessment of response by radiographic examination of the chest alone. Breur,[5] on the other hand, showed in the treatment of lung metastasis by radiotherapy that irradiation will lead to a significant, predictable reduction in tumor size, with resumption of an exponential growth following radiotherapy, the rate of which is that of the growth rate before treatment.

Carr et al.[9] examined an evaluation of x-ray changes after megavoltage treatment of 188 patients with bronchogenic carcinoma. They compared a dose of 4500 to 5000 rads in 4 to 5 weeks by continuous course with a split course of therapy in which the total dose was divided into two approximately equal fractions with a 3 to 4 week rest period. Although there were no significant differences in survival, continuous irradiation produced a slightly higher percentage of response in small-cell and large-cell undifferentiated carcinoma. Complete response or marked improvement occurred in 36% of

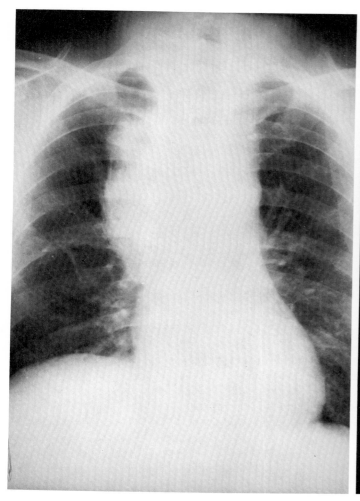
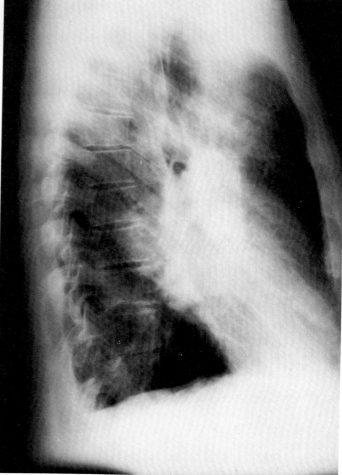

Fig. 17. Postero-anterior and left lateral chest x-ray showing large right hilar mass proven to be anaplastic carcinoma.

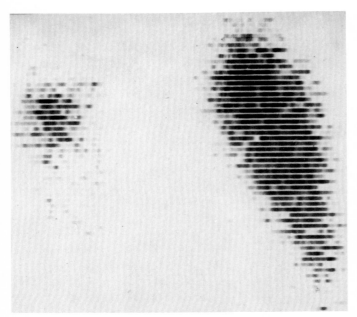

Fig. 18. Antero-posterior view of the lung scan showing impaired perfusion of the right lung (See Fig. 17).

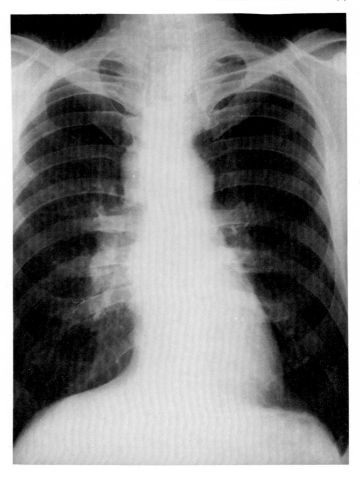

Fig. 19. The same patient after 4000 rads by cobalt teletherapy. Significant reduction in size of the mass has occurred.

epidermoid carcinomas, 82% of small-cell carcinomas, 32% of adenocarcinomas, and 25% of large-cell undifferentiated carcinomas. Slight improvement or lack of progression were shown in 58% of epidermoid carcinomas, 15% of small-cell carcinomas, 53% of adenocarcinomas, and 75% of large-cell undifferentiated carcinomas. There was no significant correlation between response and survival except in epidermoid carcinoma, in which the patients with complete clearing or marked roentgenographic improvement had a significantly longer survival rate (Fig. 21).

A postmortem study by Rissanen et al.[28] indicated that megavoltage radiation therapy of 5000 rads or more destroyed tumor in the irradiated field in 55% of epidermoid carcinomas, 50% of adenocarcinomas, 70% of large-cell undifferentiated carcinomas, and 75% of small-cell carcinomas.

A relationship of tumor regression to prognosis following x-ray therapy for lung cancer was also studied by Rubin et al.[30] Patients whose tumor did not show any response during radiation therapy had a 1-year survival of 16%, whereas patients in whom x-ray revealed a 50% regression had a 1-year survival of 25%, and those in whom the tumor responded by more than 50% as seen in decrease in size on radiographs had a 1-year survival of 66%.

SPLIT COURSE RADIATION THERAPY

A number of studies regarding a rest period between two courses of radiotherapy have been carried out to take advantage of improvement in the therapeutic ratio, based presumably on a more rapid recovery of normal tissue from radiation injury as compared to tumor tissue. Such treatment is usually administered by one course of radiation with a gap of several days to weeks in which no treatment is administered and a subsequent repeat of this cycle one or more times. Abramson and Cavanaugh[1] treated a group of 42 patients with 6000 rads for 6 weeks of five fractions per week. A comparison group consisted of 271 patients with treatment to 2000 rads tumor dose in five fractions in 1 week, followed by a 3-week rest period and an additional 2000 rads in a week. Although reactions such as nausea and esophagitis were widespread among the patients treated by the split course, late complications were not reported as disturbing. The important finding was that there was a significantly better survival rate at 1 year for the split course, 38% as compared to 14% among those patients treated with protracted irradiation. The difference in survival at 2 and 3 years

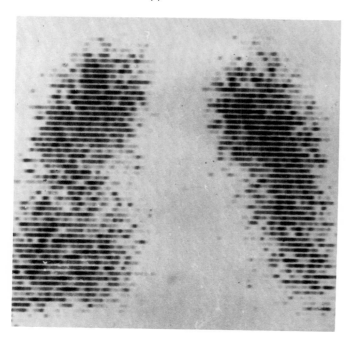

Fig. 20. Lung scan showing increased perfusion of the right lung following administration of 4000 rads cobalt teletherapy (See Fig. 19).

was less pronounced. Holsti[17] reported on split course therapy, with 5000 to 6000 rads in 5 to 6 weeks given in a continuous course of six fractions per week and compared to a split course irradiation. The split course was given by dividing the total dose into two separate courses, separated by a 2- to 3-week interval. This rest period occurred halfway through the radiation therapy. According to the authors of the study, the patients treated by a split course tolerated the radiotherapy better both subjectively and objectively. There was 42% survival at 1 year using a split course and 39% survival using continuous irradiation, compared to 15% and 12% at 2 years. The recurrence-free 1-year survival was 23% with the split course and 18% with the continuous irradiation. There was also no significant difference in intrathoracic extension, which occurred in 75% of patients with the split course treatment and in 77% of patients with continuous irradiation. Squamous cell carcinoma was separated as the only histologic subtype reported on and there was a reasonably even distribution: 37% of the patients showed this pathology among the split course group, and 41% among the continuous group.

A third report on split course therapy using a break in the middle of the treatment was reported by Ojala.[22] Patients were treated with a radiation dose up to 6400 rads. Fifty-seven patients were treated without interval and 83 patients by the split course technique. Although

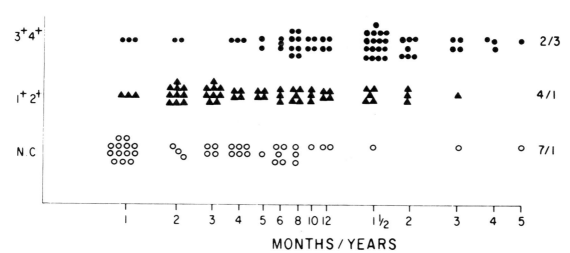

Fig. 21. Relationship between tumor regression and survival in patients with carcinoma of the lung. N. C. indicates no change, 1+ and 2+ indicate decrease in measurable size of the tumor on x-ray up to 50%. The 3+ and 4+ indicate decrease in size over 50% following radiotherapy. (Reprinted with permission from reference 30. Copyright 1970, American Cancer Society, Inc.)

TABLE 2. RESULTS OF RADIOTHERAPY FOR INOPERABLE CANCER OF THE LUNG

Study	1-Year-Survival	5-Year Survival
University of Maryland,[10] 110 patients		2.7%
Stanford University,[8] 284 patients	30%	6%
Hammersmith Hospital,[11] 513 patients	36%	6%
Columbia University,[15] 95 patients (unresectable at thoracotomy)	57.9%	7.4%
Columbia University,[15] 15 patients (incomplete resection of tumor)	25%[a]	0%
Columbia University,[15] 150 patients (inoperable, not explored)	40%	2.5%
Mount Sinai Hospital, New York[12]		
53 patients (biopsy only)		11%
21 patients (incomplete resection)		24%
Duke University[1]		
271 patients (short course)	38%	
42 patients (protracted course)	14%	
University of Turku,[17] 178 patients	31%	10%[b]
squamous cell carcinoma	33%	
adenocarcinoma	25%	
anaplastic carcinoma	36%	
University Hospital, Helsinki[22]		
74 patients, split course	42%	
33 patients, protracted course	39%	

[a] Nine-month survival.

[b] Three-year survival.

this is not a randomized study, and although changes in the patient population between groups make an interpretation of treatment results questionable, it should be noted that 42% of the patients treated by protracted irradiation survived 1 year, whereas only 28% of those treated by the split course with an interval of 2 to 4 weeks survived for this period of time.

There are many possibilities for combining treatment times and rest periods, and other authors have described modifications of treatment with a large variety of doses, fractions, and placement of the interval between series. Such treatment schemes occasionally show a slight advantage over continuous irradiation as reported by Levitt.[19] Unorthodox fractionation schemes have also been described for electron beam therapy of bronchogenic carcinoma, as mentioned in the chapter on special techniques of radiation therapy. The final results of large scale randomized studies will be necessary to show any advantage of certain dose and fractionation schedules.

REFERENCES

1. Abramson, N., and Cavanaugh, P. J.: Short course radiation therapy in carcinoma of the lung. *Radiology* 108:685–687, 1973.

2. Bignall, J. R., Martin, M , and Smithers, D. W.: Survival in 6086 cases of bronchial carcinoma. *Lancet*, 20 May, 1067–1070, 1967.

3. Bloedorn, F.: Rationale and benefit of pre-operative irradiation in lung cancer. *J. A. M. A.* 195:21–22, 1966.

4. Bloedorn, F.: Lung. In *Textbook of Radiotherapy*, G. Fletcher, Ed., Lea and Febiger, Philadelphia, 1966.

5. Breuer, K.: Growth rate and radiosensitity of human tumors. I. Growth rate of human tumors. *Eur. J. Cancer* 2:157–171, 1966.

6. Bromley, L., and Szur, L.: Combined radiotherapy and resection for carcinoma of the bronchus: experiences with 66 patients. *Lancet* 2:937–941, 1955.

7. Brouet, D., Flamant, R., and Hayat, M.: Results of a trial of radiotherapy and chemotherapy in bronchopulmonary cancer. *Eur. J. Cancer* 4:437–445, 1968.

8. Caldwell, W. L., and Bagshaw, M. A.: Indications for and results of irradiation of carcinoma of the lung. *Cancer* 22:999–1004, 1968

9. Carr, D. T., Childs, D.S., and Lee, R. E.: Radiotherapy plus FU compared to radiotherapy alone for inoperable and unresectable bronchogenic carcinoma. *Cancer* 29:375–380, 1972.

10. Cowley, R A., Wizenberg, M. J., Linberg, E. J.: The role of radiation therapy and surgery in the treatment of bronchogenic carcinoma. *Ann. Thorac. Surg.* 8:229–236, 1969.

11. Deeley, T. J.: The treatment of carcinoma of the bronchus. *Br. J. Radiol.* 40:801–822, 1967.

12. Farca, A., and Boland, J.: Lung carcinoma: radical radiotherapy. Presented at the Eleventh International Cancer Congress, Florence, 1974.

References
155

13. Fernholz, H. J., and Mueller, D.: Ergebnisse und Komplikationen der Telekobalttherapie beim Bronchialkarzinom. *Strahlenther.* **137**:381–392, 1969.

14. Fox, W., and Scadding, J.: Medical Research Council: comparative trial of surgery and radiotherapy for primary treatment of small celled or oat celled carcinoma of the bronchus. *Lancet* **2**:63–65, 1973.

15. Guttman, R.: Radical supervoltage therapy in inoperable carcinoma of the lung. *Modern Radiotherapy, Carcinoma of the Bronchus*, T. Deeley, Ed., Appleton-Century-Crofts, New York, London, 1971.

16. Hall, T. C., Dederick, M. M., and Chalmers, T. C.: A clinical pharmacologic study of chemotherapy and x-ray therapy in lung cancer. *Am. J. Med.* **43**:186–193, 1967.

17. Holsti, L. R.: Split course megavoltage radiotherapy: one year follow-up. *Br. J. Radiol.* **39**:332–337, 1966.

18 Leddy, E. T., and Moersch, H. J.: Roentgen therapy for bronchogenic carcinoma. *J. A. M. A.* **115**:2239–2242, 1940.

19. Levitt, S. H.: The split dose approach in radiation therapy. *Radiol. Clin. North Am.* **7**:291–300, 1969.

20. Mallams, J. T., Paulson, D. L., Collier, R. E., and Shaw, R. R.: Presurgical irradiation in bronchogenic carcinoma, superior sulcus type. *Radiology* **82**:1050–1054, 1964.

21. Morrison, R., Deeley, T. J., and Cleland, W. P.: The treatment of carcinoma of the bronchus. A clinical trial to compare surgery and supervoltage radiotherapy. *Lancet* **1**:683–684, 1963.

22. Ojala, A.: Results of cobalt therapy in operable carcinoma of the lung. Strahlenther. **140**:626–629, 1970.

23. Pancoast, H.: Superior pulmonary sulcus tumor. Tumor characterized by pain, Horner's syndrome, destruction of bone and atrophy of hand muscles. *J. A. M. A.* **99**:1391–1396, 1932.

24. Paulson, B.: The survival rate in superior sulcus tumors treated by pre-surgical irradiation. *J. A. M. A.* **195**:23, 1966.

25. Pereslegin, I. A.: *Radiotherapy of Lung Cancer,* Meditsina, Moscow, 1963.

26. Pierquin, B., Gravis, P., and Gelle, X.: Study of 688 cases of bronchial cancer treated by teleradiotherapy (200 kV and 22 MeV). *J. Radiol, Electrol.* **46**:201–216, 1965.

27. Preoperative irradiation of cancer of the lung. Preliminary report of a therapeutic trial. A collaborative study. *Cancer* **23**:419–429, 1969.

28. Rissanen, P. M , Tikka, U., and Holsti, L. R.: Autopsy findings in lung cancer treated with megavoltage radiotherapy. *Acta Radiol. Ther. Phys. Biol.* **7**:433–442, 1968.

29. Roswit, B., Patno, M., Rapp, R., Veinbergs, A., Feder, B., Stuhlbarg, J., and Reid, C.: The survival of patients with inoperable lung cancer: a large scale randomized study of radiation therapy versus placebo. *Radiology* **90**:688–697, 1968.

30. Rubin, P., Ciccio, S., and Setisarn, B.: The controversial status of radiation therapy in lung cancer. Sixth National Cancer Conference Proceedings, Lippincott, Philadelphia, 1970, pp. 855–866.

31. Rubin, T. H.: Lung cancer: histopathologic analysis as related to treatment policy in radiation response. *Front. Radiat. Ther. Oncol.* **9**:151–161, 1974.

32. Sicher, K.: Value of radiotherapy in inoperable bronchogenic carcinoma. *Practitioner* **180**:695–700, 1958.

33. Smart, J.: Can lung cancer be cured by irradiation alone? *J. A. M. A.* **159**:1034–1035, 1966.

Chapter Fifteen

Palliative Radiotherapy

INTRATHORACIC ADVANCED DISEASE

Once a patient's cancer extends beyond the confines described as indications for radical supervoltage radiotherapy, cure would be an unreasonable aim of treatment. These patients usually have bilateral involvement of the mediastinum on radiographic examination or mediastinoscopy, bilateral pulmonary lesions or multiple unilateral pulmonary lesions, palpable supraclavicular adenopathy over 2 cm in diameter, pleural fluid with malignant cells in the aspirate or distant metastasis. The problems of atelectasis, hemoptysis, pain, displacement of the trachea, and pneumonitis usually respond quite rapidly to radiotherapy, but it is unreasonable to expose patients with advanced disease to prolonged courses of treatment if the results of a short course of therapy are equally satisfactory. It has been our habit to treat these patients with a dose of 3000 rads in 2 weeks to all known areas of involvement and the mediastinum. Occasionally, this dose may be carried to 4000 rads in 3 weeks, if symptoms persist. Reevaluation of these patients should always include a chest x-ray to ascertain the response of the lesion, especially with oat cell carcinoma where there may be surprisingly rapid response. In our experience, improvement from palliative radiotherapy is obtained in 92% of patients with hemoptysis and in 65% of patients with cough or dyspnea.

Patients with bronchoesophageal fistula due to cancer of the lung should be treated palliatively for symptoms. The rapid destruction of the tumor by radiotherapy may lead to enlargement of the fistula or sinus tract and it remains a clinical decision to determine the need for treatment of involvement of the esophagus, dysphagia, or hemoptysis. Frequently, symptoms can be relieved by esophageal intubation or, better, gastrostomy. The patient with bronchoesophageal fistula usually has advanced disease and may be expected to develop distant metastasis rapidly, especially in the liver. One must always realize that the aim of palliative radiation therapy is not to treat the disease but to treat the patient's symptoms, and good clinical judgment is necessary to weigh the advantages of treating advanced asymptomatic disease against the symptoms which are due to the treatment itself.

SUPERIOR VENA CAVAL OBSTRUCTION

Superior vena caval obstruction is a rapidly progressive and disabling syndrome which responds consistently to appropriate radiation therapy. It always indicates mediastinal metastasis, since the tumor is usually located adjacent to the superior vena cava. Tumor involvement of this vessel may occur in up to 20% of patients at autopsy.[15] The patient's treatment classification should be made taking into consideration all previously mentioned staging characteristics.

A study involving the clinical features and results of treatment of superior vena caval obstruction has been published by Salsali and Cliffton.[23] Venous distention in the neck and upper extremities were seen in 46% of 137 patients, facial edema and swelling of the neck and trunk in 11%, and a combination of both in 37%. The syndrome occurred in 3.4% of the patients with lung cancer admitted to the reporting institution. Only one patient had superior vena caval obstruction on postmortem examination without a record of clinical symptoms. The syndrome occurred most frequently in patients with oat cell carcinoma and epidermoid carcinoma. Treatment was usually radiation therapy, sometimes associated with chemotherapy or various surgical procedures. A postmortem examination revealed complete occlusion of the vena cava in 16 of 24 patients, and in all patients there was a thrombus in the superior vena caval tributaries. The value of the combination of chemotherapy with radiotherapy for the treatment of superior vena caval obstruction was studied in a prospective randomized study by Levitt and co-authors.[13] Twenty-eight patients were randomized to a series of radiotherapy for 4000 to 5000 rads or to receive combined treatment consisting of a similar dose of radiation therapy with prior nitrogen mustard injection of 0.4 mg/kg body weight. Although the majority of the patients were men, with only one woman in each group, the distribution of histologic subtypes of carcinoma followed the general incidence. Complete relief of symptoms was achieved in 9 patients in each group. Recurrence of symptoms occurred in 40% of the patients treated by radiation therapy only, and in 60% of the patients treated by nitrogen mustard and radiation therapy. Differences in response were found in the form of a slight decrease in time of onset of relief of symptoms from start of the initial treatment if nitrogen mustard was used as part of the management. Similarly, there was a slight decrease in time for initial drop in venous pressure following start of the initial treatment if injection of nitrogen mustard was used. These differences were not significant. Patients treated by radiotherapy alone had 7.1 ± 1.5 months of relief of symptoms, whereas those treated by nitrogen mustard and radiotherapy had 6.2 ± 0.8 months' relief. According to these data therefore, the use of nitrogen mustard in association with radiotherapy produces no significant improvement in results of treatment whereas, as expected, the study showed that complications were higher in those patients in whom a combined treatment was used, especially insofar as a decreased white blood count and/or platelets in the peripheral blood is concerned. Various degrees of complications occurred in 8 of the patients treated by combined treatment, whereas only 4 of the patients treated by radiotherapy showed similar complications.

Once the histologic diagnosis is obtained in a patient with superior vena caval obstruction, treatment should commence with a relatively high dose. We have had consistent response to 3000 rads tumor dose in 2 weeks delivered by parallel opposing portals to the mediastinum and adjacent areas and also to other areas that may require treatment, such as the supraclavicular nodes. Subsequently, the treatment plan is modified according to the patient's staging. If the signs and symptoms of superior vena caval obstruction do not respond completely to 3000 rads, 4000 rads in 3 weeks or 4500 rads in 4 weeks should be the aim of the initial high dose part of the radiation therapy. Chemotherapy in combination with radiotherapy is more likely to produce significant relief of symptoms and rapid onset of relief from the shortness of breath and other disabling symptoms of superior vena caval obstruction due to oat cell carcinoma. The response to adequate treatment (4000 rads tumor dose or more) occurred in 74% of the patients treated by Longacre and Shockman.[15] Because of the advanced involvement of the mediastinum with tumor, 1-year survival is low, 12%,[23] although a few long-term survivors have been reported.

PLEURAL EFFUSION

In patients with pleural effusion, the initial step should be aspiration of the pleural fluid for diagnosis by cytology and cell block examination by the pathologist. Reaccumulation of the fluid will indicate the need for treatment unless incomplete removal had been performed at the first instance. The time interval between two aspirations, which are usually performed for pain, shortness of breath or chest x-ray findings, gives a good indication of the rapidity with which the fluid accumulates. A number of methods of treatment are possible, and it has been possible to delay the onset of reaccumulation significantly by administering radiation therapy to the hemithorax of involvement for a dose of 3000 rads in 2 weeks with open portals or, if preferred, by a modification of the moving strip therapy.

The use of intracavitary radioactive colloidal gold (50 mCi) or phosphorus (5–10 mCi) is indicated if it is easily accessible, and if the patient is expected to survive for at least 3 months, since serious problems arise from postmortem examinations done on patients containing radioactive material in the pleural cavity. If the patient is already receiving chemotherapy, the pleural administration of chemotherapeutic agents such as nitrogen mustard achieves a similar effect by delaying reaccumu-

lation of pleural fluid. Permanent eradication of tumor cells in the pleural cavity is unlikely. In our experience approximately 65% of the patients treated by radiation therapy, either by external beam or via intracavitary colloidal gold or phosphorus, will show a significant response as measured by the interval between pleural aspirations. The prognosis in these patients is invariably poor because in lung cancer pleural fluid is rarely the only manifestation of the patient's disease, and other metastatic disease becomes symptomatic and requires therapy within a short period of time.

An evaluation of treatment of pleural effusion was reported by Leininger et al.[12] who used intrapleural nitrogen mustard, usually 10 mg., through a chest tube following drainage. Of 18 patients, 11 lived 5 months or more without recurrence of the pleural effusion. Six patients died less than 5 months after treatment, apparently without need for further treatment for recurrent pleural effusion and 1 patient had no significant response. In a less selected series reported by Card et al.,[3] intracavitary installation of radioactive colloidal gold or radioactive chromic phosphate produced beneficial effects in at least 50% of patients, a percentage similar to that reported with intrapleural installation of chemotherapeutic agents, especially nitrogen mustard, in unselected patients. In patients with effusions that are resistant to this management, tube drainage of the pleural fluid with full expansion of the lung and instillation of irritants such as talc may be of value.

PERICARDIAL METASTASIS

Up to 35% of patients have involvement of the heart with metastatic carcinoma from the lung at autopsy, whereas clinical signs of involvement of the pericardium are far less frequent. The management of pericardial metastasis in lung cancer is best achieved by radiation therapy, usually using an external beam for a dose of at least 2000 rads in 2 weeks, and up to about 5000 rads in 5 weeks. At least one-half of the reported cases of pericardial effusion have been treated successfully by this method, sometimes followed by intracavitary chemotherapy according to a series reported by Lokich.[14] Intracavitary radioactive material such as radioactive gold or phosphorus is rarely used in the treatment of pericardial effusion mainly because of the poor prognosis in patients with this sign, and the problems arising from death of patients with radioactive material in body cavities.

BONE METASTASIS

The palliation of pain due to bone metastasis is very important in clinical radiotherapy because of the frequency of symptoms due to lung cancer in this site. The absorption of ionizing radiation in bone as compared to that in soft tissue shows a well-known dependence on energy. This is valid both for solid bone and for small cavities surrounded by bone. On the basis of data presented by Spiers[24] and in Handbook 62 of the International Commission on Radiological Units and Measurements,[11] the dose absorbed in bone from beams of radiation produced by an orthovoltage x-ray therapy machine is higher than that from a supervoltage machine such as a 60 cobalt teletherapy irradiator or a linear accelerator (Table 1). To determine whether there is a significant difference in palliative results of radiotherapeutic treatment of bone metastasis between super- and orthovoltage beams, a randomized clinical trial of therapy of bone metastasis was carried out at the American Oncologic Hospital.

Patients with bone metastasis from malignant tumors referred between January 1, 1970, and June 30, 1972, were randomized for the use of x-ray therapy irradiation (250 kV, 0.5 mm Cu added filter, half value thickness 1.5 mm copper, 15 mA, 50 cm TSD) or 60 cobalt teletherapy at 80 cm SSD, before they received their first palliative irradiation. The patients with even birthdates received supervoltage therapy, the others were treated by orthovoltage radiation. Usually, 1000 rads tumor dose in a single treatment were delivered followed by a similar treatment in 1 week if symptoms persisted, using a single small portal to the involved and symptomatic bone. Exceptions were in the cervical and thoracic spine, where 3000 rads in 10 treatments were administered using a single fixed portal or 140° arc rotation treating 5 days per week (NSD = 1310 rets). In weight-bearing bones, such as femur, pelvic bones, and humerus, 2000 rads were given in 5 treatments (NSD = 1150 rets). If the use of x-ray therapy was contraindicated because of the patient's condition, such as in bedridden patients with treatment of the lumbosacral region, supervoltage irradiation was used. Occasionally, patient overload on one machine required treatment on the other unit. A majority of the patients had primary breast cancer, the remainder presented with cancer of the lung, prostate, or other tumors. There were 27 patients with cancer of the breast, 9 patients with cancer of the prostate, 7 pa-

tients with cancer of the lung, 2 patients with cancer of the cervix, and 10 patients with other malignancies. A total of 59 symptomatic areas were treated, the spine in 32 patients, the femur in 10, bones of the upper extremity in 3, the skull in 3, and the pelvic bones in 11 patients (Table 2).

The patients' symptomatic response was graded at 1 to 2 weeks following the last day of a treatment series as "no relief of pain," "partial relief of pain," or "no persistent pain." The patients usually received additional therapy in the form of hormonal manipulation or chemotherapy, but no attempt was made to randomize these factors. The patients with no relief of pain continued to take a narcotic for pain control. The patients with partial relief discontinued narcotics but still used a nonnarcotic analgesic. Patients with no persistent pain discontinued all pain medications.

The results of palliative radiotherapy in the randomized patients are listed in Table 3. The rate of recurrence of pain was not influenced by the method used, although this factor was not evaluated separately because of the short life expectancy in some of these patients. Also listed are an additional 10 patients with 12 symptomatic areas who had 60 cobalt teletherapy without randomization, and an added group of 10 patients with 11 symptomatic areas who received x-ray therapy without randomization for the above-mentioned reasons. There is no significant difference between the results by modalities (t-test, $p < 0.05$) for the randomized and pooled data.

This analysis did not take into account any supplemental treatment by chemotherapy, hormonal management, or neurosurgical procedures. In any given patient the results of palliative treatment are related to the best available management, and only the use of radiation therapy was under our control and allowed for randomization. The other methods were used by several individuals with various indications that did not lend themselves to detailed analysis. In a clinical setting, radiotherapy must be administered in a pattern of referral from many sources, therefore it is felt that our results give a valid indication of the value of radiation therapy in the treatment of metastatic bone carcinoma. The results we obtained compare favorably with those reported

TABLE 1.   ENERGY ABSORPTION COEFFICIENTS AND CONVERSION FACTORS f (Rads/Roentgen)[11]

Energy MeV	Energy Absorption Coefficient				Conversion Factor		
	Water	Air	Bone	Muscle	Water	Bone	Muscle
0.01	4.89	4.66	19.0	4.96	0.920	3.58	0.933
0.10	.0252	.0231	.0386	.0252	0.957	1.47	0.957
1.0	.0311	.0280	.0297	.0308	0.974	0.927	0.965
10.0	.0155	.0144	.0159	.0154			

TABLE 2. TREATMENT SCHEDULES FOR PALLIATIVE IRRADIATION

Treatment Schedule	Orthovoltage	Supervoltage
1000 Rads tumor dose repeated after 1 week if necessary	9 patients (11 areas)	13 patients (15 areas)
2000 Rads tumor dose in 5 treatments	4 patients	5 patients
3000 Rads tumor dose in 10 treatments	9 patients	15 patients
Total patients randomized	22 (24 areas)	33 (35 areas)

by others,[1,25] who found similar results from palliative treatment of bone metastasis in patients usually treated by supervoltage radiation therapy.

Since logistics problems often lead to the administration of palliative radiation on either machine in our department, we are no longer pursuing this randomized trial. The administration of orthovoltage and supervoltage beams of radiation could be shown to be equally effective insofar as the relief of pain is concerned. The value of radiation therapy in this type of advanced malignancy could be reconfirmed.

BRAIN METASTASIS

Cerebral metastases are a frequent site of secondary spread from cancer of the lung (see page 58). They occur more frequently with adenocarcinoma and oat cell carcinoma than with squamous cell carcinoma. Usually, cerebral metastasis are multiple; however, the series of Richards and McKissock[21] indicated solitary metastasis as the only site of metastatic involvement in 27 of 303 cases (16%) and Galluzzi and Payne[6] reported 52 single brain metastases, which were associated with metastases in other sites in 17%. This has led to the surgical treatment of brain metastasis and, depending upon the interpretation of data such as the series reported by McGee,[16] the 1-year survival of 15% with an operative mortality of 26% may or may not indicate a worthwhile endeavor. It is our opinion that the mortality from

such surgery exceeds the potential benefit, although it is recognized that individual patients may survive for months or years. Montana et al.[18] reported on 15 patients with metastatic carcinoma of the lung to the brain who underwent craniotomy and subsequent radiation therapy, and 47 patients who had irradiation only. Survival for the entire group was 59% at 3 months, 28% at 6 months and 12% at 1 year. There was no difference between the surgically treated group and the group which underwent irradiation only. Neurologic objective improvement was achieved in 56% of the patients after radiation therapy.

Harr and Patterson[8] reported on 50 patients with metastatic brain tumor from previously diagnosed lung cancer who underwent craniotomy. The operative mortality was 11% in the group of 167 patients with cranial cerebral metastases from tumors of various primary sites. For patients who underwent only partial removal of their tumor, the operative mortality was 18%, whereas it was 8% in those in whom the surgeon felt the tumor was completely excised. The operative mortality was 30% if only a biopsy was obtained. Of the 167 patients, 26% of the metastases were located in the parietal region, 22% in the frontal region, 19% in the cerebellum, 13% in the temporal lobe, 8% in the occipital lobe, 2% in the dura, 8.5% in the medulla, and 7% in a combination of these classifications. Adequate survival data were available for 159 patients: 22% survived 1 year, and 7 patients survived more than 5 years. Patients with malignant melanoma, renal cell carcinoma, and carcinoma of the breast had better survival rates than those with lung cancer. Harr and Patterson feel that craniotomy is indicated in a patient with known lung cancer if after careful evaluation, including brain scanning, bilateral carotid arteriography, and possibly repeated angiography showed that the lesion was solitary. The authors believe that air studies are associated with a significant incidence of complications and should therefore be used with caution. If multiple metastatic brain tumors are present, intracranial surgery carries a substantial mortality and rarely offers significant palliation. Disregarding the surgical mortality, the category of patients in whom brain metastasis is diagnosed on craniotomy and in whom a primary

TABLE 3. RESULTS OF PALLIATIVE RADIOTHERAPY

Method	No Relief of Pain	Partial Relief	Complete Relief
60 Cobalt	5 areas: 11%	20 areas: 44.5%	20 areas: 44.5%
X-ray therapy	3 areas: 9%	16 areas: 48.5%	14 areas: 42.5%
60 Cobalt (randomized only)	4 areas: 12%	14 areas: 42.5%	15 areas: 45.5%
X-ray therapy (randomized only)	3 areas: 13.5%	10 areas: 45.5%	9 areas: 41%

tumor is questionable or not found at all has a relatively good survival. We administer a tumor dose of 4000 rads in 4 weeks to the entire cranial content with an additional 2000 rads in 2 weeks to the areas of involvement on arteriography, surgery, or brain scanning. Questionable pulmonary disease may be treated at the same time, even if positive cytology or histologic diagnosis is not obtained from this area. The evidence on clinical examination and chest x-rays should, however, be strongly indicative of a primary bronchogenic carcinoma.

A second category includes patients who have undergone treatment for bronchogenic carcinoma, either by surgery or radiotherapy, and who appear with metastatic brain disease at least 3 months after completion of their initial treatment. In these patients, there has been good relief of symptoms with 3500 rads tumor dose in 3 weeks to the entire brain. In patients who have not undergone craniotomy, the full dose should be preceded by priming doses, delivering 50 rads, 100 rads, and 200 rads before reaching a tumor dose of 300 rads/day. If metastatic disease follows closely after the treatment of the primary tumor, irradiation of the entire cranial content with 1000 rads tumor dose in a single treatment may be given. This type of treatment may be repeated about 3 weeks following the initial single increment. If there is also evidence of other metastatic sites, treatment should be as brief as possible since these patients usually follow a rapid downhill course and, as a rule, initial treatment should be in form of chemotherapy including steroids for the reduction of brain edema. Concomitant single-increment radiotherapy may be considered.

While the results of a study under the auspices of the National Cancer Institute will give statistically significant information regarding optimal radiotherapy of brain metastasis in the future, Deeley and Edwards[5] showed that 47% of the patients received significant palliation. Improvement was sufficient to enable them to return home and live a relatively normal and comfortable life for at least 1 month after completing treatment. Another significant percentage of patients had relief of troublesome symptoms without being able to return to normal life, or improvement was shown for less than 1 month. Although 5 patients among 29 reported by the above-mentioned authors survived 1 year or more, 50% of the patients had died within 6 months if significant palliation was obtained. An additional 32 survived for a few months only and were unable to return to reasonably normal activities.

The role of corticosteroids in the treatment of brain metastasis is undisputed, and they improve symptoms for a limited time, but only radiotherapy offers the probability of prolonged improvement in patients with epidermoid and adenocarcinoma. Chemotherapy may be of occasional value in the treatment of metastasis from oat cell carcinoma. We have reserved the use of corticosteroids and chemotherapy for patients with symptomatic deterioration or with side effects from radiation therapy. The superiority of radiotherapy in the management of brain metastasis was confirmed by the study of Hazra et al.[9] The median survival of patients treated by radiotherapy was 23 weeks as compared to 7 weeks for patients treated by steroids.

SPINAL CORD COMPRESSION

Compression of the spinal cord secondary to epidural metastatic deposits from lung cancer is a common condition, and physicians treating patients with cancer of the lung must be thoroughly familiar with the signs and symptoms of this metastatic site to allow early recognition and prompt treatment. Otherwise, disabling paralysis may present serious problems in management and care. Pain is the usual initial symptom in association with paresthesias. It is important to remember the saying: "When the pain is gone so is the cord." When cord compression is suspected clinically, a myelogram should be performed in any patient eligible for laminectomy, unless there is associated involvement of the adjoining bones. Treatment should always be considered as emergency therapy because actual compression of the spinal cord for more than 24 hours makes recovery of full function rare or impossible.

The surgical indications in metastatic compression of the spinal cord have been examined by White et al.[26] In a series of 226 patients 76% were followed until death and 33% were submitted to autopsy. All patients complained of back pain, which was usually the first symptom, sometimes present for several months before neurologic signs developed; 19% of the patients were ambulatory, 68% were nonambulatory but with some motor function, and 13% were paraplegic when first seen. The spinal cord was the site of compression in 83% of the patients. The most frequent primary tumor was breast cancer immediately followed by lung cancer. All patients were treated by decompression laminectomy with a 30-day postoperative mortality of 8.7%. Ambulatory status was achieved and maintained in 36% of the patients. Relief of pain and lesser degrees of improvement in neurologic function were achieved in a majority of the patients. The authors concluded from their experience that prevention remains the best therapy, and prompt treatment by radiation therapy before onset of spinal cord compression after careful physical examination and x-ray examination including possible myelography will avoid disabling paralysis. However, when paralysis is present, surgery is the primary form of treatment except in a few highly radiosensitive tumors.[27]

The radiotherapeutic treatment of epidural compression of the spinal cord without laminectomy was reported by Rubin et al.[22] The authors reported that in moderately radiosensitive or radioresponsive tumors such as lung cancer, high daily doses delivering 400 rads tumor dose on 3 successive days with subsequent reduction of the daily tumor dose to 150 to 200 rads will be effective if neurologic loss has not reached the level of complete paraplegia. In their experience there was no worsening of the patients' neurologic findings and subjective symptoms that would indicate the need for laminectomy. In patients with cancer thus treated, 40% were considered improved and the remainder showed no change in their condition.

It is important to diagnose beginning spinal cord compression early on the basis of the symptom of pain, be it localized in form of backache, or radicular. Tingling, numbness, and burning sensations indicate the presence of paresthesias. X-ray of the spine is often helpful in demonstrating involvement, possibly associated with collapse of adjacent vertebral bodies. At times, a bone scan using a radioisotope such as Sr 85 or Tc 99 m polyphosphate will demonstrate bone changes before there is evidence of radiographic changes. Myelography and examination of spinal fluid protein will prove the presence of extradural masses impinging upon the spinal canal. The majority of patients will have over 100 mg/100 ml of protein in the spinal fluid. Levels over 500 mg/100 ml are to be considered an ominous sign in cases of spinal cord compression.[26] Cell studies may not contribute to management.

Brady and co-workers[28] in their analysis of 133 patients with metastatic spinal cord tumors, in 39 of whom the primary tumor was lung cancer, were able to relate the type of symptom to the delay period before diagnosis of spinal cord compression. In patients with sensory symptoms, the average duration was 42 days, in patients with motor symptoms the average duration was 17 days, and in patients with sphincteric symptoms the average duration was 3 days. 9.8% of the patients were shown to have involvement of the cervical spinal cord, 29.3% in the T1 to T4 area, 22.5% in the T1 or L1 area, and 38.4% in the cauda equina. The return of motor function after surgery and/or approximately 3500 to 4000 rads tumor dose in a period of 25 to 30 elapsed days indicated that surgery alone produced a response in 7 of 17 patients, if the lesion was located at the T5 level or lower, whereas none of the higher lesions responded. Combination of surgery and radiation produced a response in 75% of patients with lesions in the cervical level, 61% of the lesions located at T1 to T4, 75% in

the T5 to L1 level, and 60% in the cauda equina. When radiation therapy alone was used, 50% of the patients with the cervical and T1 to T4 levels responded although only 4 were treated. Successful radiotherapy was possible in 5 of 7 patients with lesions between T5 and L1, and 2 of 8 patients with lesions in the cauda equina. Response following treatment with return of function could also be related to the duration of symptoms. Table 4 is taken from the work of Dr. Brady and co-workers.[28] The results of this study in 39 patients with primary lung cancer and metastatic spinal cord tumor also indicated that the median survival was 87 days, with a range of 9 to 167 days.

In our experience laminectomy should always be performed in patients with lung cancer when there is an indication of spinal cord compression on myelogram, and if the patient's general condition allows him to undergo the procedure. Radiotherapy should follow the laminectomy after removal of sutures and a dose from 2000 rads in 1 week (to a short segment of spinal cord) to 3000 rads in 2 weeks should be administered. This can be done either by using a direct posterior portal and calculating the depth dose at the anterior margin of the spinal canal, or better yet by posterior arc rotation if the location of lesion allows it. If radiotherapy alone is used, the dose should be at least 3000 rads in 2 weeks, and may have to be raised to 4000 rads in 3 to 4 weeks if response is unsatisfactory. Chemotherapy may be employed in oat cell carcinoma, if radiotherapy is not possible because of prior treatment and if surgery is not indicated.

PULMONARY METASTASIS FROM CANCER OF THE LUNG

The frequency with which pulmonary metastasis manifests spread of lung cancer (see page 58) has led to attempts to control pulmonary metastasis by radiation therapy. A limited series reported by Balfour et al.[2] did not, however, indicate significant benefit in a small number of patients treated by prophylactic irradiation of a hemithorax. The usual rapid appearance of pulmonary metastasis following treatment of the primary tumor, or the coexistence of metastatic disease in the lung at the time of diagnosis of the primary tumor argue against surgery. However, Rees and Cleland[20] performed

TABLE 4. METASTATIC SPINAL CORD TUMORS: DURATION OF SYMPTOMS RELATED TO RETURN OF FUNCTION FOLLOWING TREATMENT

Return of Function	Sensory	Motor	Sphincter
Good	29 days	16	1
None	42	22	4

lobectomies on 2 patients with carcinoma of the bronchus who developed metastatic disease 4 and 7 years after their original surgery. Both patients died of widespread dissemination of their tumors 3 and 5 years following resection of the assumed metastatic disease. Although resection of solitary metastasis in cancer of the testicle, kidney, breast and colon was associated with long-term survival in the series, this experience confirms the generally discouraging outlook of pulmonary metastasis from lung cancer. Other large series of patients with resection for lung metastasis[4,10,19] did not include any cases of successful surgery for metastatic lung cancer. Mincer et al.[17] reported a series of patients in whom metastatic disease in the lung was treated by total pulmonary irradiation using a modification of the moving strip technique. The few encouraging results that were mentioned did not include patients with bronchogenic carcinoma; 12 of 56 patients survived 6 months and no increase in survival of patients with metastatic bronchogenic carcinoma could be established.

The use of radioactive microspheres containing radioactive yttrium (^{90}Y) in patients with metastatic lung cancer has been described by Grady et al.,[7] without prolongation of life in the treated patients or significant palliation of symptoms from established metastasis. Early use of this method for subclinical disease has not been described.

REFERENCES

1. Allen, K. L., Johnson, T. W., Wildermuth, O., and Hibbs, G. G.: Effective bone palliation as related to various treatment regimens. Presented at the 58th Scientific Assembly and Annual Meeting of the Radiological Society of North America, November 26–December 1, 1972, Chicago, Illinois.

2. Balfour, H., Sundarsanam, A., and Charynlu, K.: En bloc radiation therapy of primary and sites of occult disease in lung cancer. Cancer. In preparation.

3. Card, R., Cole, D., and Henschke, U.: Summary of ten years of the use of radioactive colloids in intracavitary therapy. J. Nucl. Med. 1:195–202, 1960.

4. Cline, R. E., and Young, W. G.: Long-term results following surgical treatment of metastatic pulmonary tumors. Am. Surg. 36:61–68, 1970.

5. Deeley, T. J., and Edwards, J. M. Rice: Radiotherapy in the management of cerebral secondaries from bronchial carcinoma. Lancet 1:1209–1212, 1968.

6. Galluzzi, S., and Payne, P.: Brain metastasis from primary bronchial carcinoma: A statistical study of 741 necropsies. Br. J. Cancer 10:408–414, 1956.

7. Grady, E. D., Sale, W., Nicholson, W. P., and Rollins, L. C.: Intra-arterial radioisotopes to treat cancer. Am. Surg. 26:678–684, 1960.

8. Harr, F., and Patterson, R.: Surgery for metastatic intracranial neoplasm. Cancer 30:1241–1245, 1972.

9. Hazra, T., Mullins, G. M., and Lott, S.: Management of cerebral metastasis from bronchogenic carcinoma. Johns Hopkins Med. J. 130:377–383, 1972.

10. Hutchison, E. D., and Deaner, R. M.: Resection of pulmonary secondary tumors. Am. J. Surg. 124:732–737, 1972.

11. Handbook 62, International Commission on Radiological Units and Measurements (ICRU), U.S. National Bureau of Standards, Washington, D.C. 1956.

12. Leininger, B. J., Barker, W. L., and Langston, H. T.: Simplified method for management of malignant pleural effusion. J. Thorac. Cardiovisc. Surg. 58:758–763, 1969.

13. Levitt, S. H., Jones, T. K., Kilpatrick, S. J., and Bogardus, C. R.: Treatment of malignant superior vena caval obstruction. A randomized study. Cancer 24:447–451, 1969.

14. Lokich, J. J.: The management of malignant pericardial effusions. J.A.M.A. 224:1401–1404, 1973.

15. Longacre, A. M., and Shockman, A. T.: The superior vena cava syndrome and radiation therapy. Radiology 91:713–718, 1968.

16. McGee, E. E.: Surgical treatment of cerebral metastases from lung cancer. The effect on quality and duration of survival. North Neurosurg. 35:416–420, 1971.

17. Mincer, F., Botstein, C., Schwarz, G., Zacharopoulos, G., and McDougall, R.: Moving strip irradiation in the treatment of extensive neoplastic disease in the chest. Am. J. Roentgenol. Radium Ther. Nucl. Med. 108:278–283, 1970.

18. Montana, G., Mescham, W., and Caldwell, W.: Brain irradiation for metastatic disease of lung origin. Cancer 29:1477–1480, 1972.

19. Mountain, C. F.: Surgical management of pulmonary metastases. Postgrad. Med. 48:128–132, 1970.

20. Rees, G. M., and Cleland, W. P.: Surgical treatment of pulmonary metastases. Thorax 27:654–656, 1972.

21. Richards, P., and McKissock, W.: Intracranial metastasis. Br. Med. J. 1:15–18, 1963.

22. Rubin, P., Mayer, E., and Poulter, C.: Extradural spinal cord compression by tumor. High daily dose experience without laminectomy. Radiology 93:1248–1260, 1969.

23. Salsali, M., and Cliffton E. E.: Superior vena caval obstruction with carcinoma of the lung. Surg. Gynecol. Obstet. 121:783–788, 1965.

24. Spiers, F. W.: Dosage in irradiated soft tissue and bone. Br. J. Radiol. 24:365–368, 1951.

25. Vargha, Z. O., Glicksman, A. S., and Boland, J.: Single-dose radiation therapy in palliation of metastatic disease. Radiology 93:1181–1184, 1969.

26. White, W. A., Patterson, R. H., and Bergland, R. M.: The role of surgery in the treatment of spinal cord compression by metastatic neoplasm. Cancer 27:558–561, 1971.

27. Wright, R. L.: Malignant tumors in the spinal extradural space: results of surgical treatment. Ann. Surg. 157:227–231, 1963.

28. Brady, L., Antonaides, J., Prasasvinichai, S., Torpie, R. J., Asbell, S. O., Glassburn, J. R., Schatanoff, D., and Mancall, E. L.: The treatment of metastatic disease of the nervous system by radiation therapy. In Tumors of the Nervous System, Wiley, New York, 1974.

Chapter Sixteen

Special Problems and Techniques in the Radiotherapy of Cancer of the Lung

ELECTRON BEAM THERAPY

The use of new forms of radiation therapy, such as high energy electrons, has been attempted in the treatment of inoperable cancer of the lung. A large series of patients was described by Ott.[15] The author treated 294 histologically confirmed bronchogenic carcinomas, 51% of which were epidermoid carcinomas, 42% undifferentiated carcinomas, 3% adenocarcinomas, and the remainder a variety of other histologic types. The electrons had a maximum energy of 35 MeV. Treatment was given with one to two fractions of 500 to 1000 rads depth dose weekly, up to a total of approximately 6000 to 7500 rads. Although the immediate tumor response was described as very good and rapid, the 1-year survival was only 45%, not very different from a photon-irradiated series of patients. The 2-year survival was only 6.5%, and 2% of the patients survived 3 years. It is noteworthy that there were 5 patients with operable disease in form of peripheral pulmonary tumors who were not subjected to surgery for one reason or another. Of these patients, 2 survived 4 years without evidence of tumor, and all 5 lived for 3 years or more following treatment. The results of this series may be interpreted as an indication that electron beam therapy provides effective treatment for patients with lung cancer.

In another series, Schumacher[25] reported on the treatment of patients with inoperable lung cancer using the 35 MeV electron beam of the betatron. Treatment was administered using single weekly doses of 500 rads. Tumor doses were determined on the basis of histology, and 5000 rads were given for oat cell carcinoma, 6000 rads for epidermoid carcinoma and 7000 rads for adenocarcinoma. When the tumors exceeded 6 cm in greatest diameter, the dose was increased by approximately 500 to 1000 rads. Also, if there was an abscess in the lung or tumor, the first 2 treatments were given with 900 rads weekly, and these 2 weeks of treatment were followed by 1 to 3 weeks of treatment-free interval with subsequent irradiation of 500 rads per week. There was always tumor response following administration of a 3000 rad dose. No severe complications were encountered among 820 patients, and it was felt that the complication rate from pulmonary fibrosis was less than would be expected from conventional fractionation and photon beam therapy. Of the 820 patients reported, 48% had epidermoid carcinoma. The 1-year survival was 79% in Stage I, 69% in Stage II, 61% in Stage III, and 45% in Stage IV. The composite 3-year survival was 15% and the 5-year survival was 6%.

Heuss[9] reported on the technical aspects of electron beam therapy in lung cancer using a 42 MeV betatron.

The isodose distribution was determined in an Alderson Randall phantom. As expected, the inhomogeneity produced by air-containing lung was significant, approximately 3%. Special attention was drawn to a new technique of irradiation, using small-field rotational therapy which, however, has not found widespread application in electron beam therapy.

POSTOPERATIVE RADIATION THERAPY

The results of curative surgery for lung cancer in the hands of the thoracic surgeon are far from satisfactory, with more than 50 percent of the patients dying of the disease despite what appeared to be adequate surgery for early disease. Aside from local recurrence, one of the reasons is the presence of microscopic metastasis in lymph nodes in the hilum and/or mediastinum. To treat such subclinical metastastis and tumor extensions, Paterson and Russell[16] randomized 99 patients to receive surgical treatment only, and 103 patients for subsequent radiotherapy to a dose of about 4500 rads in 4 weeks using megavoltage irradiation. The survival at 3 years was 46.4% for patients who had surgery only, and 33% for patients who received postoperative radiation therapy. It is noteworthy that there was a variation of the 3-year survival between patients entered at various times of the study, extending from 29.7 to 50% for patients surviving after surgery only and from 9.1 to 45% for patients treated by postoperative radiation therapy, if these patients were divided into groups according to the calendar year during which they entered the study. No significant differences were identified, except in the first year of the study during which the patients subjected to surgery alone had a 3-year survival of 50% and only 9.1% of those treated by surgery and radiotherapy survived. Also, no significant differences were found when the patients were analyzed by cell type and by surgical procedure. An interesting result shows that among the 99 cases with surgery only, 28.3% developed distant metastasis at 3 years, whereas among the 103 patients with subsequent radiation therapy 43.7% developed distant metastasis. This is a consequence of the fact that postoperative radiation therapy prevents or delays local recurrences in the thorax, and some patients survive long enough to develop distant metastasis. This study confirms that distant metastasis is one of the major obstacles to survival of patients with lung cancer, and routine postoperative radiation therapy does not add greatly to the survival of such patients.

Postoperative radiation therapy was also administered in a randomized study by Bangma.[2] Thirty-six patients were classified to receive radiation therapy after appropriate surgery, and 37 received no irradiation. In the 1-year survival rate, there was no significant difference either for the total group or, if divided by histologic subtype or stage of disease, before surgery. The authors also found that intrathoracic recurrence was a cause of death which occurred more frequently in the patients who received no radiation therapy than in those treated with postoperative radiation therapy. Although radiation fibrosis was the verified cause of death in only 1 case of the patients under consideration, the authors felt that the advantages of postoperative irradiation therapy were counteracted by the occurrence of pulmonary fibrosis in those patients who did receive radiation therapy.

On the other hand, Kirsh et al.[12] reported their experience in patients who were selected for postoperative radiotherapy on the basis of findings on thoracotomy. A total of 48 patients out of 231 treated surgically were shown to have histologically confirmed mediastinal metastasis, and 36 of these patients underwent mediastinal irradiation in the immediate postoperative period to a dose of 5000 to 5500 rads. Indication for radiation therapy was usually the opinion of the surgeon that gross removal of all malignant tissue had not been achieved during surgery. Of the 36 patients thus treated, only 2 developed local recurrence in the thorax. Of 17 patients treated postoperatively for squamous cell carcinoma with mediastinal metastasis, 29.5% survived 5 years. Of 17 patients with adenocarcinoma of the lung and mediastinal metastasis only 1 (5.9%) survived 5 years. The total 5-year survival among the 36 patients treated postoperatively was 19.4%. Of the 12 patients treated by surgery only, none survived 5 years. Deeley[4] has also reported some benefit of postoperative radiotherapy in selected patients.

We believe that the indications for postoperative radiotherapy should be based on the finding of positive mediastinal nodes in patients with squamous cell carcinoma, oat cell carcinoma in any patient, the evidence of microscopic tumor at the margin of the resected specimen, or histologic diagnosis of an undifferentiated tumor with high probability of local nodal involvement even if such nodes are not biopsied at time of thoracotomy. Transsection of gross tumor at time of surgery is associated with poor prognosis. Guttmann[7] showed 1-year survival of only 2.5% of such patients.

Surprisingly good results were presented for postoperative radiation therapy by Pavlov et al.[19] in a report on 616 patients. The 3-year survival of patients treated postoperatively by radiotherapy was 45%, and the 5-year survival 38%. Similar survivals were found in patients treated postoperatively by chemotherapy, whereas the results of surgical treatment produced only a 32% 3-year survival and a 24% 5-year survival. Unfortunately, detailed information is not available in this work, but a dose of 4000 rads to 5500 rads is mentioned.

PREOPERATIVE RADIATION THERAPY

The lack of success of surgery is due partly to the high incidence of inoperable and unresectable tumors because of local spread in the mediastinum, either as metastasis or by direct extension. There is a theory supported by a limited number of studies that circulating cancer cells are shed during an operative procedure and lead to dissemination of the tumor during manipulation on the operating table. This correlates with the frequent tendency of bronchogenic carcinoma to spread via the blood vessels. Also, the fact that tumor cells may be seeded in the operative field at surgery is supported by the incidence of pleural effusion following surgical procedures. Attempts have been made therefore to improve survival rates by the use of radiation therapy to devitalize tumor cells before surgery. Although these attempts have been successful in some studies, they failed in a cooperative study where radiotherapy was applied routinely. The lack of success is based mainly on postoperative complications arising from high-dose radiation therapy followed by radical surgery. Delay in healing of the bronchial stump, and subsequent empyema and bronchopleural fistula are the main complications.

The largest study reported to date involved the randomized preoperative use of a radiation dose that approximates the limits of radical radiotherapy. A dose of at least 4500 rads was delivered at 1000 rads/week using 5 treatments weekly, and calculated at the level of the primary tumor and/or mediastinum. In a report on 17 medical centers,[21] 278 patients considered operable at the time of diagnosis were assigned to receive immediate surgery, while 290 similar patients were randomized to receive preoperative radiotherapy followed by surgery in 6 weeks. An additional 425 patients were initially considered inoperable because of regional spread of the cancer in the mediastinum, and they were given preoperative radiation therapy. Of these patients, 152 were considered resectable at presurgical evaluation after radiotherapy. They were assigned to either thoracotomy and resection if possible (78 patients), or to continue without further surgical treatment (74 patients). Although there were some differences among the patient groups randomized for one or the other treatment method, mainly in age incidence and histologic type, the conclusions of the study were based on a comparison of survival at 1, 4, 6, 12, 24, and 36 months following randomization for treatment. No significant difference was found between the operable patients receiving prior radiotherapy in whom $19.4 \pm 2.6\%$ survived 3 years and those who were immediately subjected to surgery, of whom $21.2 \pm 2.7\%$ survived 3 years. Among the inoperable patients because of local extension, those who received radiation therapy alone had a 3-year survival of $9.0 \pm 3.6\%$, whereas $6.0 \pm 3.4\%$ of those patients who received initial radiation therapy and subsequent operation survived. The differences between the 3-year survival figures were not statistically significant at the $p < 0.05$ level. Some of the deaths among those patients who received preoperative radiation therapy were due to complications. Of 290 patients with prior radiotherapy, 26 had evidence of bronchopleural fistula, whereas only 9 of 278 patients developed this complication following immediate surgery. There was an increase in complications among all patients who had pneumonectomy, lobectomy, or bilobectomy after radiotherapy, whereas the patients who were explored and not resected showed an incidence of complications similar to patients elected for immediate surgery but not resected. A similar lack of improvement in survival rates after unselected use of preoperative irradiation in a randomized study of lung cancer patients has been reported by Shields.[27]

Although Mercado et al.[14] initially reported encouraging results in a series of patients treated by high-dose preoperative radiotherapy, with doses up to 5500 rads delivered before radical surgery, the follow-up of their patients as published by Cowley and co-workers[3] failed to confirm the initial impression. Of 192 patients considered for preoperative irradiation in this series, 14 have survived 5 or more years for a respectable but not extraordinary survival rate of 7%. Of the 192 patients, 98 underwent surgery, and 13 survived 5 years. Five of the survivors were considered operable before radiotherapy and 8 were considered inoperable, having been rendered operable by the preoperative radiation. Approximately half of the resections actually performed in patients irradiated preoperatively were done on patients who were previously considered inoperable. Although the authors felt they had demonstrated the feasibility of combined therapy with resection in a large number of patients, the overall cure rate was not improved because of a substantial loss due to operative mortality and metastatic disease. Of the 98 patients investigated, 29 died as the result of postoperative complications.

Preoperative irradiation in a selected group of patients to a dose of 4500 to 5000 rads with subsequent limited surgery has been described by Saxena and co-workers.[23] The authors described the technique of radiation therapy and subsequent sleeve resection which permitted preservation of some of the functioning pulmonary parenchyma and resection of otherwise inoperable tu-

mors. Of the 45 patients studied, 6 later showed local recurrences. Among those receiving local preoperative radiotherapy only 2 of 31 patients had local recurrence, whereas 4 of 14 treated by sleeve resection alone showed this finding. At the end of 5 years, 14 of 32 patients treated with the combined therapies were still alive.

Although doses in excess of 4500 rads in approximately $4\frac{1}{2}$ weeks offer the possibility of sterilizing the tumor in a small number of patients with bronchogenic carcinoma, a different approach with approximately 3000 rads of preoperative radiation in 2 to 3 weeks is based on the possibility of decreasing tumor size to a minor degree and devitalizing cells that might otherwise facilitate dissemination of local or distant metastasis during surgery. Paulson[18] is the main advocate of this technique. With this dose applied in apical tumors, resections were possible in many patients, and 33% of those treated by combined preoperative radiation and subsequent surgery survived 2 years or more. Paulson and co-workers[17] also performed bronchoplastic procedures after preoperative irradiation, and 50% of the 20 patients irradiated survived 5 years, while only 30% of those who did not receive preoperative irradiation survived for this length of time. The complication rate was felt to be acceptable, and it was remarkable that only 1 of 20 patients showed recurrent cancer locally in contrast to 8 of 34 patients who did not receive preoperative irradiation. These results lend some support to the belief that a moderate dose of radiation will facilitate surgery because of a decrease in size of the tumor mass, and that a moderate dose of radiation combined with a bronchoplastic procedure will minimize the complications and death resulting from impairment of pulmonary function, either because of surgical procedures such as pneumonectomy or because of fibrosis after radiotherapy.

A third approach to preoperative radiation therapy is the use of a low dose of radiation, occasionally with up to 2400 rads given for 3 successive days. The clear distinction between low-, medium- and high-dose preoperative radiotherapy loses its significance when the biologic effect of the time-dose relationship is considered. The dose of 2400 rads in 3 successive days has to be interpreted as being in the medium-dose range, although it is unlikely to achieve the results of local control expected from the high-dose range. Groves and Rodriguez-Antunez[6] used such a dose 10 to 14 days before surgery, but results of treatment are inconclusive as to long-term survival and complications. Encouraging results with a similar dose schedule have been reported by Witz and co-workers[29] who reported improved 8-year survival among patients treated in this manner.

At present the value of preoperative radiation therapy in controlling lung cancer must be considered questionable. Since local control of large tumor masses by radiotherapy is difficult, a combination of moderate dose radiation to 3000 rads with subsequent surgery and preservation of pulmonary function may prove useful. The routine use of preoperative radiation therapy must however be discouraged, as has been shown in the nationwide study mentioned earlier. Some of the results of preoperative radiotherapy are of value because they indicate that a dose of 5500 to 6000 rads sterilized at least 53% of the lymph nodes initially diagnosed as positive by biopsy and about 35% of the primary tumors.[14] The use of azygograms might lead to a further definition of indications for surgery after radiation therapy, although this study has found a lesser degree of acceptance since the introduction of mediastinal biopsies. Encouraging results using this study as a preoperative sign of operability, including preoperative radiation, have been reported by Wolfel and co-workers[30] and Rinker and Templeton.[22]

ENDOBRONCHIAL RADIATION THERAPY

Schlungbaum et al.[24] reported on the use of radioactive cobalt beads which are threaded on a metal sound and introduced into major and minor bronchi. Usually, 6 to 8 mCi of cobalt are used and left in place for about 3 to 4 hr. The authors estimated that 6 to 8 beads of 4 to 6 mm in diameter left in place for 1 hr produced about 1000 rads at 3 mm from the surface of the beads. It is necessary for the patient to be anesthetized during the procedure. Although the authors indicated that the method was mainly used in patients with advanced bronchogenic carcinoma as an adjunct to other treatment, if significant symptoms arose from endobronchial tumor growth, they found that the use of endobronchial therapy in stump recurrence may offer the possibility of cure and described at least 1 patient in whom endobronchial therapy controlled a lesion, as well as 45 of 109 patients with "remarkable palliative success." This type of treatment has not been used widely.

INTERSTITIAL IMPLANTATION IN THE TREATMENT OF BRONCHOGENIC CARCINOMA

As in other sites of malignancy, the advantages of a high dose in a limited volume have been best realized by the use of interstitial implantation. In this country, the group of radiation therapists at the Memorial Hospital in New York have popularized the procedure in a number of papers. Martini and co-workers[13] and Hilaris et al.[10] reported their experience with inoperable patients or patients in whom incomplete surgery was carried out. Radioactive seeds containing ^{222}Rn or ^{125}I were used in a group of 90 patients, 54 of whom had no remaining di-

sease at thoracotomy, while residual tumor was implanted in 32 cases. Of these, 3 (9.4%) were alive and free of disease for 5 years. Of 16 patients who received external beam radiation therapy postoperatively for disease of limited extent, none survived for 5 years. In a group of 38 patients with unresectable apical lung cancer, 6 (16%) survived 5 years or more after interstitial irradiation at thoracotomy when resection of the tumor could not be carried out. Of 16 patients who had incomplete resection and implantation, 3 are alive 5 years following treatment. The authors stated that only with interstitial implantation could they give a dose high enough for probable sterilization of the tumor. These are doses two or three times higher than those administered by external beam radiation and they have not produced significant side effects. Technically, volume implants are usually attempted as described by Henschke et al.,[8] and the dose of radiation delivered to the tumor has been calculated as 10,000 to 15,000 rads. The authors compared their technique by randomization to patients treated by external beam radiation only and found that interstitial implantation offers a better chance of survival for these patients.

In Great Britain, Gibbons and Baker[5] reported on a series of 198 patients suffering from inoperable lung cancer who were treated by interstitial implantation of radioactive gold seeds. The gold seeds had an activity of between 3.5 and 5 mCi each. The technique used by the authors delivered a dose of about 18,000 rads to a tumor 2.5 cm in diameter when gold seeds with an activity of 3.5 mCi were used. They estimated that a majority of the patients received between 5,000 and 15,000 rads from an average of 20 to 40 gold seeds implanted in a regular fashion. Indications for the procedure were defined by the authors as follows: (1) growth not resectable at thoracotomy; (2) resectable growth but poor respiratory reserve; (3) supplement to surgery and partially resected growth; (4) endobronchial implantation of inoperable carcinomas.

The last mentioned method was applied in tumors involving the carina or trachea, and occasionally in recurrences at the suture line of previous resection. The authors felt that multiple pulmonary and pleural metastases were contraindications to interstitial irradiation. The 2-year survival among 169 patients thus treated was 20%, whereas among 29 patients treated by endobronchial implantation 10% survived 2 years. This compared favorably with the result of 101 patients explored and not resected without further treatment, among whom 10% survived 2 years, whereas among 47 patients who received external beam radiotherapy following thoracotomy only 6% survived 2 years.

Although supplemental external beam radiation therapy could be administered, the authors felt that palliation of cough, pain, and malaise were more effective by interstitial irradiation in their series. They also stated that they rarely encountered postoperative complications such as empyema. The main disadvantage of the treatment was the exposure to radiation of the staff administering the implantation, but Gibbons and Baker felt that if due precautions were taken, this hazard did not warrant discontinuing this form of treatment. It should be mentioned here that the first successful pneumonectomy performed in the United States at the Memorial Hospital in New York by Dr. Evards Graham on April 5, 1933, was supplemented by the implantation of radon seeds at the margins of resection. The patient, a dentist, outlived Dr. Graham.

LOW-DOSE RATE IRRADIATION

Pierquin and Baillet[20] have made use of irradiation at very low-dose rates (2–3 rads per minute) in advanced cancers of the head and neck and other sites. Their results have been encouraging and have shown that the tumoricidal effect is equal to that at conventional dose

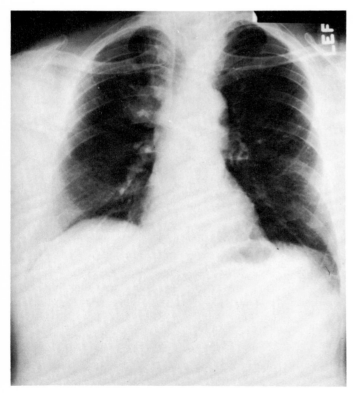

Fig. 1. Patient H. L. Posteroanterior x-ray of the chest after previous radiotherapy of the mediastinum for lymphoma to 3500 rads tumor dose. Epidermoid carcinoma was diagnosed in the right mediastinum on mediastinal biopsy.

rates (about 100 rads/min), whereas the normal tissue effects seem to decrease.

In a limited series of patients treated for lung cancer, with 5500 to 6000 rads tumor dose by conventional fractionation at approximately 20 rads/min and at 200 rads/min at the American Oncologic Hospital, this observation could not be confirmed. In 14 patients who were matched by treatment regimen, histologic diagnosis, T stage, sex, and age decade, with 7 patients each treated by high and low dose rates, there was no significant difference in survival, dysphagia, and pulmonary fibrosis 1 to 3 months after the end of radiotherapy. Local tumor response on x-rays obtained at 4000 rads tumor dose also did not differ significantly. All 6 patients with complete response at this dose level had oat cell carcinoma. One patient each with adenocarcinoma and epidermoid carcinoma treated with the high dose rate had partial response, and one patient with epidermoid carcinoma treated with low dose rate had complete response.

BRONCHOGENIC CARCINOMA AS PART OF MULTIPLE CANCERS

Bilateral bronchogenic carcinoma poses a problem of its own from both a diagnostic and a therapeutic point of view. The appearance of an apparently solitary lesion in the lung in a patient previously treated for cancer of the lung or recently diagnosed as having untreated lung cancer has a significant influence on prognosis and management. Whether metastatic disease or multiple simultaneous bronchogenic carcinomas are present is a difficult question to answer. Even pathologic examination of a specimen from the tumor does not resolve this problem because squamous cell carcinomas look alike under the microscope unless they are distinguished by significant differences in histopathologic pattern.

The importance of the biologic behavior of multiple pulmonary malignant disease has been emphasized by Ishihara et al.,[11] who examined the tumor growth rate in 77 patients with pulmonary metastasis. A detailed analysis of the relationship between survival following surgical or chemotherapeutic treatment for the metastatic disease and the doubling time indicated that the major factor leading to successful treatment of the metastatic disease was a long interval between treatment of the primary tumor and appearance of metastasis. Patients with tumor doubling times of less than 30 days had a mean interval of 12 months between primary treatment and detection of pulmonary metastasis. Patients with tumor doubling times of 30 days or more had a mean interval of 38 months between primary operation and detection of pulmonary metastasis. Five 5-year survivors were treated by various combinations of surgery

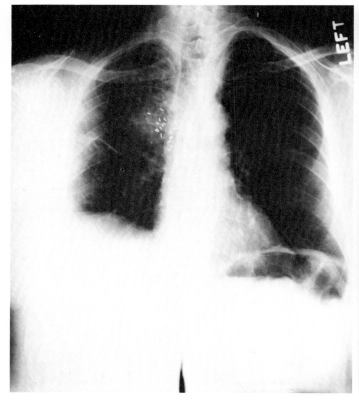 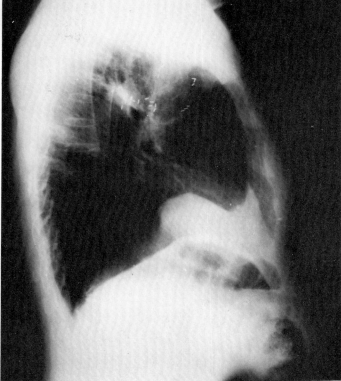

Fig. 2. Same patient, after placement of radon seeds in the tumor during thoracotomy. A tumor dose of 2000 to 5000 rads was delivered in the known tumor-bearing area. Additional treatment was administered by external beam cobalt teletherapy for 3000 rads in 3 weeks. Patient died of metastatic tumor 20 months later.

radiotherapy, and chemotherapy for their metastatic disease. The interval between primary operation and detection of pulmonary metastasis for these few patients ranged from 14 months to 10 years.

The largest series of bilateral primary bronchogenic carcinoma with results of treatment was described by Struve-Christensen,[28] who reported on a total of 40 synchronous and 30 asynchronous, bilateral primary bronchogenic carcinomas. In 24 patients the diagnosis was established at autopsy, in 18 patients on surgical specimens and autopsy, and in 28 patients on surgical specimens. Twenty-four patients with synchronous, bilateral bronchogenic carcinomas had an identical histology of their tumors, and 16 patients had a different histology. Among the asynchronous bronchogenic carcinomas, 21 patients had identical histology and 9 had a different histology. The interval between diagnosis of the first and second tumors in asynchronous cancers varied from 13 months to 10 years. The usual interval was from 1 to 3 years. In this series of 10 patients from the author's personal experience and 60 patients from the literature, follow-up information was available on 20: 14 patients died postoperatively and up to 29 months following the second operation, and 6 patients have survived for 10 to 24 months.

The clinical approach to a patient with what appears to be either solitary metastasis or multiple primary bronchogenic carcinoma is best decided on the basis of the statement of Shields et al.,[26] who emphasized in their study that whenever doubt prevails in case of suspected second primary tumor, the suspicion must benefit from the doubt, and thoracotomy should be performed on all patients able to tolerate the operation. This approach has also been supported by Adkins and co-workers[1] who reported on 50 patients submitted to thoracotomy for questionable second bronchogenic malignancies. Thirty-two were shown to have metastatic disease, and 18 had new primary lung tumors. The average survival after pulmonary resection was 39 months, ranging from 27 to 68 months in patients with metastatic cancer originating from primary cancer of the breast and an average of 24 months (range: 2 to 120 months) following genitourinary malignancy. Among patients diagnosed as having second bronchogenic primary tumors, an average survival of 20.2 months was noted, with a range of 1 to 48 months.

It has been our policy to consider all patients in whom

doubt exists about the presence of a new bronchogenic primary tumor or metastatic disease as patients who have primary lung cancer and to treat them according to the staging of this new cancer. The figures mentioned earlier support the value of this treatment, although we have not encountered any 5-year survivors.

REFERENCES

1. Adkins, P. C., Wesselhoeft, C. W., Jr., Newman, W., and Blades, B.: Thoractomy on the patient with previous malignancy: metastasis or new primary? *J. Thorac. Cardiovasc. Surg.* **56**: 351–360, 1968.

2. Bangma, P. J.: Post-operative radiotherapy. In *Carcinoma of the Bronchus*, T. Deeley, Ed., Appleton-Century-Crofts, London, New York, 1971.

3. Cowley, R. A., Wizenberg, M. J., and Linberg, E. J.: The role of radiation therapy and surgery in the treatment of bronchogenic carcinoma. *Ann. Thorac. Surg.* **8**:229–236, 1969.

4. Deeley, T. J.: The treatment of carcinoma of the bronchus. *Br. J. Radiol.* **40**:801–822, 1967.

5. Gibbons, J. R. P., and Baker, R.: Treatment of carcinoma of the bronchus by interstitial irradiation. A study of 198 patients. *Thorax* **24**:451–456, 1969.

6. Groves, L. K., and Rodriguez-Antunez, A.: Treatment of carcinoma of esophagus and lung with concentrated radiation followed by surgery. *Ann. Thorac. Surg.* **6**:154–162, 1968.

7. Guttmann, R. J.: Results of radiation therapy in patients with inoperable carcinoma of the lung whose status was established at exploratory thoracotomy. *Am. J. Roentgenol. Radium Ther. Nucl. Med.* **93**:99–103, 1965.

8. Henschke, U. K., Hilaris, B. S., Mahan, G. D., and Wright, F. E.: Interstitial implantation of radioactive seeds during thoracotomy. In *Lung Cancer*, W. L. Watson, Ed., C. V. Mosby, St. Louis, 1968.

9. Heuss, K.: Beitrag zur Bestrahlungsplanung bei der Elektronentherapie des Bronchialkarzinoms. *Strahlenther.* **141**:25–31, 1971.

10. Hilaris, B. S., Luomanen, R. K., and Beattie, E. J.: Integrated irradiation and surgery in the treatment of apical lung cancer. *Cancer* **27**:1369–1373, 1971.

11. Ishihara, T., Keiichi, K., Ikeda, T., Yamazaki, S.: Metastatic pulmonary diseases: biologic factors and modes of treatment. *Chest* **63**:227–232, 1973.

12. Kirsh, M. M., Kahn, D. R., Gago, O., Lampe, I., Fayos, J. V., Prior, M., Moores, W. Y., Haight, C., and Sloan, H.: Treatment of bronchogenic carcinoma with mediastinal metastasis. *Ann. Thorac. Surg.* **12**:11–21, 1971.

13. Martini, N., Hilaris, B. S., and Beattie, E. J.: Interstitial vs. external irradiation combined with pulmonary resection in lung cancer. *Cancer* **26**:638–641, 1970.

14. Mercado, R., Bloedorn, F. G., Cuccia, C. A., and Cowley, R. A.: Combined radical radiotherapy and surgery in the treatment of bronchogenic carcinoma. *Radiology* **74**:97–98, 1960.

15. Ott, A.: Fuenf Jahre Strahlenthe rapie des Bronchuscarcinomas mit hochenergetischen Electronen. *Strahlenther.* **141**:141–145, 1971.

16. Paterson, R., and Russell, M. H.: Clinical trials in malignant disease: IV. lung cancer. *Clin. Radiol.* **13**:141–144, 1962.

17. Paulson, D. L., Urschel, H. C., McNamara, J. J, and Shaw, R. R.: Bronchoplastic procedures for bronchogenic carcinoma. *J. Thorac. Cardiovasc. Surg.* **59**:38–47, 1970.

18. Paulson, D : The role of pre-operative radiation therapy in the surgical management of carcinoma in the superior pulmonary sulcus. In *The Interrelationship of Surgery and Radiation Therapy in the Treatment of Cancer*, University Park Press, Baltimore, 1970.

19. Pavlov, A., Priogov, A., Trachtenberg, A., Volkova, M., Maximov, T., and Matveeva, T.: Results of combination treatment of lung cancer patients: surgery plus radiotherapy and surgery plus chemotherapy. *Cancer Chemother. Rept.* (Pt. 3) **4**:133–135, 1973.

20. Pierquin, B., and Baillet, F.: La Teleradiotherapie Continue et de Faible *Debit. Ann. Radiol.* **14**:617–629, 1971.

21. Preoperative irradiation of cancer of the lung. Preliminary report of a therapeutic trial. A collaborative study. *Cancer* **23**:419–429, 1969.

22. Rinker, C. T., and Templeton, A. W.: Pre- and post-irradiation azygography: its value in determining surgical resectability in pulmonary carcinoma. *Am. J. Roentgenol. Radium Ther. Nucl. Med.* **105**:83–85, 1969.

23. Saxena, V. S., Hendrickson, F. R., Jensik, R. J., and Faber, P.: Conservative surgery following pre-operative radiation therapy of lung cancer. *Am. J. Roentgenol. Radium Ther. Nucl. Med.* **114**:93–98, 1972.

24. Schlungbaum, W., Blum, H., and Brandt, H. J.: Results of endobronchial irradiation in bronchogenic carcinoma. *Radiol. Austriaca* **13**:201–214, 1962.

25. Schumacher, W.: Radiotherapy of cancer of the lung. Presented at the Eleventh International Cancer Congress, Florence, 1974.

26. Shields, T. W., Drake, C. T., and Sherrick, J. C.: Bilateral primary bronchogenic carcinoma. *J. Thorac. Cardiovasc. Surg.* **48**:401–417, 1964.

27. Shields, T.: Preoperative radiotherapy in the treatment of bronchial carcinoma. *Cancer* **30**:1388–1394, 1972.

28. Struve-Christensen, E : Diagnosis and treatment of bilateral primary bronchogenic carcinoma. *J. Thorac. Cardiovasc. Surg.* **61**:501–513, 1971.

29. Witz, J. P., Herdly, J., Miech, G., and Morand, G.: Modalites d'association irradiation preoperatoire et chirurgie dans le traitement du cancer du poumon. *Ann. Chir. Thorac. Cardiol.* **7**:475–478, 1968.

30. Wolfel, D. A, Linberg, E. J., and Light, J. P.: The abnormal azygogram—an index of inoperability. *Am. J. Roentgenol. Radium Ther. Nucl. Med.* **97**:933–938, 1966.

Chapter Seventeen

Specific Medical Management of Cancer of the Lung

Chemotherapy for bronchogenic carcinoma can be given either as the only form of treatment, usually in an unfavorable group of patients with widely disseminated disease, or it may be given as an adjunct to surgery or radiotherapy.

Carter[1] summarized the results of chemotherapy and indicated that nitrogen mustard was the most frequently used drug, which produced some response in 30% of 1,123 patients. The best results were obtained with cyclophosphamide to which 33% of 509 patients responded, a similar figure was obtained for methotrexate and busulfan in a significantly smaller number of patients. Table 1 summarizes a large number of chemotherapeutic series. Among the drugs under clinical investigation at present, adriamycin has shown a 20% response in a total of 147 patients treated. Hexamethylmelamine showed a 21% response in 202 patients, while bis-chloroethyl-nitrosourea (BCNU) and chloroethyl-cyclo-hexyl-nitrosourea (CCNU) are currently under investigation with some promise of effectiveness. Takita and Brugarolas[18] using CCNU were able to show a response rate of 36% in 50 patients, some of whom had previously failed to respond to other chemotherapy. Among patients with squamous cell carcinoma and adenocarcinoma 46% responded, whereas those with anaplastic and oat cell carcinoma showed a lower response rate. Unfortunately, survival is still measured in weeks, with a mean survival for the nonresponding patients of 9.5 weeks, and a mean survival for the responders of 17.8 weeks. Among the patients who showed more than 50% regression on objective findings, remission lasted from 3 months to 1 year.

The result of combination chemotherapy of multiple drugs in bronchogenic carcinoma has been summarized by Selawry.[17] At present, the best combinations for various cell types are procarbazine and fluorouracil, which elicited a response in 55% of 11 patients with epidermoid carcinoma, 44% of 9 patients with small cell carcinoma, 83% of 6 patients with adenocarcinoma, and 40% of 10 patients with large cell undifferentiated carcinoma. A combination of procarbazine, cytoxan, methotrexate and vincristine produced 39% response in epidermoid carcinoma, and 69% response in 16 patients with small cell carcinoma. A combination of cytoxan, methotrexate, and CCNU produced a median survival of 250 days in patients with small cell carcinoma and 240 days in patients with adenocarcinoma. In addition, there are many studies which fail to exhibit evidence of significant improvements in response or survival rate from combination chemotherapy, and a great number of ongoing studies are using the available drugs as well as newly discovered drugs in a multitude of combinations. An interesting combination of treatment modalities in which multiple drug chemotherapy forms the mainstay of treatment of small cell undifferentiated carcinoma and low dose radiotherapy added to this regimen has been described by Eagen et al.[9] Cyclic monthly courses of high dose cyclophosphamide, vincristine, procarbazine and methotrexate are used, and radiotherapy (3200 rads) is administered to the primary tumor as part of the sched-

TABLE 1. CUMULATIVE DATA ON THE ACTIVITY OF STANDARD CHEMOTHERAPEUTIC AGENTS AGAINST BRONCHOGENIC CARCINOMA[a]

Drug	Number of Patients Treated	Number of Responses	Percent Response
Nitrogen Mustard (Mustargen)	1123	334	30
Cyclophosphamide (Cytoxan®)	509	168	33
Chlorambucil (Leukeran®)	23	3	8
Phenylalanine mustard (Alkeran®)	38	4	10.5
Busulfan (Myleran)	19	6	32
Methotrexate (Methotrexate®)	167	56	33
5-Fluorouracil (Fluorouracil®)	158	12	7.5
6-Mercaptopurine (Purinethol®)	95	4	9
Arabinosyl cytosine (Cytosar®)	60	0	0
Vincristine (Oncovin®)	43	4	9
Vinblastine (Velban®)	109	12	11
Actinomycin D (Cosmegen)	16	0	0
Mithramycin (Mithracin®)	13	0	0
Mitomycin C	135	29	21
Hydroxyurea (Hydrea®)	36	4	11
Procarbazine (Matulane®)	172	26	15

[a] Compiled by the Cancer Therapy Evaluation Branch.[4]

uled management of these patients. Seventeen of 19 patients thus treated had an objective tumor response (89%). The mean survival of these patients was 6 months at the time of this report. Six of the 8 living patients were free of demonstrable disease and they are being followed. The response of these patients was significantly higher than the 50% expected from cyclophosphamide alone. On the other hand, the authors gained the impression that concomitant radiotherapy and chemotherapy lead to severe hematologic toxicity, and therefore advise against this concomitant use.

CHEMOTHERAPY AS AN ADJUNCT TO OTHER MODES OF TREATMENT

The use of cytotoxic drugs in combination with surgical resection has been disappointing. None of the large cooperative studies has shown significant improvement in long-term survival using nitrogen mustard or cytoxan with standard surgical therapy. The only exception has been a substantial increase in survival in patients with oat cell carcinoma who had surgical resection followed by the administration of cyclophosphamide. In a report by Higgins,[12] 181 patients who had curative surgery were randomized to receive cytoxan. Among the treated group with oat cell carcinoma, 16% survived 4 years, while the control group with surgery only had a 4-year survival of 4%. Among a group of other undifferentiated carcinomas, treatment with cytoxan and surgery produced a 3-year survival of 35%, while the control group with surgery only had 4-year survival of 31%. On the other hand, Brunner and co-workers[3] reported that among patients who were treated by cytoxan intermittently following surgery, recurrence and death from cancer during the first 2 years of observation were significantly higher than in those patients who did not receive the drug. The possibility that cytoxan acts as an immunosuppressor must be taken into consideration.

The use of chemotherapy in association with radiation therapy for cancer of the lung has been attempted using vinblastine,[7] cyclophosphamide,[2] 5-fluorouracil and actinomycin D,[11] procarbazine,[14] and nitrogen mustard[8] without much difference in survival compared to patients treated by radiation therapy alone. Bergsagel et al.[1] recently reported on a series of patients with nonresectable lung cancer confined to the thorax who were treated by radiotherapy to 4000 to 5000 rads, or by radiotherapy followed by four to eight courses of high-dose intermittent cyclophosphamide. Although the drug was only minimally effective in the treatment of this disease, the interval to progression of tumor was 190 days for 80 patients receiving chemotherapy as compared to 114 days for the 43 patients treated by radiotherapy only.

The majority of the patients had epidermoid carcinoma; however, there were 41 patients with oat cell carcinoma. The median survival was 306 days for the patients treated by chemotherapy and radiotherapy, as compared to 216 days for the patients treated by radiotherapy only. The authors felt that this indicated a minimally effective drug in the form of cyclophosphamide, the use of which should be explored further.

Similar results were reported by Brouet.[2] The 1-year survival among 46 patients receiving radiation therapy to 6000 rads in 6 weeks and cyclophosphamide was 35%, and the 1-year survival with radiation therapy only to 6000 rads in six weeks, 31%.

Intraarterial Chemotherapy

A special technique of chemotherapy is bronchial artery perfusion, either by selective catheterization of bronchial arteries or by perfusion of a segment of the aorta from which the bronchial arteries arise. Patients were selected for this form of treatment if no other form of treatment appeared possible. Palliation was obtained in 13 of 21 patients, or 62%. Dyspnea improved in 12 of 18, cough improved in 80 or 16%, and hemoptysis improved in most. Pain improved in 60%, and was relieved almost completely in 2 patients. An objective response in the form of a decrease of visible tumor occurred in 33% of the patients. Complications included injury of blood vessels during the catheter advancement, aortic rupture by rapid balloon inflation, and balloon fragmentation with rupture. The method has not been applied extensively.[6]

IMMUNOTHERAPY OF BRONCHOGENIC CARCINOMA

The use of immune manipulation as part of the treatment of bronchogenic carcinoma is based on the experience that the immunologic competence of patients with various types of cancer including bronchogenic carcinoma may be deficient (see page 61). Clinical trials with immunotherapy have been carried out in patients with advanced disease in whom no specific curative treatment was indicated. Cheema and Hersh[5] injected metastatic tumors including bronchogenic carcinoma into the subcutaneous tissue with autochthonous lymphocytes activated in vitro with phytohemagglutinin or with nonactivated in vitro incubated autochthonous lymphocytes, and observed the response of these tumors by measurement. Twenty-seven of 29 tumors showed regression 1 week following injection without associated treatment by chemotherapy or other means. Four of 14 tumors continued to regress over a period of 6 weeks without any further chemotherapy or immune manipulation. Ten of the 14 tumors occurred in patients who subsequently needed chemotherapy, and 8 of these 10 continued to maintain regression under the circumstances.

Regression occurred in 93% of the 29 tumors injected with activated lymphocytes, in 39% of the 18 tumors injected with nonactivated lymphocytes, and in only 7% of the tumors either injected with saline or without treatment. The authors assumed that the effect of tumor regression was produced at least in part by release of cytotoxin from activated lymphocytes. This effect depends upon cell contact.

Israel and Halpern[15] reported on 20 patients with advanced bronchogenic carcinoma who were treated by palliative chemotherapy and weekly injections of a suspension of corynebacterium parvum. Twenty-seven patients received only palliative chemotherapy. The median survival of the patients treated by chemotherapy and immunotherapy was 9.5 months compared to 5 months for those treated by chemotherapy only, with an average survival of 9.25 months versus 5.85 months. The authors also made the interesting observation that the 1-year survival among the patients who had positive tuberculin tests and who were treated by immunotherapy was 53%, compared to 16% in those who were tuberculin negative and treated by immunotherapy. Patients not receiving immunotherapy and treated by chemotherapy only had a 1-year survival of 25% if their tuberculin test was positive, and of only 5% if their tuberculin test was negative. The authors concluded that one may expect a prolongation of life from immune therapy in appropriately selected patients. They also concluded that the place of immunotherapy cannot be determined until patients with less advanced disease are evaluated after deactivation of the major portion of their tumor burden by either radiotherapy or surgery. It is likely that the effect of this new manipulation is based on patient's increased tolerance to chemotherapy. Studies are in progress to determine whether immunotherapy itself has an antitumor effect.

As part of such investigation, studies involve the inhalation of BCG (bacille Calmette Guérin). To date, however, no results have been reported from this clinical trial. On the other hand, nonspecific immune stimulation with BCG via a vaccination technique, usually starting 10 to 14 days after the end of cytotoxic treatment for cancer of the lung, or after radiotherapy, revealed a 10% disease-free 1-year survival among the controls as compared to 50% among the BCG treatment patients in a small series reported by Pines.[16]

Humphrey and co-workers[13] reported on 43 patients with inoperable or metastatic cancer of the lung who were treated by active immunization with a tumor homogenate followed by the simultaneous exchange of plasma white blood cells. In 1 of 20 patients with primary cancer of the lung, reduction of the tumor size was observed for 18 months. In 6 of 23 patients with metastatic disease there was a demonstrable decrease in size of the lesion for periods of 2 to 18 months.

REFERENCES

1. Bergsagel, D. E., Jenkins, R. D. T., Pringle, J. F., White, D. M., Fetterly, J. C. M., Klassen, D. J., and McDermot, R. S. R.: Lung cancer: clinical trial of radiotherapy alone vs. radiotherapy plus cyclophosphamide. *Cancer* **30**:621–627, 1972.

2. Brouet, D. G.: Resultats d'un essai therapeutique clinique sur une association radiotherapie et chimiotherapy dans les cancers bronco-pulmonaires. Groupe Cooperative d'essais therapeutics sur les cancers bronco pulmonaires. *Eur. J. Cancer* **4**:437–445, 1968.

3. Brunner, K., Marthalen, T., and Muller, W.: Unfavorable effects of long term adjuvant chemotherapy with endoxan in radically operated bronchogenic carcinoma. *Eur. J. Cancer* **7**: 285.288, 1971.

4. Carter, S.: New drugs on the horizon in bronchogenic carcinoma. *Cancer* **30**:1402–1409, 1972.

5. Cheema, A. R., and Hersh, E. M.: Local tumor immunotherapy with in vitro activated autocthonous lymphocytes. *Cancer* **29**: 982–986, 1972.

6. Cliffton, E. E.: Bronchial artery perfusion for treatment of advanced lung cancer. *Cancer* **23**:1151–1157, 1969.

7. Coy, P.: Randomized study of irradiation and Vinblastine in lung cancer. *Cancer* **26**:86–88, 1970.

8. Durrant, K. R., Ellis, F., Black, J. M., Berry, R. J., Ridehalgh, F. R.: and Hamilton, W. S.: Comparison of treatment policies in inoperable bronchial carcinoma *Lancet* **1**:715–719, 1971.

9. Eagan, R. T., Maurer, L. H., Forcier, R. J., and Tulloh, M.: Combination chemotherapy and radiation therapy in small cell carcinoma of the lung *Cancer* **32**:371–379, 1973.

10. Elias, E. G., and Brugarolas, A.: The role of heparin in the chemotherapy of solid tumors: preliminary clinical trial in carcinoma of the lung. *Cancer Chemother. Rep.* **56**:783–785, 1972.

11. Hall, T.: A clinical pharmacologic study of chemotherapy and x-ray therapy in lung cancer. *Am. J. Med.* **43**:186–193, 1967.

12. Higgins, G.: Use of chemotherapy as an adjuvant to surgery for bronchogenic carcinoma. **30**:1383–1387, 1972.

13. Humphrey, L. J., Osler, A., Logan, W., Murray, D. R., and Hatcher, C. R., Jr.: Immunal therapy of cancer in man: five studies of patients with primary and metastatic tumors of the lung. *Am. Surg.* **38**:418–421, 1972.

14. Hussey, D. H., Landgren, R. C., Leary, W. V., and Samuels, M. L.: A randomized study of radiotherapy compared to radiotherapy plus procarbazine in inoperable bronchogenic carcinoma. Presented at the 58th Scientific Assembly and Annual Meeting of the Radiological Society of North America, Chicago, November 26–December 1, 1972.

or atelectasis which prohibited accurate evaluation of the pulmonary parenchyma.

Chest x-rays were graded either as showing no evidence of pulmonary fibrosis, or as showing minimal, moderate, or severe fibrosis. No evidence of fibrosis indicated that there was no appreciable change following the initial preirradiation chest x-ray, either in the bronchovascular markings or in the pulmonary parenchymal appearance. When there was a discernible increase in the pulmonary markings in the treated areas, it was called minimal fibrosis. Patients who were graded as showing moderate fibrosis showed opacification of lung parenchyma, usually fluffy in nature and with definite areas of aeration within the opacified zone. Sometimes there was slight loss of volume of the affected lung. Severe fibrosis was evident on the chest x-ray by dense opacification with coalescence of the above-mentioned areas, usually without areas of aeration within the densely opacified areas, and frequently with partial atelectasis, volume loss of the lung, elevation, and later tenting of the diaphragm. In no case was pulmonary fibrosis seen in the lung outside the direct beam of radiation.

The changes on the chest x-ray were correlated with the patient's symptomatology, and the symptoms were graded as absent, mild, or severe. Mild symptoms consisted of slight cough and slight shortness of breath, which required no medication other than a cough rem-

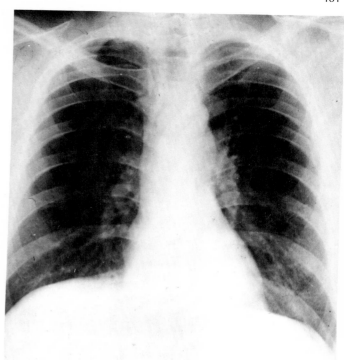

Fig. 2. The same patient following administration of 4000 rads cobalt teletherapy showing decrease in tumor mass and minimal changes of radiation fibrosis of the lung.

edy. Generally, these patients continued their normal activities. Severe symptoms were shortness of breath at rest or during mild exertion, coughing, and elevation of temperature. The changes were indications for treatment with antibiotics, steroids, or a combination of the two, and expectorants or cough preparations, and the patients had to change their normal way of life. In no case was radiation fibrosis severe enough to cause death. An evaluation of the patients treated for Hodgkin's disease is given in Table 1. Patients treated for bronchogenic carcinoma, who were treated to a higher dose of radiation, showed a similar incidence of radiation fibrosis (Table 2).

Comparison of these figures indicates that the patients with Hodgkin's disease developed pulmonary fibrosis slightly earlier than those with bronchogenic carcinoma,

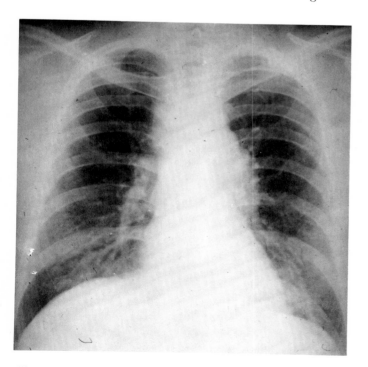

Fig. 1. Chest x-ray of a patient with epidermoid carcinoma of the left main stem bronchus before radiotherapy.

TABLE 1. PATIENTS WITH HODGKIN'S DISEASE

	3 Months	6 Months	12 Months
Pulmonary fibrosis, minimal	25%	30%	23%
Pulmonary fibrosis, moderate	37%	38%	38%
Pulmonary fibrosis, severe	12%	23%	30%
Mild symptoms	25%	20%	15%
Severe symptoms	5%	20%	10%

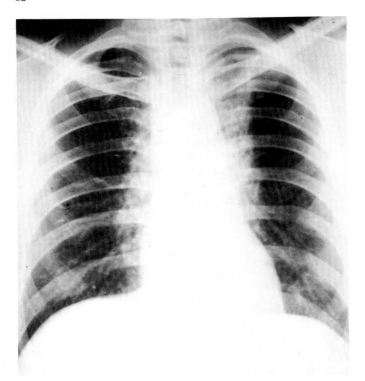

Fig. 3. The same patient three months following administration of an additional 2000 rads by small field rotational therapy. Pulmonary fibrosis has progressed to moderately severe radiographic findings. The patient was entirely asymptomatic.

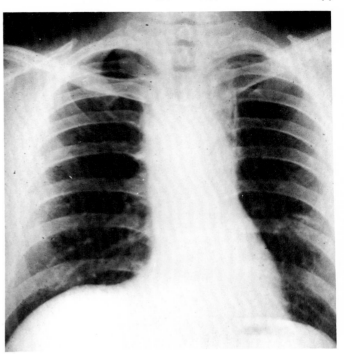

Fig. 4. The same patient one year following treatment, with severe changes on the radiograph due to pulmonary fibrosis. Although the patient had occasional cough which required a nonnarcotic antitussive he continued to work full time and had not shown any evidence of recurrent or metastatic tumor.

although the overall incidence is approximately similar. Only 8% of both groups did not show any evidence of pulmonary fibrosis. One year following radiation the symptoms of pulmonary fibrosis were much more severe and frequent among patients who underwent treatment for bronchogenic carcinoma. It is not possible to exclude entirely late tumor recurrence or metastasis in these patients. One must also realize that there is not only a difference in dose and volume of radiation, but also in natural history of the tumor and age incidence.

It should be stressed that although symptoms were frequent, pulmonary fibrosis did not produce any fetal sequelae in the patients under observation. Since the fibrosis is irreversible, extreme care should be taken in

TABLE 2. PATIENTS WITH BRONCHOGENIC CARCINOMA

	3 Months	6 Months	12 Months
Pulmonary fibrosis, minimal	40%	25%	17%
Pulmonary fibrosis, moderate	20%	50%	50%
Pulmonary fibrosis, severe	13%	6%	25%
Mild symptoms	25%	30%	30%
Severe symptoms	0%	25%	30%

treatment designs to protect normal lung, using appropriate portal arrangements and secondary blocking if cobalt irradiation is used.

The physiologic changes which take place in the lung during the course of radiation reaction have been related to the volume dose in megagram rads in the lung parenchyma by Germon and Brady.[4] They noted a significant decrease in arterial pulmonary perfusion due to the tumor and its treatment. The vital capacity increased up to 1 month after treatment and decreased thereafter. Diffusion capacity gradually decreased after treatment because of the associated pulmonary changes due to preexisting lung disease, associated smoking, and similar. No relationship to radiation dose could be established for this study of pulmonary physiologic parameters. This study differs from other reports.

Table 3 lists the results of a study carried out under the supervision of the Steering Committee on Pre-operative Irradiation in Cancer of the Lung.[13] The physiologic changes were expressed in terms of change in vital capacity and forced expiratory volume. Predisposing factors for severe pulmonary fibrotic changes on chest x-ray and the subsequent decrease in pulmonary physiologic parameters included infection, tuberculosis, bronchiec-

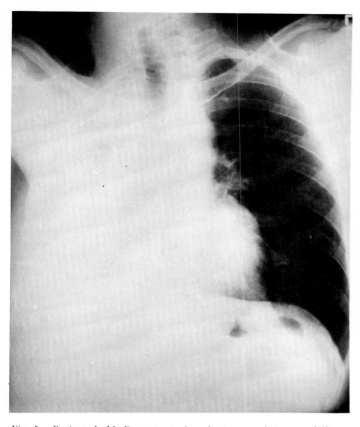

Fig. 5. Patient J. M. Posteroanterior chest x-ray 4½ years following thoracotomy with biopsy of a lesion of the right lower lobe of the lung involving the pleura. Histologic diagnosis: epidermoid carcinoma. Treated by 4000 rads to the right hemithorax with an additional dose of 2000 rads to the known area of tumor involvement in the right lower lobe. There is opacification and volume loss of the right hemithorax. The patient is short of breath on exertion. He pursues his occupation as bookkeeper. There has been no evidence of recurrent or metastatic disease.

tasis, empyema, abscess and emphysema. Although the reduction in tumor mass increased the respiratory capacity, underlying lung disease of the above-mentioned type had to be carefully evaluated before radiation therapy could be initiated.

For supervoltage portals using parallel opposing technique with a field size up to approximately 150 cm^2, a dose of 3000 rads in 3 weeks produces radiographic evidence of minimal lung fibrosis. As the radiation dose exceeds this limit, the degree of pulmonary fibrosis increases. This has been evaluated by Phillips and Margolis[12] who noted that no pneumonitis occurred in patients treated with less than 2650 rads to the whole lung in 20 fractions (nominal standard dose[3] NSD = 900 rets). With concomitant administration of actinomycin D for metastatic disease, this complication-free dose was lowered to 2050 rads in 20 fractions (NSD = 700 rets). Pneumonitis may be expected in 50% of treated patients for doses of 1040 rets without and 840 rets with actinomycin D. There is a lower incidence and severity of radiation fibrosis in patients treated by the split-course method.[6]

Pathophysiologic changes that take place in the lung following irradiation can be shown on lung scans as a slight decrease in pulmonary perfusion approximately 7 weeks after the administration of 3000 rads to the whole lung. As radiographic findings of progressive pulmonary pneumonitis and fibrosis occur, the lung scan indicates a progressive decrease in perfusion of the involved areas.[5]

Since pulmonary fibrosis requires at least 6 months and sometimes even several years to fully manifest itself, long-term survival after treatment for malignancy is necessary. Most patients with pulmonary parenchymal changes on chest x-ray after irradiation are relatively asymptomatic, and severe symptoms of shortness of

TABLE 3. CHANGE IN VITAL CAPACITY AND FORCED EXPIRATORY VOLUME ONE YEAR AFTER TREATMENT[13]

Type of resection	Treatment group	Number	Change in VC[a] as Percent of Predicted VC		Change in FEV[b] as Percent of Predicted FEV	
			Mean	SE	Mean	SE
No resection	Prior radiotherapy	11	−15%	4.2	−17%	4.4
	Immediate surgery	9	−13	4.6	−10	5.0
Pneumonectomy	Prior radiotherapy	51	−27	2.7	−16	2.9
	Immediate surgery	38	−29	2.8	−21	3.0
Lobectomy	Prior radiotherapy	40	−24	2.1	−13	2.4
	Immediate surgery	38	− 9	1.9	− 7	3.7

[a] VC: Vital capacity.
[b] FEV: Forced expiratory volume.

breath usually respond rapidly to corticosteroid therapy. When the fibrosis is well established, steroids give symptomatic relief but do not reverse the histopathologic changes in the lung parenchyma.[14] Antibiotics are of value for secondary infection. Although some studies suggest the prophylactic value of corticosteroids in pulmonary fibrosis of animals, the growth-promoting effect of steroids on human malignant disease does not warrant their routine use. A clear definition of the target volume and protection of normal pulmonary parenchyma consistent with good radiotherapeutic technique are necessary to avoid disabling pulmonary fibrosis as far as possible.

HEART

Radiation damage to the heart is felt to be secondary to damage to the cardiac blood vessels and the pericardium. The myocardium, consisting of a stable cell population without mitotic arcivity, is very radioresistant and direct radiation injury of the muscle fiber is a minor factor.

Pericarditis is the major heart-related complication of radiotherapy in patients with long survival. Acute pericarditis leading to chronic constrictive pericarditis in 6 to 48 months after radiation does not occur often in a population whose 1-year survival is as low as that of patients with bronchogenic carcinoma. Acute pericarditis is diagnosed by symptoms of fever, tachycardia, substernal pain, and pericardial friction rub. Effusion is frequent and tamponade should be ruled out. Some patients will show recurrence under treatment or will develop chronic constrictive pericarditis.

Although studies with fractionated doses of radiation between 2000 and 10,000 rads in 20 to 100 days did not produce electrocardiographic (ECG) changes indicative of myocardial damage in humans after 2-year follow-up, Stewart and Fajardo[18] reported 8 patients with pericardial damage among 120 patients treated by radiation therapy for Hodgkin's disease. Among 84 patients treated with 3500 and 4500 rads, 4 patients developed serious pericarditis and 1 developed myocardial infarction. Among 13 patients treated with more than 4500 rads, 1 patient developed heart disease. The sporadic reports in the literature have not yet permitted a determination of time/dose/volume relationship for the incidence of serious pericardial damage; however, limitation of the radiation to the cardiac and pericardial volume should be achieved whenever it is compatible with the treatment of the patient's tumor.

Lawson et al.[9] reported on 4 patients with radiation pericarditis among a group of 98 patients treated by radiation therapy for lung cancer. When 4500 to 5000 rads were given in 4 to 5 weeks to at least half of the heart volume, 4 patients presented 1 year later with fever, dyspnea, and pericardial effusion; 1 patient had a well-defined rub, and in 3 the jugular venous pressure was raised. ECG changes were nonspecific with low voltage. All patients had enlargement of their cardiac silhouette. Two patients died with myocardial infarction, 1 after anterior parietal pericardectomy; 1 patient died of tumor recurrence, and 1 is alive and well after drainage of the pericardium.

SPINAL CORD

Dynes and Smedal[2] reported on 800 patients treated by supervoltage radiation therapy for malignancies in the head and neck, mediastinum, and lung. There were 10 cases of radiation myelitis, 6 of which occurred in patients with lung cancer. All patients received at least 6000 rads tumor dose to the spinal cord, usually over fairly long segments. More recent data, especially those of Lindgren[10] and Phillips and Buschke[11] indicate the importance of limiting irradiation of long segments of spinal cord to 4500 to 5000 rads at a fractionation of approximately 800 to 1000 rads/week. Thus in order to deliver a cancerocidal dose of about 6000 rads to the tumor, it is necessary to limit the beam of radiation by the use of rotational therapy or small-field cross-firing arrangements for at least one-quarter of the dose. A combination of large-field irradiation to 4500 rads in 4½ to 5 weeks, and subsequent limitation of field arrangements that deliver no more than about 5000 rads to a short segment of spinal cord, will avoid the major complication of radiation myelitis. The data of Phillip and Buschke indicate that a nominal standard dose (NSD)[3] of approximately 1600 rets for long segments and 1800 rets for short segments of spinal cord will produce radiation myelitis in less than 3% of patients.

Again, as in cardiac damage, the short life expectancy of patients with bronchogenic carcinoma masks the true incidence of this complication, since 6 to 12 months are required for evidence of spinal cord damage. Transitory signs, such as Lhermitte's syndrome, are occasionally observed after treatment of the spinal cord. This syndrome of transient myelopathy manifests itself in peripheral sensory changes, best described by the patient as the feeling of an electric shock extending along the body on sharply flexing the head forward. It is a self-limiting entity and usually disappears after a number of weeks or months without specific treatment.

REFERENCES

1. Deeley, Thomas, J.: The effect of radiation on the lungs in the treatment of carcinoma of the bronchus. *Clin. Radiol* **11**:33–39, 1960.

2. Dynes, J. B., and Smedal, M. I.: Radiation myelitis. *Am. J. Roentgenol. Radium Ther. Nucl. Med.* **83**:78–87, 1960.

3. Ellis, F.: Dose, time and fractionation: a clinical hypothesis. *Clin. Radiol.* **20**:1–7, 1969.

4. Germon, Patricia, A., and Brady, L. W.: Physiological changes before and after radiation treatment for carcinoma of the lung. *J. A. M. A.* **206**:809–814, 1968..

5. Goldman, S. M., Freeman, L. M., Ghossein, N. A., and Sanfilippo, L. J.: Effects of thoracic irradiation on pulmonary arterial perfusion in man. *Radiology* **93**:289–296, 1969.

6. Holsti, L. B., and Vuorinen, P.: Radiation reaction in the lung after continuous and split-course megavoltage radiotherapy of bronchial carcinoma. *Br. J. Radiol.* **40**:280–284, 1967.

7. Holt, J. A. G.: Letter to the editor. *Br. J. Radiol.* **18**:638, 1965.

8. Lacassagne, A.: Action des rayons du radium sur les muqueuses de l'oesophage et de la trachee chez le lapin. *C. R. Soc. Biol.* **84**:26–27, 1921.

9. Lawson, R. A. M., Ross, W. M., Gold, R. G., Blesovsky, A., and Barnsley, W. C.: Postradiation pericarditis: report on four more cases with special reference to bronchogenic carcinoma. *J. Thorac. Cardiovasc. Surg.* **63**:841–847, 1972.

10. Lindgren, M.: On tolerance of brain tissue and sensitivity of brain tumors to irradiation. *Acta Radiol. Suppl.* 170:1–73, 1958.

11. Phillips, T. L., and Buschke, F.: Radiation tolerance of the thoracic spinal cord. *Am. J. Roentgenol. Radium Ther. Nucl. Med.* **105**:659–664, 1969.

12. Phillips, T., and Margolis, L.: Radiation pathology and the clinical response of lung and esophagus. In *Radiation Effect and Tolerance, Normal Tissue,* University Park Press, Baltimore, 1972.

13. Preoperative irradiation of cancer of the lung. Preliminary report of a therapeutic trial. A collaborative study. *Cancer* **23**: 419–429, 1969.

14. Rubin, P., and Andrews, J.: Response of radiation pneumonitis to corticoids. *Am. J. Roentgenol, Radium Ther. Nucl. Med.* **79**:453–464, 1968.

15. Seydel, H. G., and Maun, J.: Pulmonary fibrosis following radiotherapy for bronchogenic carcinoma and Hodgkin's Disease. *Md. State Med. J.* **18**:61–62, 1969.

16. Smith, J. C.: Radiation Pneumonitis: a review. *Am. Rev. Respir. Dis.* **87**: 647–655, 1963.

17. Smith, J. C.: Radiation pneumonitis: case report of bilateral reaction after unilateral irradiation. *Am. Rev. Respir. Dis.* **89**:264–269, 1964.

18. Stewart, J., and Fajardo, L.: Radiation-induced heart disease. In *Radiation Effect and Tolerance, Normal Tissue,* University Park Press, Baltimore, 1972.

19. Taylor, R. M.: The somatic effects of radiation. *Can. Med. Assoc. J.* **86**:521–525, 1962.

20. Whitfield, A. G. W., Bond, W. H., and Kunkler, P. B.: Radiation damage to thoracic tissues. *Thorax* **18**:371–380, 1963.

21. Wiernick, G.: Radiation pneumonitis following a low dose of cobalt teletherapy. *Br. J. Radiol.* **38**:312–314, 1965.

Chapter Nineteen

Radiation Dosimetry in the Treatment of Cancer of the Lung

The dosimetry of the radiation dose delivered to lung tumors and surrounding tissues is complicated by the wide variety of tissue densities that occupy the space between skin and tumor. Lung tissue absorbs significantly less radiation than equivalent volumes of muscle, fat, or bone (see Table 1). Since the size of the thorax is greatly increased in patients with emphysema, the skin tumor distance is large and an even greater proportion of the beam entering through the skin will traverse lung tissue. Much inaccuracy is produced if central axis isodoses are used according to measurements in a water phantom. On the other hand, atelectatic lung, mediastinum, and tumor in the lung itself transmit beams of ionizing radiation similar to waterlike material. Although transverse tomography has become more available thus making it possible to define the thickness of various tissue types in a transverse cross section of the patient with reasonable accuracy, it is not possible at present to use this method routinely in the planning of radiotherapy for lung cancer. Heuss[5] has found that dosimetry is even more complex in electron beams.

The effect of lung tissue on absorbed and transmitted dose from photon beams is less complex than that arising at a bone tissue interface, where the change in atomic number results in the loss of electron equilibrium. The density of lung in a living subject is by no means uniform, but it can be generally assumed for purposes of dosimetry to be about 0.3 g/cm³ (Fowler and Young[2]). Since lung is similar to normal tissue in atomic composition, electron equilibrium established in front of the slab of lung tissue will be maintained within and there are no discontinuities in the dose because of build-up or build-down effects at the interfaces. However, when bone enters the picture, the electron equilibrium will be significantly disturbed.

Although in parallel opposing treatment a large amount of bone in the form of the spinal column is placed in the beam of radiation, it is possible and even desirable to protect the spinal cord, and therefore only the effect of lung tissue on the dose distribution will be considered here. This protection of the spinal cord can be achieved either by placement of a midline shield or by the use of portals avoiding the spinal column.

There are several methods for experimental measurement on patients to determine the dose to regions in the lung, the simplest being the measurement of transit doses. Holt and Laughlin[6] measured the transmission of radiation by a series of narrow beams covering the region to be treated by the therapy beam, and used this information to estimate the cross-field radiation due to non-unit density tissue. Transit dose can also be measured in the central axis of a therapy beam with a suitable instrument placed on the patient's skin. If densitometer readings are obtained for films exposed at a constant distance from the source of radiation, compensators may be constructed from such measurements that will allow a homogeneous dose of radiation to be delivered.[1] However, these methods will only give indirect information about the dose distribution at the tumor. Better information may be obtained by measurement through introduction of *in vivo* dosimeters into the esophagus or bronchus. These techniques are quite time consuming, uncomfortable, and require accurate localization of the dosimeter in the isodose to allow comparison of the measured and computed or calculated dose.

Stewart and Greene[7] have shown how one can approximate the lack of absorption of the beam of radiation produced by a 4 MeV linear accelerator or by a 60 cobalt teletherapy device by shifting the normal isodose curve forward by 0.4 times the thickness of the lung traversed by the beam of ionizing radiation. This method provides and accuracy of ±2% for megavoltage radiation. For orthovoltage x-rays, the isodose lines have to be shifted 0.5 times the thickness of lung traversed in the direction of the beam. Stewart and Greene have published a table which allows correction of a tumor dose as obtained from unit density material calculation, if the tumor is irradiated through 6 cm of lung tissue (see Table 2).

In vivo dosimetry can be performed using lithium fluoride dosimeters in the esophagus, but the measurements are not representative of the dose delivered to a peripheral lung lesion. The mediastinal dose, especially when treated by a relatively narrow portal, can be

TABLE 1. ENERGY ABSORPTION COEFFICIENTS[4]

Energy (MeV)	Water	Air	Bone	Muscle
0.01	4.89	4.66	19.0	4.96
0.10	.0252	.0231	.0386	.0252
1.0	.0311	.0280	.0297	.0308
10.0	0.155	.0144	.0159	.0154

TABLE 2. CORRECTIONS TO BE APPLIED TO THE DOSE IN A TUMOR IRRADIATED THROUGH 6 CM OF LUNG TISSUE[a]

Radiation	FSD	Correction for 6 cm of Lung
300 kv	50 cm	+40%
60 Cobalt	80 cm	+20%
4 MV	100 cm	+15%
8 MV	100 cm	+10%

[a] Corrections are to be applied to central axis data read from standard tables.[7]

measured effectively using dosimeters in the esophagus, and the measurements show that no significant correction is necessary for parallel opposing portals because of the dense tissue in the mediastinum. On the other hand, when rotation is employed, or when narrow cross-firing portals are centered on a peripheral lung tumor, transmitted dosimetry as described by Holt and Laughlin[6] may be of value.

Worsnop[8] surveyed data on the national cooperative study on preoperative irradiation and measured radiation dose in the phantom, duplicating the treatment set up as a basis for his analysis. He found that the average dose to the primary tumor was 16% higher at the University of Maryland than the dose calculated for unit density material. In other institutions participating in the same study, doses were found to be up to 28% higher than those calculated for unit density material. For the dose delivered in the lung 2 cm inside the margin of the 60 cobalt treatment portal, the corresponding figures were +4% for the University of Maryland and +13% to −13% in other institutions. The normal lung 2 cm outside the margin of the beam of radiation received 7%

of the calculated dose at the University of Maryland and 4 to 21% at other institutions.

Goldenberg et al.[3] reported their results of intraluminal measurements during the treatment of esophageal cancers with an increase of measured dose over the calculated dose between 6 and 27%, depending on the anatomy of the patient and the extent of the tumor. Our own measurements using small *in vivo* thermoluminescent dosimeters revealed that the dose to the mediastinum is 5 to 20% higher than that calculated for unit density material, and the dose in the periphery of the lung may be expected to be higher yet.

At present there is no simple way to allow for tissue inhomogeneity short of computer dosimetry based on transverse tomography. The dose of megavoltage radiation delivered to a tumor in the periphery of the lung may be up to 25% higher than that calculated from unit density material, whereas the dose delivered in the mediastinum, in enlarged mediastinal nodes or atelectatic lung is fairly well described by a dosimetry which considers the volume of tumor and the traversed tissue as consisting of unit density material.

REFERENCES

1. Ellis, F., and Lescrenier, C.: Combined compensation for contours and heterogeneity. *Radiology* **106**:191–194, 1973.

2. Fowler, J. F., and Young, A. E.: The average density of healthy lung. *Am. J. Roentgenol. Radium Ther. Nucl. Med.* **81**:312–315, 1959.

3. Goldenberg, D. B., Gopala, U. V., Lott, S., and Digel, J.: Dosimetric considerations in cobalt 60 rotational therapy for esophageal lesions. A comparison of transit and intraluminal dose measurement. *Am. J. Roentgenol. Radium Ther. Nucl. Med.* **105**:518–522, 1969.

4. Handbook 62, International Commission on Radiological Units

and Measurements (ICRU). U.S. National Bureau of Standards, Washington, D.C., 1956.

5. Heuss, K.: Beitrag zur Bestrahlungsplanung bei der Elektronentherapie des Bronchialkarzinoms. Strahlenther. **141**:25–31, 1971.

6. Holt, J. G., and Laughlin, J. S.: Practical method of obtaining density distribution within patients. *Radiology* **93**:161–168, 1969.

7. Stewart, J. G., and Greene, D.: Dose distribution in lung treatments. In *Modern Radiotherapy. Carcinoma of the Bronchus*, T. J. Deeley, Ed., Appleton-Century-Crofts, New York, 1971.

8. Worsnop, B. R.: Phantom thermoluminescent dosimeter comparison for a cooperative radiotherapy trial. *Radiology* **91**:545–551, 1968.

Epilogue

Although it appears odd to use the term "treatment" with reference to "lung cancer" except possibly for the resection of small peripheral lesions, the review presented in this volume indicates that advances are being made even though they are measured in mean survival times of a few months. Human nature being what it is, it is unlikely that we will be able to alter the smoking habits of the U.S. population. Therefore our most important step in combating the increasing mortality of cancer of the lung is prevention through public education to foster a preference for low-tar cigarettes in those unable to abstain from consuming the deadly weed. Along with this effort there should be progress in decreasing man's exposure to environmental carcinogens. Other avenues of research might be directed toward the control of carcinogen activation, or toward the enhancement of inactivation of carcinogens.

From an economic point of view, treatment will be most successful if it is directed toward a high-risk population. Continuing research toward identification of such patient groups will help to reveal the most advanced treatment available upon diagnosis of lung cancer. One can speculate that in such a group of highly susceptible individuals drug therapy might be used to inhibit the activation or to enhance the inactivation of chemical oncogens. A new avenue for further investigation may be the attempt to reverse the neoplastic lesions which precede invasive cancer of the lung.

Bronchogenic carcinoma is truly a disease of civilization, born out of the technological advances man has achieved over the last two centuries. Longer life spans make it possible for individuals to attain an age at which they develop mucosal alterations, which we diagnose as lung cancer. At the same time, technological advances and the tendency toward self-gratification such as smoking have made our environment increasingly dangerous. It is possible and probable that civilization in a positive sense will also provide us with the tools to avoid morbidity and decrease mortality from this scourge of mankind.

Index